The U.S. RDA is the Recommended Daily Allowance of nutrients suggested by the Federal Food and Drug Administration. It is obviously not an absolute figure, but rather a very educated estimate of how much of a certain kind of food is required on a daily basis to keep people healthy. For example, when it comes to proteins . . .

Some Super Sources of Protein

Food	Amount	% of U.S. RDA
Chicken, light meat, stewed	1 cup	100
Chicken liver, chopped	1 cup	80
Peanuts	1 cup	80
Salmon	7¾ oz. can	100
Sardines	7½ oz. can	80
Seeds, pumpkin and sunflower	1 cup	80–90
Tuna fish	6½ oz. can	100

THE BRAND-NAME NUTRITION COUNTER

BY JEAN CARPER

Revised Edition

BANTAM BOOKS
NEW YORK · TORONTO · LONDON · SYDNEY · AUCKLAND

ACKNOWLEDGMENTS

I wish to thank the many food companies which sent me the nutritional information on their products. My thanks also to Elizabeth Brooks for her research help in collecting the data and compiling the charts and the U.S. Department of Agriculture for the information on fresh foods.

THE BRAND-NAME NUTRITION COUNTER
A Bantam Book / June 1975
Bantam revised edition / November 1985
8 printings through August 1990

ISBN 0-553-25267-4

Published simultaneously in the United States and Canada

PRINTED IN THE UNITED STATES OF AMERICA

OPM   18   17   16   15   14   13   12   11   10   9

CONTENTS

INTRODUCTION
by Jean Carper

There are superfoods, junk foods, and just plain nutritious foods. Which are which? And how much of which nutrients do they really contain? How much salt? How much carbohydrate? How much fat? Calories? Protein? Vitamin A, vitamin C, vitamins B_1, B_2, niacin, calcium, and iron? This is information everyone should have—for it is just possible it could revolutionize eating habits. The author can attest to the fact that compiling the many charts in this book radically changed her food choices.

No one wants intentionally to cheat him or herself—and certainly not growing children—of vital nutrients. But for too long, too many of us have been nutritional innocents wandering in a foodmaker's paradise, forced to make choices on insufficient nutritional knowledge and on lack of handy comparative information. Though the nutritionists' advice to choose a variety of foods and eat a "balanced" diet is certainly sound, it is increasingly difficult to follow in the age of calorie watching and processed and fabricated foods. A person who takes the "variety" advice literally might come home with a bagful of Tang, potato chips, Cool Whip, cake mixes, soft drinks—all of which are nutritionally marginal and would not support life for long.

Our forefathers had an easier time getting proper nutrients, for they could load up on many different types of food for insurance. If they didn't get a nutrient in one food, they could get it in another, and count on hard work to burn off excess calories. But in our age of lower expenditures of energy we can no longer afford caloric sprees in our search for adequate intake of nutrients. We must make each calorie count—pack it as full of nutrients as possible. In modern life empty caloric bubbles of sugar and fat present a definite health hazard—both by making us fat and starving us of nutrients obtainable from more wholesome foods.

Essential to calorie-conscious eaters are the nitty-gritty nutritional specifics, so we don't have to guess wildly about what nutrients we are—or aren't—getting. To make wise choices and

1

comparisons we must have the actual nutritional counts on certain foods—by brand name when applicable. Nothing can substitute for having the figures right in front of you. Although more food companies than ever before are providing such information on their labels, many best-selling food products still contain no nutrient labeling. Many food labels leave out sodium. And it is difficult to make intelligent comparisons of food labels at the same time you are rushing around the supermarket. It is far better to make your nutritional choices before you go food shopping.

That is what this book is about. It is a handbook of nutritional tables where you can look up how much protein, fat, carbohydrate, calories, sodium (in most cases), vitamins A, C, thiamine (B_1), riboflavin (B_2), niacin, calcium, and iron are contained in the servings of more than 3000 brand-name foods, fresh foods, and fast foods. The precise meaning of the figures is explained on page 3, and I urge everyone to read that section thoroughly before using the information, so that there will be no misunderstandings.

But first—a few words about protein, the major vitamins and minerals, sodium, fats and sugar, and the rapidly changing field of nutritional knowledge.

It is encouraging to note that since the first edition of this book was published in 1975, the nation's relentless slide toward poor nutrition has been interrupted. The state of the nation's nutritional health no longer seems as grim as it once was. True, many Americans are still eating junk foods, but many others have become much more nutrition-conscious, and nutritional knowledge is spreading. For example, physicians, once lacking in nutritional information, are becoming much more sophisticated and knowledgeable about sound nutrition. Numerous scientific studies are confirming the role of nutrition in any number of chronic diseases, including heart disease, cancer, diabetes, and kidney disease.

Nutrition, not so long ago considered the purview of fringe practitioners, has now moved center stage. Scientific conferences, meetings, and panels made up of the country's most prominent researchers and policy makers are commonplace. Recommendations on how to eat to remain healthy have been made by several government bodies. The nation is increasingly becoming more conscious of the need to eat well to stave off disease and stay fit. High-fat foods are out; complex carbohydrates are in. Food manufacturers are increasingly paying attention to nutrition, and creating some new products lower in fat, sugar, and calories. Some fast-food outlets, although still offering food oozing with fat, have at least set up salad bars.

There is still much to be regretted in the nation's dietary habits. There are still nutritional deficiencies and abuses that should not exist. Several nutrients have been designated "problem nutrients" by the U.S. Department of Agriculture; they are those in which the American diet is likely to be deficient. You should pay special attention to make sure you are getting enough of these nutrients. They are: calcium and iron (especially among females), vitamins A and C.

Still, more people seem to be concerned about good nutrition and how to find it. That makes this book all the more important. Letters have confirmed the need for the information in this book. After seven printings, it has been revised by popular demand.

What the Figures Mean

Most important, the nutritional figures in this revised edition are totally new. They include many of the food items in the previous edition and many new items that have come on the market since then. We went back to all the manufacturers included in the first version and asked for the nutritional content of all their current food products. Almost all the food companies we contacted replied promptly. Thus, you will find in the book nearly all the major manufacturers of food products.

All of the nutrients for the various food items are listed in the format required by the Food and Drug Administration for companies using nutritional labeling. This includes number of calories, grams of carbohydrate, grams of fat, and percentages of the U.S. Recommended Daily Allowances for protein, vitamins A, C, thiamine (B_1), riboflavin (B_2), niacin, and calcium and iron. We have added the content of sodium whenever it was available.

Here are the U.S. Recommended Daily Allowances as designated by the Food and Drug Administration. The nutrients are listed in the order they must be listed by food companies. If a company lists one it must list at least the first eight—through iron—and may also list other nutrients at its option.

U.S. RDAs
For Adults and Children over Age Four

NUTRIENT	U.S. RDA
Protein	45 grams (high quality)
	65 grams (lower quality)
Vitamin A	5000 IU (international units)
Vitamin C	60 mg (milligrams)
Thiamine (B_1)	1.5 mg
Riboflavin (B_2)	1.7 mg
Niacin	20 mg
Calcium	1 gram
Iron	18 mg
Vitamin D	400 IU
Vitamin E	30 IU
Vitamin B_6 (pyridoxine)	2 mg
Folic acid	0.4 mg
Vitamin B_{12}	6 mcg (micrograms)
Phosphorus	1 gram
Iodine	150 mcg
Magnesium	400 mg
Zinc	15 mg
Copper	2 mg
Biotin	0.3 mg
Pantothenic acid	10 mg

The FDA also drew up U.S. RDAs for children under four and for infants. They are:

NUTRIENT	INFANTS	UNDER AGE FOUR
Protein	18 grams (high quality)	20 grams
	25 grams (lower quality)	28 grams
Vitamin A	1500 IU	2500 IU
Vitamin C	35 mg	40 mg
Thiamine (B_1)	0.5 mg	0.7 mg
Riboflavin (B_2)	0.6 mg	0.8 mg
Niacin	8 mg	9 mg
Calcium	600 mg	800 mg
Iron	15 mg	10 mg
Vitamin D	400 IU	400 IU
Vitamin E	5 IU	10 IU
Vitamin B_6	0.4 mg	0.7 mg
Folic acid	0.1 mg	0.2 mg
Vitamin B_{12}	2 mcg	3 mcg
Phosphorus	500 mg	800 mg
Iodine	45 mcg	70 mcg
Magnesium	70 mg	200 mg

NUTRIENT	INFANTS	UNDER AGE FOUR
Zinc	5 mg	8 mg
Copper	0.6 mg	1 mg
Biotin	0.15 mg	0.15 mg
Pantothenic acid	3 mg	5 mg

Important

To avoid confusion and to enable consumers to make accurate comparisons, the appropriate figures in this book follow the FDA's format for nutritional labeling. The figures are expressed in percentages of the U.S. RDA. All of the foods in the book follow the U.S. RDAs for adults—except for baby foods, which are calculated on the infant U.S. RDA. Note especially that protein is also expressed in percentage of RDA, not in grams. So if a product is shown with protein of 50, that means one serving of the food supplies one-half or 50 percent of the recommended daily allowance of protein. It does not mean the food has 50 grams of protein, which would be about all an adult would need in a day.

Also, in figuring the RDA for protein, companies take into consideration how much "high quality" and "lower quality" protein the food has. High quality protein is generally regarded as animal and dairy protein, and lower quality as protein from vegetables, grains, or nuts.

It must also be pointed out that the figures are based on calculations or analyses of *average samples* of specific products; there may be nutritional variations from batch to batch from the same manufacturer. Nutritional values may be influenced by such factors as soil composition and climatic conditions. Some companies have also asked us to note that if there is a discrepancy between the figures in this book and those on a food label, the food has been modified and the label reflects the latest food formulation. For further clarification you can contact the company.

In the tables, NA means "not available."

Unless otherwise noted, figures for pudding mixes, cake mixes, condensed soups, and the like are for the final product prepared *according to package directions*. Obviously, if you depart from these the nutritional values change.

Before noting the major nutrients and why you need them, here is a reminder from the National Academy of Sciences against the misuse of the RDAs. The Academy defines the RDAs

5

as "the levels of intake of essential nutrients considered in the judgment of the Food and Nutrition Board on the basis of available scientific knowledge to be adequate to meet the known nutritional needs of practically all healthy persons." Thus, the RDAs are intended to provide a statistical base, gleaned from both human and animal studies, which applies to the population at large. However, the scientists cautiously point out that some persons may require more or less than the allowances suggested because of genetic makeup or "biochemical individuality," as scientist Dr. Roger Williams, author of *Nutrition Against Disease*, called it. Also, a person may require more of certain nutrients under certain conditions: stress, disease or infection, use of birth-control pills, pregnancy, after menopause. Recognizing there is no way of predicting whose needs are high and whose are low, the Academy says its RDAs are set deliberately high to exceed the requirements of most individuals. The FDA, in slightly modifying the Academy's RDAs, came up with the U.S. RDAs, which are slightly higher.

The U.S. RDAs, then, are a guide to what scientists believe most people need in the light of present knowledge. They are not absolute for everyone—and to an extent you must depend on your own "body wisdom"—which some experts believe each of us has—in deciding how much you need. Eating slightly less or more than 100 percent of the U.S. RDAs for each nutrient probably won't damage your health. However, it is not advisable to eat the same foods constantly. The key to healthful eating, as nutritionists endlessly stress, is obtaining nutrients from a variety of wholesome foods—as insurance against all the things we don't know.

Certainly no one should overeat—or overfeed babies—just to get the 100 percent daily quota of nutrients. If it comes to that, you would be much better off to supplement your diet with vitamin pills. Obviously, vitamin and mineral supplements are not substitutes for wholesome food, but sometimes may be advisable in addition to good food—as insurance against the vagaries of "biochemical individuality" and any nutritional surprises that scientists may turn up in the future.

Protein

Protein is vital; you could not survive on a pure diet of carbohydrates and fat, for amino acids that are essential to life would be missing. Protein is necessary for the replacement and building of tissues—for example, hair, fingernails, skin, muscles. The hormones, enzymes, and hemoglobin of the body that keep life going are proteins. Without protein the body could not manufacture antibodies to fight off infection. About 20 percent of the body is protein and it must be replenished constantly. Protein cannot be stored for long periods like some nutrients.

Protein foods are not all of the same quality—equally nourishing for the body. They are made up of varying patterns of amino acids, some of which do not correspond perfectly with those our bodies need. We have twenty-two amino acids—eight of which we cannot synthesize but must obtain from food. These are called the *essential* amino acids; they all must be present in precise amounts to make protein synthesis "complete." Foods that meet this requirement are called "complete" protein foods; they are foods of animal origin—meat, fish, poultry, cheese, eggs, milk—and are the highest quality protein. Proteins from vegetables, nuts, and grains are of lower quality because they lack enough of certain amino acids.

Dr. Isaac Asimov explains it this way: "Suppose the protein in the food we eat contains all the amino acids in the same proportion that is found in the protein of our tissues except that one of the essential amino acids—lysine, for instance—is present in only half the expected supply. This means that when the body begins to rearrange the absorbed amino acids in our own tissue protein, it will run out of lysine when only half the amino acids have been arranged. The body cannot form protein molecules without lysine, nor can it make the lysine from anything else. Nor can it store the remaining amino acids and wait till some more lysine comes along. What the body does is burn the remaining amino acids for fuel." In other words the protein is wasted when the body could better burn fats and carbohydrates for fuel. In "complete" proteins very little of the protein is wasted.

Thus you actually get more protein value from meat and dairy products, but lower-quality protein foods can be combined to bring up their total protein value. When you eat rice and beans together, or milk and cereal, some of the missing amino acids from one are supplied by the other, and much less protein is wasted. The book *Diet for a Small Planet* by Frances Moore Lappe is a superb account of how to mix proteins to get the greatest value.

7

SOME SUPER SOURCES OF PROTEIN

	AMOUNT	PERCENT OF U.S. RDA
Beef, steaks, roasts, ground lean	3 oz	60
Bluefish	3 oz	50
Chicken	½ breast	60
Chicken, light meat, stewed	1 cup	100
Clams	1 cup	60
Cottage cheese	1 cup	70
Frozen dinner, chicken, boneless (Swanson Hungry-Man)	1 dinner	100
Legumes, dried, cooked	1 cup	35
Liver, chicken, chopped	1 cup	80
Milk	1 cup	20–25
Oysters, Pacific	1 cup	60
Parmesan cheese	1 oz	25
Peanuts	1 cup	80
Peanut butter (Skippy)	2 tbsp	15
Salmon	7¾-oz can	100
Sardines	7½-oz can	80
Seeds, pumpkin and sunflower	1 cup	80–90
Tunafish	6½-oz can	100
Turkey, roasted	3 oz	60
Yogurt, plain	1 cup	30

Vitamin A

Though the ancient Egyptians did not know specifically why night blindness occurred, they did know what cured it: roast ox liver, according to a 3500-year-old Egyptian medical textbook. It was not until early in this century that vitamin A—the crucial curative in liver—was identified and named.

Still today a first sign of vitamin A deficiency is night blindness—inability to see in subdued light or slow recovery of vision when exposed to a bright light, such as car headlights. When the deficiency is severe the major danger is "dry eye" (xerophthalmia), which is a major public-health problem among young children in the Orient. Amazingly, at least 80,000 children in the world below the age of four go blind every year—and 50 percent of them die—because of lack of vitamin A.

Studies on vitamin A show it is essential not only for vision but in complex metabolic processes—especially cell growth—though its role is not yet fully understood. Vitamin A contributes to the health and development of teeth, bones, skin, hair, and the urinary and gastrointestinal tracts. Deficiencies can cause skin eruptions, impairment of healing and bone formation, birth defects, abortion, and infertility. Insufficient vitamin A may be linked to enlargement of the thyroid gland, perhaps even goiter. Lower stores of vitamin A may lessen a person's ability to fight off infection. Recent studies show that vitamin-A-like substances called retinoids, as well as carotene, may help prevent the development of certain types of cancer. Some experts recommend at least half a cup of carrots a day as a possible preventive for lung cancer.

Ninety percent of the body's vitamin A is stored in the liver, where if there is enough it may last for three months or even a year or more. Since it accumulates you don't have to eat vitamin A every day to keep stocks replenished; three ounces of beef liver, for example, contains enough vitamin A to meet the U.S. RDA requirements for nine days. However, the state of your health determines how rapidly your stores of vitamin A disappear. Rapid depletion occurs during infections, such as pneumonia, chronic nephritis, urinary tract infection, and prostate disease.

Also, vitamin A, like other vitamins, is not independent. Without sufficient vitamin E, the absorption and storage of vitamin A by the liver is impaired. Too little fat and protein can do the same thing—but deficiencies in these two are not much to worry about in this country.

A warning about excessive doses of vitamin A due to abuse of vitamin pills is appropriate. The Eskimos for years have shunned polar bear liver because its enormous vitamin A content is toxic. Symptoms of too much vitamin A are hard tender lumps in the arms and legs, hair loss, dry skin, fatigue, insomnia, joint pain, and jaundice—in general much the same symptoms as those caused by a deficiency. Since a toxic dose of vitamin A is high—from 50,000 to 100,000 international units a day—the chance of getting an overdose from food is of no concern. However, doses in vitamin pills are sometimes 25,000 international units; only two of these a day could be potentially dangerous.

Sources: As the charts show, the richest sources of vitamin A are fat-storage foods—milk, butter, eggs, liver—as well as leafy green vegetables and the roots of plants such as carrots and sweet potatoes. In vegetables, notably carrots, the vitamin A is locked in the cellular structure, which must be broken down for full access to the vitamin. That is why only cooked carrots fully release the nutrient.

SOME SUPER SOURCES OF VITAMIN A

	AMOUNT	PERCENT OF U.S. RDA
Apricots, dried	10 med. halves	80
Beet greens, cooked	1 cup	150
Cantaloupe	½ 5″ diam. melon	180
Carrots, cooked	1 cup	330
Chicken stew (Swanson)	7⅝ oz	110
Collard greens, cooked	1 cup	300
Grapefruit sections, fresh	1 cup	140
Liver, beef	3 oz	910
Liver, chicken	1 cup	340
Pumpkin (Del Monte)	1 cup	1200
Sirloin burger soup (Campbell's)	10¾ oz	100
Turnip greens, fresh	1 cup	200

Vitamin C (Ascorbic Acid)

For many years vitamin C's best claim to fame was in eliminating that dread disease of seventeenth-century seamen—scurvy. As these hapless sailors discovered, without vitamin C from fresh fruits and vegetables, their teeth fell out, their gums became inflamed, wounds refused to heal, and bone and cartilage grew abnormally.

Scurvy has occurred both accidentally and in controlled clinical experiments in Americans. It is not to be expected unless one is on a diet that is extremely vitamin C deficient, and such cases have occurred recently. Nevertheless, scientists have little knowledge of the effects of longer-term chronic deficiencies of vitamin C that exist in this country. Vitamin C is called a "problem nutrient" in the United States, because, according to a recent major study by U.S. Department of Agriculture scientists, from one-fourth to one-third of those surveyed consumed under 70 percent of the recommended daily allowance of vitamin C.

Theories have been advanced that an insufficiency of vitamin C may be linked with arthritis, infections, pernicious anemia, cholesterol buildup, duodenal ulcer, and cancer to name a few. Increased intakes of vitamin C in this century, due to refrigeration and widespread distribution of citrus fruits and other high vitamin-C-content fruits and vegetables, are thought to have contributed greatly to the decrease of stomach cancer in the U.S. Vitamin C, for one thing, blocks the formation in the stomach of potent cancer-causing chemicals called nitrosamines. Nitrosamines are the byproducts of nitrite-cured meats, such as hot dogs, salami, and ham. It is still unclear what the role of vitamin C is in other chronic diseases.

SUPER SOURCES OF VITAMIN C

	AMOUNT	PERCENT OF U.S. RDA
Bright & Early	6 fl oz	180
Broccoli, cooked	1 stalk	270
Brussels sprouts	7–8	230
Cantaloupe	½ of 5″ diam. melon	150
Collard greens, cooked	1 cup	300
Hi-C, all flavors	6 fl oz	100
Mango, raw	1	120
Orange, fresh, sections	1 cup	150
Orange juice	8 fl oz	210
Orange Plus	6 fl oz	100
Peppers, red	1	250
Strawberries, fresh	1 cup	150
Tang	6 fl oz	100

Thiamine (Vitamin B₁)

Thiamine and other B vitamins are known as the ''nerve'' vitamins, though they affect other parts of the body too. The credit for discovering B_1 goes to a Dutch physician, Christiaan Eijkman. Working in Java in 1898, he found that chickens fed ''polished'' rice became weak and developed other signs of the dread disease beriberi, which also afflicted patients Eijkman was treating in the military hospital. When he fed the hens polishings from the rice—which contained B_1—the symptoms disappeared. Thus he knew that something in the germ or outer

11

coating of the rice had cured the disease. That something, which he thought was an amino acid, was named thiamine and later vitamin B₁.

Although beriberi is still a scourge in parts of the world where rice is polished and not enriched, it is rare in the United States. Much of the thiamine is removed in the milling and processing of wheat for flour and rice in this country. However, rice and bread are enriched with B_1.

The need for thiamine fluctuates depending on your condition. For example, consumption of sugar and other carbohydrates increases the need for thiamine; thiamine aids in the metabolism of carbohydrates. A person under stress or with a hyperactive thyroid also demands more thiamine. Increased thiamine requirements also occur in adolescents, the aged, and women during the last trimester of pregnancy.

Signs of vitamin B_1 deficiency embrace almost all the ills of the human condition. This makes the shortage difficult to spot. Early signs of thiamine inadequacy are fatigue, loss of weight, loss of appetite—and later, gastrointestinal and neurological symptoms: tingling and pain. Symptoms also include nausea, vomiting, constipation, irregular heartbeat, paleness, chills, irregular menstruation, frequent colds, shortness of breath, headache, inability to concentrate, irritability and depression, and vision problems. (Thiamine given with vitamin A has cleared up night blindness better than vitamin A alone.)

It is useless to ingest more vitamin-B_1-rich foods than your body can use. Being water soluble, the vitamin is not stored in the body, but is excreted.

SOME SUPER SOURCES OF THIAMINE (VITAMIN B₁)

	AMOUNT	PERCENT OF U.S. RDA
Bacon, Canadian (Oscar Mayer)	2 slices	26
Brazil nuts	1 cup	90
Ham, roasted, lean	3 oz	35
Pecans	1 cup	60
Pork chop, lean, broiled	2 oz	40
Pork loin, lean	3 oz	60
Product 19	1 cup	100
Sunflower seeds	1 cup	190
Total	1¼ cups	100

Riboflavin (Vitamin B_2)

It is difficult to separate the symptoms of riboflavin deficiency from those of the other B vitamins, because they are similar. Some that have been spotted in B_2-deficient humans are sore throat, inflammation and lesions of the mucous membranes, dermatitis, and eye changes such as cataracts. Animal studies indicate riboflavin deficiencies are somehow associated with birth defects and cancer, but precisely how is unknown. At present scientists are still investigating riboflavin for clues to the extent of its true role. The consequences of inadequate dietary intake may be quite complex.

Although in general vitamin B_2 deficiency is not a problem in this country (mainly because of the enrichment of white flour with the vitamin) it could affect those on fad or restricted diets.

SOME SUPER SOURCES OF RIBOFLAVIN (VITAMIN B_2)

	AMOUNT	PERCENT OF U.S. RDA
Almonds	1 cup	80
Carnation Slender	1 can	25
Cottage cheese	1 cup	35
Heart, beef	3 oz	60
Kidney, beef	3 oz	240
Liver, beef	3 oz	210
Liver, chicken	1 cup	90
Liverwurst spread (Underwood)	4¾-oz can	100
Milk	1 cup	25
Product 19	1 cup	100
Roe, herring, canned	3 oz	40
Total	1 cup	100
Yogurt, plain	1 cup	30

Niacin

When an epidemic of pellagra struck a mental hospital in Alabama in 1907, medical authorities were stunned: pellagra—or *pelle agra* (rough skin)—was thought to be a disease endemic to Italy and Spain but not found in the United States. As it turned out, pellegra, a disease of corn-eating regions, was widespread in the South until corn was fortified with niacin, also called nicotinic acid and sometimes vitamin B_3.

It is said that a niacin shortage results in the three D's—dermatitis, diarrhea, and dementia. At first, symptoms of deficiency are inflammation of the mouth and tongue, and burning sensations throughout the body. Later the skin becomes hard, dry, and scaly, or "sunburned," with blisters that refuse to heal. Some victims are apprehensive, irritable, forgetful, unable to sleep, and mildly paranoid. Indeed, niacin is used by some physicians in treating schizophrenia. Studies also have shown that niacin in large doses may help reduce blood cholesterol and other fats, including triglycerides, in humans.

SOME SUPER SOURCES OF NIACIN

	AMOUNT	PERCENT OF U.S. RDA
Beef liver	3 oz	70
Chicken	½ breast	60
Peaches, dried	1 cup	45
Peanuts	1 cup	120
Peanut butter (Skippy)	2 tbsp	20
Pork loin, lean	3 oz	30
Product 19	1 cup	100
Rabbit, stewed	3 oz	50
Salmon	7¾-oz can	70
Sunflower seeds	1 cup	40
Total	1 cup	100
Tunafish	6½-oz can	120

Calcium

Presumably, nearly everyone knows that calcium is needed for bone growth, but probably few realize how astonishingly versatile this nutrient is—essential for numerous processes in the body. It regulates muscle contraction and is essential in blood clotting, the formation of intercellular cement, and the maintenance of capillary integrity. It activates certain enzyme systems and is necessary for the absorption of vitamin B_{12} and other vitamins and the proper functioning of chemical neurotransmitters in the brain. Calcium intake has also been linked to high blood pressure and is important in preventing osteoporosis, a "softening" of the bones that affects the elderly, mostly women. High intake of calcium—1500 milligrams a day—is recommended for postmenopausal women not taking estrogen. Young women need between 1000 and 1500 milligrams of calcium a day to help prevent osteoporosis in later years. Yet, studies show that the intake of calcium, especially among females, is shockingly low. The average American woman consumes only about 500 milligrams of calcium daily. Of those over age 35, about 75 percent do not consume the recommended daily allowance for calcium.

Only about 20 to 30 percent of the calcium in the diet is absorbed; in order for it to be absorbed adequately, the body must have sufficient vitamin D and phosphorus.

Women during pregnancy and lactation need more calcium. About 1000 milligrams (100 percent of the U.S. RDA for calcium) are depleted every day just through a mother's milk.

Though vegetables and grains contain some calcium, the richest source is milk. About 85 percent of the calcium intake in this country is from milk and dairy products. If you are worried about the high fat content of dairy products, skim milk and skim-milk products contain as much calcium as the high-fat dairy products. Thus skim milk can be used as a substitute.

SOME SUPER SOURCES OF CALCIUM

	AMOUNT	PERCENT OF U.S. RDA
Blackstrap molasses	¼ cup	60
Cheddar cheese	1 oz	20
Collard greens	1 cup cooked	35
Cottage cheese	1 cup	25
Ice cream	1 cup	20–25
Macaroni and cheese, frozen (Stouffer's)	6 oz	25
Milk	1 cup	30–35
Parmesan cheese	1 oz	40
Pudding, most flavors (Jell-O)	1 cup	30
Salmon	7¾-oz can	70
Sardines (Underwood)	3¾-oz can	25
Yogurt, plain	1 cup	40

Iron

Of all nutrients, iron is one of those least consumed. A recent major study by the U.S. Department of Agriculture showed that about 60 percent of the population gets less than 100 percent of the RDA for iron. Only about 5 percent of women of menstruating age get 100 percent of the recommended amount of iron. On the other hand, over 80 percent of American adult males take in 100 percent or more of the recommended daily allowance for iron. Especially worrisome are the low levels of iron in the diets of teenagers, both males and females, and infants and pregnant women.

The result of iron deficiency can be anemia, which can be easily spotted by tests, as well as preanemic conditions that are not easily diagnosed and consequently go overlooked for years. Iron deficiency causes fatigue, weakness, breathlessness, and eventually heart problems; without adequate iron, the blood's hemoglobin cannot carry enough oxygen to the tissues.

It is difficult to get enough iron in the diet without going overboard on calories. Our usual diet provides only 0.6 milligram of iron for every 100 calories. To get the recommended 18 milligrams daily from such food you have to consume 3000 calories—which is too high for many people. However, with the help of charts in this book, you can select foods high in iron and low in calories.

As a rule of thumb only about 10 percent of the iron ingested is absorbed by the body. How much is absorbed depends on several things. If you're well nourished, you absorb less iron—about 5 to 10 percent—than if your body is deficient and needs more iron. Iron is absorbed more easily from meat than from beans and green leafy vegetables like spinach. But food combinations release iron that would ordinarily be unobtainable. Studies show that the vitamin C in orange juice increases the absorption of iron from some foods. Eating beans and meat together increases absorption.

SOME SUPER SOURCES OF IRON

	AMOUNT	PERCENT OF U.S. RDA
Almonds	1 cup	35
Beans, baked (B & M)	1 cup	35
Beef heart	3 oz	30
Blackstrap molasses	¼ cup	80
Kidney, beef	3 oz	60
Lima beans, dried, cooked	1 cup	35
Liver, calf	3 oz	70

	AMOUNT	PERCENT OF U.S. RDA
Liver, chicken	1 cup	70
Liverwurst spread (Underwood)	4¾-oz can	50
Oysters, Atlantic	1 cup	70
Peaches, dried	1 cup	60
Product 19	1 cup	100
Pumpkin seeds	1 cup	90
Sunflower seeds	1 cup	60

Sodium

Sodium is in vast supply and, unlike other nutrients, it is nearly impossible not to get enough of it. The danger is in getting too much. Americans typically consume from one to three teaspoons of salt per day, about twice as much sodium as even conservative medical experts recommend. (Salt is about 40 percent sodium.) The American Medical Association and the Food and Nutrition Board of the National Academy of Sciences–National Research Council both say that sodium should be restricted to about 1100 to 3300 milligrams per day, which would cut the average American's consumption of sodium at least in half.

Although recent research suggests that the relationship between sodium and hypertension (high blood pressure) is perhaps more complex and mysterious than previously thought, most experts still insist that cutting down on sodium is advisable for many Americans, notably those with a predisposition to high blood pressure.

Numerous studies show that blood pressure in populations throughout the world is often related to sodium consumption. For example, Japan, the world's number one consumer of high-sodium soy sauce, also has the highest mortality rate from high blood pressure. In many developing countries where salt is not a staple on the table, high blood pressure is not a prominent killer, and in fact, often does not even rise with age as it does in the United States and other industrialized countries. However, when people who have not grown up eating salt do so, their blood pressure often rises. Similarly, when people cut back on salt their blood pressure often sinks. It has been well demonstrated that many Americans are extra sensitive to salt, or are ''salt reactors''; their blood pressure falls or rises depending on sodium intake. About 60 million Americans have high blood pressure.

Researchers doubt that sodium is the only cause of high blood pressure. Recent research indicates that an intricate metabolic balance of sodium, calcium, and potassium may be involved. Some research, mainly that by Dr. David McCarron and colleagues at the Oregon Health Sciences University, has suggested that some individuals with high blood pressure are deficient in calcium and potassium and even sodium. Preliminary studies by Dr. McCarron and a few other blood-pressure experts have found that dietary supplements of calcium have lowered blood pressure in some patients, especially those with low blood levels of ionized calcium and high sodium consumption. The researchers cautioned that those who cut back on sodium should not inadvertently also reduce their intake of calcium and potassium below recommended daily allowances.

Despite new evidence indicating that the relationship between diet and high blood pressure may not be as simple as many once thought, most experts, including Dr. McCarron, still believe that cutting down on sodium intake is an important nondrug way to control hypertension for many people. Some who do reduce sodium intake see almost immediate beneficial results. Many people who have used this book tell us they pay special attention to the sodium values in the charts.

You will want especially to check the sodium content in baby foods. About five years ago Gerber and Beech-Nut stopped their practice of adding salt as well as MSG (monosodium glutamate) to processed foods for infants. However, canned foods for toddlers may still contain alarmingly high amounts of sodium. For example, one jar of Gerber's junior chunky beef and egg noodles with vegetables contains 514 milligrams of sodium. That could exceed the limit recommended by the National Academy of Sciences Committee on Dietary Allowances. They noted that children from one to three years of age needed at most 325 to 975 milligrams of sodium daily.

Dietary Fat

Since this book was first published, the evidence against high-fat foods has skyrocketed. The health dangers of too much fat, both saturated (animal fats) and unsaturated (vegetable fats), are increasingly being confirmed, as well as the benefits of cutting down on fats. Fat, including cholesterol, is associated with our high incidence of heart disease, and possibly cancer. According to Dr. Antonio M. Gotto, a professor of medicine at Baylor College of Medicine in Houston and president of the American Heart Association, about half of all adult Americans have blood cholesterol levels of about 210 mg/dl (milligrams per deciliter of blood). At this point, he says, the risk of heart disease rises dramatically, and generally the higher the blood cholesterol level, the greater the risk of heart attack, although other factors, such as cigarette smoking, obesity, and high blood pressure, are also important.

Even children, as a result of high-fat diets, often have alarmingly high levels of cholesterol, according to some prominent medical experts. A panel of experts convened by the American Health Foundation agreed that 25 to 30 percent of Americans between the ages of 5 and 18 have high blood cholesterol levels that could lead to an epidemic of heart attacks in later life. They recommend that youngsters be put on lifelong low-fat diets starting at ages one or two. That, they said, would mean a shift from whole to low-fat or skim milk and to soft margarine and a diet lower in red meat and higher in fish and chicken. At the same time there is new evidence that some of the fatty acids in fish (generally low in fat) actually protect against heart disease by reducing blood clotting and lowering blood cholesterol.

Many researchers also believe that cancer, notably colon and breast cancer, is related to eating too much fat. The theory is that although a high-fat diet may not initiate the cancer, it may promote the growth of the cancerous tissue culminating in a tumor. Studies in animals show that vegetable oils (mostly unsaturated fat) can produce a high incidence of certain kinds of cancer.

Numerous studies show that populations consuming a high-fat diet (especially rich in dairy and meat products) have a higher rate of certain cancers. The National Cancer Institute, the American Cancer Society, and the National Academy of Sciences have all recognized the possible role of dietary fat in cancer and recommended reducing fat intake as one way to help prevent cancer. In fact, the National Cancer Institute estimated that diet is connected with 38 percent of all cancers, making it the single most important cause.

Because of this growing evidence against fat, experts recommend that Americans reduce their fat intake to at least 30 percent of calories. The American Heart Association notes that some should go to an extremely low-fat diet—only 20 percent of calories. Americans now take in 40 percent of their calories in fats. A major study by the National Heart, Lung, and Blood Institute concluded definitively that fatal heart attacks are prevented when levels of cholesterol in the blood are lowered. Although the cholesterol lowering in that study was done by drugs, the experts said that lowering cholesterol by diet would also drastically reduce the risk of heart attack. They noted that every 1 percent reduction in blood cholesterol meant a 2 percent reduction in heart-disease risk. That means, according to Dr. Robert Levy, a cardiologist at Columbia University, that if everyone lowers his cholesterol by 10 to 15 percent, heart-attack deaths will decrease by 20 to 30 percent.

WHERE DO WE GET OUR DIETARY FAT?

FOOD	PERCENT FAT INTAKE
Meat	23
Milk products	16
Fat and oils	16
Desserts and sweets	8
Grain products	6
Mixed protein dishes	5
Fruits and vegetables	5
Eggs	5
Cheese	3
Poultry	2
Salty snacks	2
Soups	2
Sugar products	2
Legumes and nuts	2
Fish and shellfish	1
Other	2

Source: Health and Nutrition Examination Survey, 1981. National Center for Health Statistics

Sugar

There is no question that processed foods are heavily dosed with sugar. "Hidden sugar" is everywhere: in cereals, bakery products, candy, soft drinks, as well as in unexpected foods such as peanut butter, catsup, bread, soups, bouillon cubes, and salad dressing. The consumption of sugar has increased dramatically so that today the average American eats 25 percent of his or her daily calories in sugar. Each of us consumes about 130 pounds of sugar a year, an astounding one-third of a pound a day. In contrast, in the 1750s in England, the average person ate only four pounds of sugar per year. Furthermore, at the turn of the century, 75 percent of the sugar came from family kitchens. Today only 25 percent of our sugary intake originates at home; we get the rest from processed foods.

The contribution of sugar to dental decay is well documented. Sugar also provides "empty calories" (calories with no nutritional value except energy) and is a prime culprit in obesity. Consumption of sugar has also been linked to diabetes, hypoglycemia, atherosclerosis, heart disease, and high blood pressure.

Some ready-to-eat cereals are so heavily coated with sugar that some experts believe they should be more accurately called candy. For example, Sugar Smacks is 56 percent sugar. You can look on the labels of such cereals and often see sugar of various kinds as the first ingredient, meaning it contains more sugar than any other ingredient, including the grain from which it was made. Such cereals are often also very heavily fortified with vitamins and minerals, which allows one serving of the cereal to meet all of the daily requirements for the major nutrients. However, one could also get the same nutritional value by eating any cereal and taking a multivitamin pill. To say that you have to eat four times as much Raisin Bran to get the same nutritional value as from Total (as Total's TV commercial claims) is accurate, but does not tell the whole story.

SUGAR CONTENT OF READY-TO-EAT CEREALS

PRODUCT	PERCENT DRY WEIGHT
All-Bran	19.1
Alpha-Bits	37.8
Apple Jacks	52.4
Cap'n Crunch	40.4
Cap'n Crunch's Crunch Berries	44.2
Cap'n Crunch's Peanut Butter	32.2
Cheerios	3.0
Cocoa Krispies	44.6
Cocoa Pebbles	42.1
Cookie-Crisp (chocolate chip and vanilla wafer)	42.3
Corn Chex	4.5
Corn Flakes (Kellogg's)	7.1
Cracklin' Bran	28.6
40% Bran Flakes (Post)	12.5

PRODUCT	PERCENT DRY WEIGHT
Froot Loops	48.9
Frosted Mini-Wheats	26.1
Frosted Ricekrinkles	42.2
Frosted Krispies	38.1
Fruity Pebbles	41.8
Golden Grahams	29.4
Grape-Nuts	7.0
Grape-Nuts Flakes	12.9
Heartland Natural	
With coconut	22.3
With raisins	26.0
Honeycomb	37.0
Kix	4.3
Life, plain and with cinnamon	17.9
Lucky Charms	42.4
Oat flakes, fortified	18.3
100% Bran	22.2
100% Natural (Quaker)	
Plain	21.6
With apples and cinnamon	25.2
With raisins and dates	28.4
Product 19	10.4
Quisp	40.7
Raisin Bran (Kellogg's)	29.7
Raisin Bran (Post)	30.3
Rice Chex	5.1
Rice Krispies	8.2
Rice, puffed	.3
Special K	7.6
Sugar Corn Pops	46.5
Sugar Frosted Flakes (Kellogg's)	39.2
Sugar Smacks	55.8
Super Sugar Crisp	45.2
Team	15.8
Toasties	5.4
Total	8.2
Wheat Chex	4.5
Wheat, puffed, plain	2.5
Wheat, shredded	.5
Wheaties	8.2

Source: U.S. Department of Agriculture

THE TABLES

Alcoholic Beverages	Amt.	Pro-tein	A	C	B_1	B_2	Nia-cin	Cal-cium	Iron	Sodium (mg)	Fat (g)	Carbohy-drate (g)	Calories
						% U.S. RDA							
Beer	8 fl oz	2	*	*	*	4	6	2	*	17	0	9	100
Gin, Rum, Vodka, Whiskey													
80 Proof	1 fl oz	*	*	*	*	*	*	*	*	0	0	0	70
86 Proof	1 fl oz	*	*	*	*	*	*	*	*	0	0	0	70
90 Proof	1 fl oz	*	*	*	*	*	*	*	*	0	0	0	70
94 Proof	1 fl oz	*	*	*	*	*	*	*	*	0	0	0	80
100 Proof	1 fl oz	*	*	*	*	*	*	*	*	0	0	0	80
Wine, Dessert	1 fl oz	*	*	*	*	*	*	*	*	1	0	3	40
Wine, Table	1 fl oz	*	*	*	*	*	*	*	*	1	0	2	25
Baby Foods:[1] Baked Goods													
Biscuits (Gerber)	1 biscuit	4	*	*	4	8	4	*	2	30	1	9	50
Cookies, Animal Shaped (Gerber)	2 cookies	6	*	*	20	35	15	*	2	25	2	9	60
Cookies, Arrowroot (Gerber)	2 cookies	4	*	*	8	4	4	*	2	42	2	8	50
Pretzels (Gerber)	2 pretzels	6	*	*	10	6	8	*	6	31	0	10	50
Zwieback Toast (Gerber)	2 toasts	4	*	*	6	4	4	*	2	33	2	10	60
Baby Foods: Cereal, Dry													
Barley (Beech-Nut Stage 1)[2]	½ oz	6	*	*	45	45	45	20	45	NA	0	10	50

		% U.S. RDA										
Barley (Gerber)	4 tbsp	6	*	*	45	45	25	15	45	4	1	11	60
Barley (Heinz)	½ oz	6	*	*	45	45	45	45	45	NA	1	10	50
Hi-Protein (Beech-Nut Stage 2)	½ oz	20	*	*	45	45	45	20	45	NA	1	7	50
High Protein (Gerber)	4 tbsp	20	*	*	45	45	25	15	45	3	1	6	50
Hi-Protein (Heinz)	½ oz	20	*	*	45	45	45	45	45	NA	1	6	50
High Protein w Apple and Orange (Gerber)	4 tbsp	15	*	*	45	45	25	15	45	15	1	8	60
Mixed (Beech-Nut Stage 2)	½ oz	8	*	*	45	45	45	20	45	NA	1	10	50
Mixed (Gerber)	4 tbsp	8	*	*	45	45	25	15	45	4	1	10	60
Mixed (Heinz)	½ oz	8	*	*	45	45	45	45	45	NA	1	10	60
Mixed w Banana (Gerber)	4 tbsp	6	*	*	45	45	25	15	45	13	1	11	60
Oatmeal (Beech-Nut Stage 1)	½ oz	8	*	*	45	45	45	20	45	NA	1	9	50
Oatmeal (Gerber)	4 tbsp	10	*	*	45	45	25	15	45	4	1	9	50
Oatmeal (Heinz)	½ oz	8	*	*	45	45	45	45	45	NA	1	9	50
Oatmeal w Banana (Gerber)	4 tbsp	8	*	*	45	45	25	15	45	14	1	10	60

[1]Note: All of nutrients for baby foods are based on the U.S. RDAs for infants (not young children who may need more).

[2]Beech-Nut

Stage 1 (0–6 months) 4½-oz jar
Stage 2 (6–9 months) 4½-oz jar
Stage 3 (9 months and up) 7½-oz jar
Table Time (1 year and up) 12-oz jar

25

Baby Foods: Cereal, Dry	Amt.	Pro-tein	A	C	B$_1$	B$_2$	Nia-cin	Cal-cium	Iron	Sodium (mg)	Fat (g)	Carbohy-drate (g)	Calories
								% U.S. RDA					
Rice (Beech-Nut Stage 1)	½ oz	4	*	*		45	45	20	45	NA	1	11	60
Rice (Gerber)	4 tbsp	4	*	*	45	45	25	15	45	4	1	11	60
Rice (Heinz)	½ oz	4	*	*	45	45	45	45	45	NA	1	11	60
Rice w Banana (Gerber)	4 tbsp	4	*	*	45	45	25	15	45	11	1	11	60
Baby Foods: Strained Cereal, Canned													
Mixed w Applesauce and Bananas (Beech-Nut Stage 2)	1 jar	8	*	45	45	45	45	2	45	NA	0	18	80
Mixed w Apples and Bananas (Heinz)	1 jar	6	*	45	45	45	45	2	45	NA	1	22	100
Mixed w Applesauce and Bananas (Gerber)	1 jar	8	*	45	45	45	45	*	45	3	1	18	90
Oatmeal w Apples and Bananas (Heinz)	1 jar	8	*	45	45	45	45	2	45	NA	1	22	100
Oatmeal w Applesauce and Bananas (Beech-Nut Stage 2)	1 jar	8	*	45	45	45	45	2	45	NA	1	17	90
Oatmeal w Applesauce and Bananas (Gerber)	1 jar	8	*	45	45	45	45	*	45	3	1	15	80
Rice w Applesauce and Bananas (Beech-Nut Stage 2)	1 jar	8	*	45	45	45	45	6	45	30	0	20	90

		% U.S. RDA											
Rice w Apples and Bananas (Heinz)	1 jar	4	*	45	45	45	45	45	2	45	NA	1	24	110
Rice w Applesauce and Bananas (Gerber)	1 jar	6	2	45	45	45	45	45	2	45	8	1	22	100
Baby Foods: Strained Desserts														
Apple Betty (Beech-Nut Stage 2)	1 jar	*	*	45	2	8	*	2	2	2	15	0	22	90
Banana Apple Dessert (Gerber)	1 jar	4	2	45	2	2	2	*	*	2	3	0	23	100
Cottage Cheese w Pineapple (Beech-Nut Stage 2)	1 jar	15	2	45	4	10	*	6	*	6	30	2	21	110
Dutch Apple Dessert (Gerber)	1 jar	*	4	25	2	2	*	*	*	*	27	2	22	110
Dutch Apple Dessert (Heinz)	1 jar	*	*	45	*	2	*	*	2	2	NA	0	23	90
Fruit Dessert (Beech-Nut Stage 2)	1 jar	*	15	45	2	4	*	*	2	2	25	0	24	100
Fruit Dessert (Gerber)	1 jar	*	10	4	4	2	2	*	*	*	13	1	23	100
Fruit Dessert (Heinz)	1 jar	*	15	45	2	2	*	2	*	*	NA	1	22	90
Hawaiian Delight (Gerber)	1 jar	8	2	45	6	10	2	8	*	8	23	1	25	120
Mixed Fruit Yogurt (Beech-Nut Stage 2)	1 jar	4	4	45	4	10	*	*	2	4	25	1	25	110
Peach Cobbler (Gerber)	1 jar	2	4	40	2	2	4	*	*	4	9	1	23	100

Baby Foods: Strained Desserts	Amt.	% U.S. RDA								Sodium (mg)	Fat (g)	Carbohy- drate (g)	Calories
		Pro- tein	A	C	B₁	B₂	Nia- cin	Cal- cium	Iron				
Peach Cobbler (Heinz)	1 jar	2	6	45	4	2	*	2	*	NA	1	21	110
Peaches and Yogurt (Beech-Nut Stage 2)	1 jar	6	25	45	2	10	4	6	*	25	1	22	100
Pineapple Dessert (Beech-Nut Stage 2)	1 jar	*	*	45	6	10	*	6	*	25	0	25	100
Pineapple-Orange (Heinz)	1 jar	*	*	45	2	2	*	2	2	NA	0	23	90
Pudding, Apple Custard (Beech-Nut Stage 2)	1 jar	6	*	45	2	10	*	4	2	40	1	20	100
Pudding, Banana (Heinz)	1 jar	4	4	45	2	6	2	2	2	NA	3	23	120
Pudding, Banana Custard (Beech-Nut Stage 2)	1 jar	6	*	45	4	10	*	2	2	40	1	18	90
Pudding, Cherry Vanilla (Gerber)	1 jar	*	*	2	2	2	*	*	2	9	1	22	100
Pudding, Chocolate Custard (Gerber)	1 jar	10	4	4	2	15	*	10	4	31	2	20	110
Pudding, Custard (Heinz)	1 jar	15	*	*	4	20	*	10	*	NA	2	17	100
Pudding, Orange (Gerber)	1 jar	6	6	25	6	10	2	6	*	28	2	24	120
Pudding, Vanilla Custard (Beech-Nut Stage 2)	1 jar	10	4	*	2	15	*	10	*	45	1	20	100
Pudding, Vanilla Custard (Gerber)	1 jar	10	6	2	2	15	*	10	2	31	2	21	110
Raspberry Dessert w Non- fat Yogurt (Gerber)	1 jar	6	*	*	4	10	*	8	*	29	0	20	80

Food	Serving														
		% U.S. RDA													
Tutti-Frutti (Heinz)	1 jar	2	8	45	6	2	*	2	*	2	*	NA	1	22	100

Baby Foods: Strained Fruit

Food	Serving														
Apples and Apricots (Heinz)	1 jar	*	45	45	2	8	2	2	2	2	2	NA	1	15	70
Apple Blueberry (Gerber)	1 jar	*	2	45	4	8	2	*	*	*	4	4	1	17	80
Apples and Cranberries w Tapioca (Heinz)	1 jar	*	*	45	2	2	4	*	*	*	*	NA	1	20	90
Apples and Grapes (Beech-Nut Stage 2 Fruit Supreme)	1 jar	*	8	45	4	4	*	*	4	*	4	NA	0	27	110
Apples, Oranges, and Bananas (Beech-Nut Stage 2 Fruit Supreme)	1 jar	*	6	45	4	6	*	*	*	*	*	NA	0	22	90
Apples, Peaches, and Strawberries (Beech-Nut Stage 2 Fruit Supreme)	1 jar	*	10	45	2	4	2	*	2	*	*	NA	0	24	100
Apples and Pears (Heinz)	1 jar	*	4	45	2	4	2	*	2	*	2	NA	1	18	80
Apples, Pears, and Bananas (Beech-Nut Stage 2 Fruit Supreme)	1 jar	*	2	45	2	6	*	*	*	*	*	NA	0	24	100
Apples, Pears, and Pineapples (Beech-Nut Stage 2 Fruit Supreme)	1 jar	*	2	45	4	4	*	*	*	*	*	NA	0	24	100
Apples and Strawberries (Beech-Nut Stage 2 Fruit Supreme)	1 jar	*	2	45	4	6	2	*	2	*	*	NA	0	24	100

Baby Foods: Strained Fruit	Amt.	% U.S. RDA Protein	A	C	B_1	B_2	Niacin	Calcium	Iron	Sodium (mg)	Fat (g)	Carbohydrate (g)	Calories
Applesauce (Gerber)	1 jar	*	2	45	2	6	*	*	*	3	1	15	70
Applesauce (Heinz)	1 jar	*	*	45	2	4	2	2	*	NA	1	16	70
Applesauce and Apricots (Beech-Nut Stage 2)	1 jar	*	25	45	2	4	*	*	*	NA	0	14	60
Applesauce and Apricots (Gerber)	1 jar	*	15	45	2	6	2	*	*	3	1	17	80
Applesauce and Bananas (Beech-Nut Stage 2)	1 jar	*	2	45	4	6	*	*	*	NA	0	15	60
Applesauce and Cherries (Beech-Nut Stage 2)	1 jar	*	4	45	4	6	*	*	2	NA	0	17	70
Applesauce, Golden Delicious (Beech-Nut Stage 1)	1 jar	*	*	45	2	6	*	*	*	0–10	0	14	60
Applesauce w Pineapple (Gerber)	1 jar	*	*	45	4	6	*	*	*	3	0	16	60
Apricots w Tapioca (Beech-Nut Stage 2)	1 jar	*	60	45	*	2	2	2	2	25	0	20	80
Apricots w Tapioca (Gerber)	1 jar	2	50	45	*	2	4	*	2	5	1	22	100
Apricots w Tapioca (Heinz)	1 jar	*	70	45	*	2	2	2	*	NA	0	19	80
Bananas (Beech-Nut Stage 1)	1 jar	4	10	45	4	10	4	*	2	0–10	0	24	100
Bananas w Tapioca (Gerber)	1 jar	2	2	45	*	4	2	*	*	17	1	21	100

				% U.S. RDA								
Bananas w Tapioca (Heinz) 1 jar	2	2	45	4	2	2	2	2	NA	1	24	110
Bananas and Pineapple w Tapioca (Beech-Nut Stage 2) 1 jar	*	2	45	2	8	2	2	2	NA	0	19	80
Bananas w Pineapple and Tapioca (Gerber) 1 jar	*	2	45	2	4	2	*	*	6	1	15	70
Bananas and Pineapple w Tapioca (Heinz) 1 jar	*	2	45	2	2	2	*	2	NA	0	22	90
Guava w Tapioca (Beech-Nut Stage 2) 1 jar	*	6	45	2	2	2	*	*	NA	0	25	100
Island Fruits (Beech-Nut Stage 2) 1 jar	*	20	45	6	2	*	*	*	NA	0	22	90
Mango w Tapioca (Beech-Nut Stage 2) 1 jar	*	70	45	4	2	2	*	*	NA	0	22	90
Peaches (Gerber) 1 jar	2	15	45	2	4	10	*	*	5	1	23	100
Peaches (Heinz) 1 jar	2	10	45	2	6	8	*	2	NA	0	12	50
Peaches (Beech-Nut Stage 1) 1 jar	2	30	45	4	6	8	*	*	0–10	0	14	60
Pears (Gerber) 1 jar	2	2	45	2	4	2	2	2	4	1	15	70
Pears (Heinz) 1 jar	*	*	45	4	4	*	*	2	NA	0	17	70
Pears, Bartlett (Beech-Nut Stage 1) 1 jar	*	*	45	2	6	2	2	2	0–10	0	16	70
Pears and Pineapple (Beech-Nut Stage 2) 1 jar	*	2	45	6	10	2	4	2	NA	0	25	100

Baby Foods: Strained Fruit	Amt.	Protein	A	C	B₁	B₂	Niacin	Calcium	Iron	Sodium (mg)	Fat (g)	Carbohydrate (g)	Calories
						% U.S. RDA							
Pears and Pineapple (Gerber)	1 jar	2	2	45	4	4	2	2	*	3	1	16	80
Pears and Pineapples (Heinz)	1 jar	2	*	45	2	4	2	2	2	NA	0	18	80
Plums w Tapioca (Beech-Nut Stage 2)	1 jar	*	15	15	2	6	2	2	2	10	0	25	100
Plums w Tapioca (Gerber)	1 jar	2	4	*	*	4	4	*	*	5	1	22	100
Prunes w Tapioca (Beech-Nut Stage 2)	1 jar	2	30	*	4	10	8	2	2	NA	0	24	100
Plums w Tapioca (Heinz)	1 jar	*	8	45	4	2	*	2	*	NA	0	20	80
Prunes w Tapioca (Gerber)	1 jar	4	20	20	4	20	8	2	2	13	1	24	110
Prunes w Tapioca (Heinz)	1 jar	4	20	45	4	10	6	4	2	NA	0	27	120
Baby Foods: Strained Fruit Juices													
Apple (Beech-Nut Stage 1)	1 jar	*	*	120	*	*	*	*	2	NA	0	14	60
Apple (Beech-Nut Stage 2)	4 fl oz	*	*	120	*	*	*	*	2	NA	0	14	60
Apple (Gerber)	1 can	*	*	120	*	2	*	*	2	3	0	16	60
Apple (Heinz)	1 can	*	*	120	*	*	*	*	4	NA	0	15	60
Apple-Apricot (Heinz)	1 can	*	35	120	*	2	2	2	4	NA	0	16	70
Apple-Banana (Gerber)	1 can	*	*	120	2	2	2	*	2	4	0	15	60

32

Food	Serving	% U.S. RDA									Calories
Apple Cherry (Beech-Nut Stage 2)	1 jar	*	120	*	2	*	4	NA	0	12	50
Apple-Cherry (Gerber)	1 can	*	120	2	4	*	2	0-1	0	16	60
Apple-Cherry (Heinz)	1 can	*	120	*	*	*	*	NA	0	15	60
Apple Cranberry (Beech-Nut Stage 2)	1 jar	8	120	*	2	*	4	NA	0	14	60
Apple Grape (Beech-Nut Stage 2)	1 jar	*	120	2	4	*	2	NA	0	14	60
Apple-Grape (Gerber)	1 can	*	120	2	4	*	2	3	0	16	60
Apple-Grape (Heinz)	1 can	*	120	2	2	2	2	NA	0	16	70
Apple Peach (Beech-Nut Stage 2)	1 jar	8	120	*	2	*	4	NA	0	15	60
Apple-Peach (Gerber)	1 can	4	120	*	2	*	2	4	0	15	60
Apple-Peach (Heinz)	1 can	*	120	*	*	*	4	NA	0	15	60
Apple-Pineapple (Heinz)	1 can	*	120	2	*	2	2	NA	0	15	60
Apple-Plum (Gerber)	1 can	2	120	2	6	*	2	4	0	16	60
Apple-Prune (Gerber)	1 can	*	120	*	10	*	2	5	0	16	60
Apple-Prune (Heinz)	1 can	*	120	*	4	*	6	NA	0	16	70
Grape (Beech-Nut Stage 1)	1 jar	*	120	2	2	2	4	NA	0	19	80
Juice Plus (Beech-Nut Stage 2)	4 fl oz	*	120	2	8	*	30	10	0	15	60
Mixed Fruit (Beech-Nut Stage 2)	1 jar	8	120	2	2	*	4	NA	0	15	60

Baby Foods: Strained Fruit Juices

	Amt.	Pro-tein	A	C	B₁	B₂	Nia-cin	Cal-cium	Iron	Sodium (mg)	Fat (g)	Carbohy-drate (g)	Calories
						% U.S. RDA							
Mixed Fruit (Gerber)	1 can	2	2	120	8	2	2	*	2	3	0	16	70
Mixed Fruit (Heinz)	1 can	*	6	120	4	2	2	2	2	NA	0	17	70
Orange (Beech-Nut Stage 2)	1 jar	2	10	120	10	4	2	2	*	NA	0	14	60
Orange (Gerber)	1 can	2	4	120	15	6	4	2	*	4	1	14	70
Orange (Heinz)	1 can	2	*	120	15	8	2	2	2	NA	0	14	60
Orange-Apple (Gerber)	1 can	2	6	120	8	4	2	*	*	5	1	15	70
Orange-Apple-Banana (Heinz)	1 can	*	2	120	6	4	2	2	4	NA	0	16	60
Orange-Apricot (Gerber)	1 can	4	20	120	15	6	4	*	*	8	1	15	70
Orange-Pineapple (Gerber)	1 can	2	4	120	15	4	4	2	*	0-1	1	17	80
Pear (Beech-Nut Stage 1)	1 jar	*	*	120	2	4	2	2	*	NA	0	14	60
Tropical Blend (Beech-Nut Stage 2)	4 fl oz	*	2	120	2	6	2	2	2	NA	0	15	70
Beef Dinner Supreme (Beech-Nut Stage 2)	1 jar	15	150	15	2	15	15	2	2	50	7	12	120
Baby Foods: Strained Main Dishes													
Beef and Egg Noodles (Heinz)	1 jar	15	20	*	6	6	6	*	2	NA	2	10	60
Beef Egg Noodle Dinner w Vegetables (Beech-Nut Stage 2)	1 jar	10	210	10	6	8	8	4	2	35	4	10	90

Food	Serving						% U.S. RDA						
Beef and Egg Noodles w Vegetables (Gerber)	1 jar	15	45	4	6	8	10	*	2	19	3	12	90
Beef w Vegetables (Gerber High Meat Dinner)	1 jar	45	30	6	6	15	20	*	6	30	6	8	120
Beef w Vegetables (Heinz High Meat Dinner)	1 jar	40	60	2	15	20	20	2	6	NA	5	6	100
Cereal and Egg Yolk (Gerber)	1 jar	10	6	2	4	10	2	6	2	17	2	10	70
Chicken and Noodles (Gerber)	1 jar	10	45	6	6	8	10	6	2	20	2	12	80
Chicken Noodle Dinner (Heinz)	1 jar	15	40	*	15	10	6	6	2	NA	3	10	70
Chicken Noodle Dinner w Vegetables (Beech-Nut Stage 2)	1 jar	10	180	10	6	10	8	4	4	40	3	12	80
Chicken Rice Dinner w Vegetables (Beech-Nut Stage 2)	1 jar	10	150	10	6	8	8	6	4	40	3	12	90
Chicken w Vegetables (Gerber High Meat Dinner)	1 jar	45	60	6	2	10	15	15	6	33	7	8	130
Chicken w Vegetables (Heinz High Meat Dinner)	1 jar	45	15	2	25	25	30	15	6	NA	6	7	110
Chicken Soup (Heinz)	1 jar	10	45	*	6	6	2	4	2	NA	2	10	70
Chicken Soup, Cream of (Gerber)	1 jar	10	30	4	2	6	6	8	2	29	3	11	80

Baby Foods: Strained Main Dishes	Amt.	Protein	A	C	B₁	B₂	Niacin	Calcium	Iron	Sodium (mg)	Fat (g)	Carbohydrate (g)	Calories
		|			% U.S. RDA			|					
Cottage Cheese w Pineapple (Gerber High Meat Dinner)	1 jar	45	2	4	10	20	2	10	*	194	2	19	130
Ham w Vegetables (Gerber High Meat Dinner)	1 jar	45	25	6	15	15	20	*	4	18	4	9	100
Macaroni and Cheese (Gerber)	1 jar	15	2	4	10	15	8	10	2	102	3	11	90
Macaroni, Tomato, and Beef (Beech-Nut Stage 2)	1 jar	10	180	6	8	10	10	4	4	55	3	13	90
Macaroni-Tomato w Beef (Gerber)	1 jar	10	50	6	8	6	10	2	2	18	2	13	80
Macaroni, Tomatoes, and Beef (Heinz)	1 jar	15	25	*	25	15	15	4	4	NA	1	11	70
Turkey Dinner Supreme (Beech-Nut Stage 2)	1 jar	15	90	8	2	10	10	10	4	45	5	10	100
Turkey and Rice w Vegetables (Gerber)	1 jar	10	40	4	*	8	10	4	2	23	3	10	80
Turkey Rice Dinner w Vegetables (Beech-Nut Stage 2)	1 jar	10	80	6	4	4	10	6	2	45	2	11	70
Turkey Rice Dinner w Vegetables (Heinz)	1 jar	10	30	*	4	6	4	6	2	NA	1	10	60
Turkey w Vegetables (Gerber High Meat Dinner)	1 jar	45	55	6	2	15	20	10	6	37	7	8	130

Food	Serving	% U.S. RDA											
Turkey w Vegetables (Heinz High Meat Dinner)	1 jar	20	35	*	4	10	6	10	4	NA	8	9	120
Veal w Vegetables (Gerber High Meat Dinner)	1 jar	45	6	6	4	15	25	*	4	27	2	8	80
Vegetables and Bacon (Gerber)	1 jar	10	50	4	6	6	10	2	2	79	5	11	100
Vegetables w Bacon (Heinz)	1 jar	10	120	*	15	4	4	2	2	NA	3	10	80
Vegetable Beef Dinner (Beech-Nut Stage 2)	1 jar	10	150	10	4	10	10	2	2	40	3	12	90
Vegetables and Beef (Gerber)	1 jar	10	70	4	4	4	10	*	2	17	3	11	80
Vegetables and Beef (Heinz)	1 jar	20	160	2	6	8	8	2	2	NA	2	8	70
Vegetable Chicken Dinner (Beech-Nut Stage 2)	1 jar	15	120	10	4	8	6	10	2	50	3	13	90
Vegetables and Chicken (Gerber)	1 jar	10	50	2	4	4	4	4	2	14	2	9	70
Vegetables, Dumplings, and Beef (Heinz)	1 jar	15	30	*	8	8	8	4	4	NA	2	11	70
Vegetables, Egg Noodles, and Chicken (Heinz)	1 jar	20	60	*	10	8	8	6	4	NA	3	13	90
Vegetables, Egg Noodles, and Turkey (Heinz)	1 jar	8	60	*	6	8	4	6	2	NA	2	10	60

Baby Foods: Strained Main Dishes	Amt.	Pro-tein	A	C	B₁	B₂	Nia-cin	Cal-cium	Iron	Sodium (mg)	Fat (g)	Carbohy-drate (g)	Calories
		% U.S. RDA											
Vegetable Ham Dinner (Beech-Nut Stage 2)	1 jar	10	190	8	8	10	10	2	2	50	2	13	80
Vegetables and Ham (Gerber)	1 jar	10	45	4	6	4	8	*	2	15	3	11	80
Vegetables and Ham (Heinz)	1 jar	15	45	*	6	6	4	6	4	NA	1	9	60
Vegetable Lamb Dinner (Beech-Nut Stage 2)	1 jar	8	150	10	2	6	8	2	2	35	3	12	80
Vegetables and Lamb (Gerber)	1 jar	10	70	4	4	8	8	*	2	15	3	10	80
Vegetables and Lamb (Heinz)	1 jar	15	140	*	8	4	4	4	4	NA	1	9	60
Vegetables and Liver (Gerber)	1 jar	10	120	10	6	50	20	*	20	19	1	10	60
Vegetables and Turkey (Gerber)	1 jar	10	50	4	2	4	8	2	2	20	2	10	70
Baby Foods: Strained Meat and Eggs													
Beef (Gerber)	1 jar	70	4	6	2	20	40	*	8	51	4	1	90
Beef and Beef Broth (Beech-Nut Stage 1)	1 jar	70	*	*	2	20	30	*	8	75	8	1	120
Beef and Beef Broth (Heinz)	1 jar	70	*	*	*	15	25	*	8	NA	8	0	130

						% U.S. RDA							
Beef w Beef Heart (Gerber)	1 jar	70	6	6	2	60	40	*	15	53	4	1	90
Beef Liver (Gerber)	1 jar	80	1940	50	6	260	100	*	30	46	3	3	90
Chicken (Gerber)	1 jar	80	2	4	*	20	40	10	6	39	9	1	140
Chicken and Chicken Broth (Beech-Nut Stage 1)	1 jar	70	*	*	2	25	35	6	8	70	6	1	110
Chicken and Chicken Broth (Heinz)	1 jar	70	*	*	4	15	40	10	6	NA	8	0	130
Egg Yolks (Gerber)	1 jar	50	25	6	10	35	*	10	20	45	16	1	180
Ham (Gerber)	1 jar	70	2	4	20	25	30	*	6	40	6	1	110
Lamb (Gerber)	1 jar	80	*	*	2	35	30	*	10	50	4	1	100
Lamb and Lamb Broth (Beech-Nut Stage 1)	1 jar	70	*	*	4	20	30	*	10	75	8	1	130
Lamb and Lamb Broth (Heinz)	1 jar	70	*	*	2	15	20	*	10	NA	11	0	150
Liver and Liver Broth (Heinz)	1 jar	80	1670	60	8	240	90	*	25	NA	3	2	90
Pork (Gerber)	1 jar	70	*	4	20	25	25	*	6	38	6	1	110
Turkey (Gerber)	1 jar	80	2	8	2	30	40	2	6	55	7	1	120
Turkey and Turkey Broth (Beech-Nut Stage 1)	1 jar	70	*	*	4	20	30	4	6	60	7	1	120
Turkey and Turkey Broth (Heinz)	1 jar	80	4	6	4	20	40	2	4	NA	7	0	120
Veal (Gerber)	1 jar	80	2	6	2	25	45	*	6	51	4	0	90

Baby Foods: Strained Meat and Eggs	Amt.	Protein	A	C	B₁	B₂	Niacin	Calcium	Iron	Sodium (mg)	Fat (g)	Carbohydrate (g)	Calories
					% U.S. RDA								
Veal and Veal Broth (Beech-Nut Stage 1)	1 jar	70	*	*	2	20	25	*	6	70	7	1	120
Veal and Veal Broth (Heinz)	1 jar	70	2	4	4	20	40	*	6	NA	8	0	130
Baby Foods: Strained Vegetables													
Beets (Gerber)	1 jar	6	*	*	2	6	2	2	2	119	0	11	50
Beets (Heinz)	1 jar	6	2	4	2	4	2	2	2	NA	0	10	50
Carrots (Gerber)	1 jar	4	120	15	4	8	4	4	2	47	0	7	35
Carrots (Heinz)	1 jar	4	1050	15	6	4	*	4	2	NA	0	6	25
Carrots, Royal Imperial (Beech-Nut Stage 1)	1 jar	4	590	30	4	10	6	4	*	130	0	8	40
Corn, Creamed (Beech-Nut Stage 2)	1 jar	6	6	10	*	10	6	2	2	15	0	15	70
Corn, Creamed (Gerber)	1 jar	10	2	6	2	8	10	4	*	11	1	17	90
Corn, Creamed (Heinz)	1 jar	4	50	*	*	4	6	2	2	NA	1	19	90
Garden (Beech-Nut Stage 2)	1 jar	8	170	20	8	15	10	4	4	60	0	11	60
Garden (Gerber)	1 jar	10	200	25	15	15	10	6	6	28	1	7	50
Green Beans (Gerber)	1 jar	6	20	15	6	15	6	8	4	4	0	7	40
Green Beans (Heinz)	1 jar	6	30	10	6	10	2	6	4	NA	0	8	40

40

							% U.S. RDA						
Green Beans, Mohawk Valley (Beech-Nut Stage 1)	1 jar	6	45	25	25	20	4	10	8	0-10	0	8	40
Mixed (Beech-Nut Stage 2)	1 jar	6	220	8	6	6	8	2	2	45	0	12	50
Mixed (Gerber)	1 jar	6	120	6	6	4	6	2	2	27	1	10	60
Mixed (Heinz)	1 jar	6	120	*	6	4	2	4	*	NA	0	10	60
Peas (Gerber)	1 jar	15	30	25	20	10	15	2	8	4	1	10	60
Peas, Creamed (Heinz)	1 jar	10	25	*	15	10	8	4	4	NA	3	12	80
Peas, Sweet, Tender (Beech-Nut Stage 1)	1 jar	20	40	30	10	10	15	6	8	0-10	0	12	70
Peas and Carrots (Beech-Nut Stage 2)	1 jar	10	300	25	10	10	10	6	4	50	0	11	60
Spinach, Creamed (Gerber)	1 jar	10	120	15	6	20	4	20	8	49	2	7	60
Squash (Beech-Nut Stage 1)	1 jar	4	110	25	*	10	4	4	*	0-10	0	7	30
Squash (Gerber)	1 jar	4	90	25	2	6	6	4	2	5	1	8	40
Squash (Heinz)	1 jar	4	210	8	4	6	6	6	2	NA	0	9	45
Sweet Potatoes (Beech-Nut Stage 1)	1 jar	4	380	20	4	6	4	4	2	60	0	16	70
Sweet Potatoes (Gerber)	1 jar	6	120	35	4	8	6	2	*	24	0	19	80
Sweet Potatoes (Heinz)	1 jar	6	900	15	10	8	6	6	4	NA	0	21	90
Baby Foods, Junior: Cereal, Canned													
Mixed w Applesauce and Bananas (Gerber)	1 jar	10	2	45	45	45	45	2	30	8	2	28	140

41

Baby Foods, Junior: Cereal, Canned	Amt.	Protein	A	C	B₁	B₂	Niacin	Calcium	Iron	Sodium (mg)	Fat (g)	Carbohydrate (g)	Calories
		% U.S. RDA											
Oatmeal w Applesauce and Bananas (Gerber)	1 jar	15	2	45	45	45	45	2	30	4	2	24	130
Rice w Mixed Fruit (Gerber)	1 jar	10	*	45	45	45	45	6	30	18	1	37	170
Baby Foods, Junior: Desserts													
Banana Dessert (Beech-Nut Stage 3)	1 jar	*	4	45	6	10	4	4	4	NA	0	40	160
Banana-Apple Dessert (Gerber)	1 jar	6	4	45	6	6	4	*	2	9	1	39	170
Cottage Cheese w Pineapple (Beech-Nut Stage 3)	1 jar	30	6	45	6	20	*	8	2	50	3	31	180
Dutch Apple Dessert (Gerber)	1 jar	*	6	45	2	4	*	*	*	46	2	36	160
Dutch Apple Dessert (Gerber Chunky)[1]	1 jar	*	*	45	*	*	4	*	*	45	2	30	140
Dutch Apple Dessert (Heinz)	1 jar	*	*	45	*	4	*	2	2	NA	0	37	150
Fruit Dessert (Beech-Nut Stage 3)	1 jar	*	60	45	2	6	2	2	2	80	0	42	170
Fruit Dessert (Gerber)	1 jar	2	15	6	6	6	4	2	2	18	1	39	170
Fruit Dessert (Heinz)	1 jar	2	25	45	2	2	*	4	*	NA	1	38	160
Hawaiian Delight (Gerber)	1 jar	10	4	45	15	15	4	10	2	40	1	42	190

	Serving	% U.S. RDA										
Mixed Fruit Yogurt (Beech-Nut Stage 3)	1 jar	8	8	45	6	15	8	4	40	1	41	180
Peach Cobbler (Gerber)	1 jar	4	6	45	6	4	*	*	20	1	38	160
Peach Cobbler (Gerber Chunky)	1 jar	2	15	45	2	4	8	2	17	1	31	140
Pineapple-Orange (Heinz)	1 jar	2	*	45	4	2	*	2	NA	0	34	140
Pudding, Banana Custard (Beech-Nut Stage 3)	1 jar	8	2	45	4	20	4	4	55	1	38	170
Pudding, Cherry Vanilla (Gerber)	1 jar	2	*	4	4	2	*	2	17	1	36	160
Pudding, Custard (Heinz)	1 jar	25	*	*	6	30	20	*	NA	4	30	170
Pudding, Vanilla Custard (Beech-Nut Stage 3)	1 jar	15	8	*	4	25	20	2	70	2	29	150
Pudding, Vanilla Custard (Gerber)	1 jar	20	6	6	4	20	15	2	51	4	35	190
Raspberry Dessert w Nonfat Yogurt (Gerber)	1 jar	10	*	2	6	20	10	2	51	1	34	150
Tutti-Frutti (Heinz)	1 jar	4	25	45	4	8	2	2	NA	1	35	150
Baby Foods, Junior: Fruit												
Apples and Apricots (Heinz)	1 jar	2	80	45	4	15	2	2	NA	1	25	110
Apple-Blueberry (Gerber)	1 jar	2	6	45	6	15	*	2	6	1	28	120
Apples and Cranberries w Tapioca (Heinz)	1 jar	*	*	45	4	4	6	*	NA	1	33	140

43

¹U.S. RDA for Gerber Chunky products is for children 1-4 yrs. old

Baby Foods, Junior: Fruit	Amt.	Protein	A	C	B₁	B₂	Niacin	Calcium	Iron	Sodium (mg)	Fat (g)	Carbohydrate (g)	Calories
			% U.S. RDA										
Apples and Grapes (Beech-Nut Stage 3 Fruit Supreme)	1 jar	*	15	45	6	8	2	*	8	NA	0	44	190
Apples, Mandarin Oranges, and Bananas (Beech-Nut Stage 3 Fruit Supreme)	1 jar	*	10	45	8	10	2	2	2	40	0	37	150
Apples, Peaches, and Strawberries (Beech-Nut Stage 3 Fruit Supreme)	1 jar	*	20	45	4	8	4	2	2	40	0	40	160
Apples and Pears (Heinz)	1 jar	2	6	45	4	8	4	2	2	NA	1	30	130
Apples, Pears, and Bananas (Beech-Nut Stage 3 Fruit Supreme)	1 jar	*	4	45	4	10	2	2	2	40	0	40	160
Apples, Pears, and Pineapples (Beech-Nut Stage 3 Fruit Supreme)	1 jar	*	4	45	8	8	2	2	2	40	0	40	160
Apples and Strawberries (Beech-Nut Stage 3 Fruit Supreme)	1 jar	*	4	45	6	10	2	2	2	40	0	40	160
Applesauce (Gerber)	1 jar	*	4	45	6	10	2	*	*	2	1	24	100
Applesauce (Heinz)	1 jar	*	2	45	6	6	2	2	*	NA	1	26	110
Applesauce and Apricots (Beech-Nut Stage 3)	1 jar	*	40	45	6	8	2	2	2	40	0	23	90

Food	Serving	% U.S. RDA										
Applesauce and Apricots (Gerber)	1 jar	2	35	6	10	4	2	2	6	1	24	110
Applesauce and Bananas (Beech-Nut Stage 3)	1 jar	*	4	45	6	10	2	2	*	NA	0	26	110
Applesauce and Apple Bits (Beech-Nut Stage 3)	1 jar	*	2	45	6	10	*	2	*	40	0	24	100
Applesauce and Cherries (Beech-Nut Stage 3)	1 jar	*	8	45	8	10	2	2	4	40	0	28	110
Apricots w Tapioca (Beech-Nut Stage 3)	1 jar	*	90	45	2	4	4	4	4	40	0	33	140
Apricots w Tapioca (Gerber)	1 jar	4	80	45	2	4	6	2	4	9	1	38	160
Apricots w Tapioca (Heinz)	1 jar	*	90	45	2	2	4	2	2	NA	0	36	150
Bananas w Tapioca (Beech-Nut Stage 3)	1 jar	*	2	45	2	10	4	4	2	40	0	32	130
Bananas w Tapioca (Gerber)	1 jar	4	2	45	2	10	6	*	2	28	1	35	150
Bananas w Tapioca (Gerber Chunky)	1 jar	2	*	45	2	4	4	*	2	16	1	29	130
Bananas w Tapioca (Heinz)	1 jar	4	4	45	6	4	4	4	4	NA	2	39	180
Bananas w Pineapple and Tapioca (Gerber)	1 jar	2	4	45	6	6	4	2	*	8	1	27	120
Bananas and Pineapple w Tapioca (Heinz)	1 jar	*	*	45	4	2	2	2	*	NA	1	36	150
Island Fruits (Beech-Nut Stage 3 Fruit Supreme)	1 jar	*	30	45	4	4	2	2	*	NA	0	37	150

Baby Foods, Junior: Fruit	Amt.	Protein	A	C	B₁	B₂	Niacin	Calcium	Iron	Sodium (mg)	Fat (g)	Carbohydrate (g)	Calories
		%%% U.S. RDA											
Peaches (Beech-Nut Stage 3)	1 jar	2	110	45	4	10	15	2	4	NA	0	37	150
Peaches (Gerber)	1 jar	4	20	45	4	10	15	*	2	7	1	37	160
Peaches (Heinz)	1 jar	4	20	45	4	10	15	*	4	NA	1	21	90
Pears (Gerber)	1 jar	2	4	45	4	8	4	2	2	6	1	26	120
Pears (Heinz)	1 jar	*	2	45	6	6	2	4	*	NA	1	30	120
Pears, Bartlett (Beech-Nut Stage 3)	1 jar	*	*	45	6	10	4	4	4	NA	0	35	140
Pears, Bartlett, and Pineapple (Beech-Nut Stage 3)	1 jar	*	4	45	10	15	4	6	4	NA	0	40	160
Pears and Pineapple (Gerber)	1 jar	2	4	45	10	6	4	2	2	4	1	26	120
Plums w Tapioca (Gerber)	1 jar	2	4	*	2	10	6	2	2	9	1	39	170
Prunes w Tapioca (Gerber)	1 jar	6	35	25	6	30	10	4	4	20	1	42	180
Baby Foods, Junior: Fruit Juices													
Apple (Gerber Toddler Juices, 7-oz jar)	4 fl oz	*	*	100	*	*	*	*	2	1	0	15	60
Apple-Cherry (Gerber Toddler Juices, 7-oz jar)	4 fl oz	*	*	100	2	2	*	*	4	2	0	14	60
Apple-Grape (Gerber Toddler Juices, 7-oz jar)	4 fl oz	*	*	100	2	*	*	*	2	2	0	15	60

		% U.S. RDA											
Mixed Fruit (Gerber Toddler Juices, 7-oz jar)	4 fl oz	*	*	100	6	2	2	*	2	1	0	15	60
Baby Foods, Junior: Main Dishes													
Beef Dinner Supreme (Beech-Nut Stage 3)	1 jar	20	210	10	6	20	25	4	8	95	9	20	190
Beef and Egg Noodles w Vegetables (Gerber)	1 jar	25	80	10	10	10	15	2	6	36	4	20	140
Beef and Egg Noodles w Vegetables (Gerber Chunky)	1 jar	25	30	10	10	10	15	2	8	514	4	15	120
Beef Noodle Dinner w Vegetables (Beech-Nut Stage 3)	1 jar	15	300	10	10	15	15	4	8	75	4	21	140
Beef Stew (Beech-Nut Table Time)	6 oz	30	60	25	4	15	15	4	10	660	4	15	130
Beef w Vegetables (Gerber High Meat Dinner)	1 jar	45	60	4	4	15	20	2	6	36	7	9	130
Beef w Vegetables and Cereal (Heinz High Meat Dinner)	1 jar	40	180	*	20	20	20	*	4	NA	8	7	130
Cereal and Egg Yolk (Gerber)	1 jar	15	8	4	4	15	4	8	4	25	4	15	110
Chicken and Noodles (Gerber)	1 jar	20	70	8	10	8	15	6	4	28	3	19	120
Chicken Noodle Dinner (Heinz)	1 jar	20	60	*	20	15	10	10	2	NA	5	23	150

Baby Foods, Junior: Main Dishes	Amt.	% U.S. RDA								Sodium (mg)	Fat (g)	Carbohydrate (g)	Calories
		Protein	A	C	B1	B2	Niacin	Calcium	Iron				
Chicken Noodle Dinner w Vegetables (Beech-Nut Stage 3)	1 jar	20	170	15	10	15	10	6	8	55	3	21	130
Chicken w Vegetables (Gerber High Meat Dinner)	1 jar	50	100	8	2	10	15	15	8	33	7	8	130
Chicken w Vegetables (Heinz High Meat Dinner)	1 jar	45	60	*	25	25	30	6	6	NA	6	10	120
Chicken Soup, w Stars, Hearty (Beech-Nut Table Time)	6 oz	15	240	10	4	10	10	6	6	630	10	17	180
Egg Noodles and Beef (Heinz)	1 jar	25	50	*	15	8	15	4	4	NA	3	18	120
Ham w Vegetables (Gerber High Meat Dinner)	1 jar	50	40	8	20	15	20	*	4	24	4	10	110
Macaroni and Cheese (Gerber)	1 jar	25	6	6	15	20	15	20	4	168	4	19	140
Macaroni Tomato Beef (Beech-Nut Stage 3)	1 jar	20	340	15	10	20	15	8	8	85	4	24	150
Macaroni-Tomato w Beef (Gerber)	1 jar	20	100	10	10	15	15	4	6	34	2	22	130
Macaroni, Tomatoes, and Beef (Heinz)	1 jar	20	45	*	35	15	25	4	6	NA	3	16	110

48

								% U.S. RDA						
Noodles and Chicken w Carrots and Peas (Gerber Chunky)	1 jar	25	75	8	10	8	20	2	8	452	3	14	110
Pasta Squares in Meat Sauce (Beech-Nut Table Time)	6 oz	25	50	35	8	15	15	6	10	660	4	22	150
Spaghetti Rings in Meat Sauce (Beech-Nut Table Time)	6 oz	25	110	10	6	15	15	10	8	660	4	22	150
Spaghetti, Tomato, and Beef (Beech-Nut Stage 3)	1 jar	20	200	10	10	20	15	6	6	90	4	22	150
Spaghetti, Tomato Sauce, and Beef (Gerber)	1 jar	20	110	10	15	20	25	6	6	57	3	25	150
Spaghetti, Tomato Sauce, and Meat (Heinz)	1 jar	25	45	*	20	20	15	6	8	NA	3	22	130
Split Peas w Ham (Gerber)	1 jar	30	100	8	15	15	10	6	6	36	3	24	150
Turkey Dinner Supreme (Beech-Nut Stage 3)	1 jar	25	170	8	6	20	15	25	8	80	6	24	180
Turkey and Rice w Vegetables (Gerber)	1 jar	20	120	6	2	10	15	6	4	36	5	18	140
Turkey Rice Dinner w Vegetables (Beech-Nut Stage 3)	1 jar	15	270	6	6	10	10	8	6	60	3	20	120
Turkey Rice Dinner w Vegetables (Heinz)	1 jar	20	35	*	6	10	6	10	2	NA	3	18	110

49

Baby Foods, Junior: Main Dishes	Amt.	Pro-tein	A	C	B₁	B₂	Nia-cin	Cal-cium	Iron	Sodium (mg)	Fat (g)	Carbohy-drate (g)	Calories
						% U.S. RDA							
Turkey w Vegetables (Gerber High Meat Dinner)	1 jar	45	80	8	4	15	25	10	6	40	7	8	130
Turkey w Vegetables (Heinz High Meat Dinner)	1 jar	25	30	*	4	10	6	15	4	NA	8	9	130
Veal w Vegetables (Gerber High Meat Dinner)	1 jar	45	70	8	6	15	25	*	4	31	2	10	90
Vegetables and Bacon (Gerber)	1 jar	20	170	10	15	10	10	4	4	121	8	20	170
Vegetables w Bacon (Heinz)	1 jar	15	220	*	15	15	8	6	6	NA	4	17	130
Vegetable Bacon Dinner (Beech-Nut Stage 3)	1 jar	10	310	15	10	10	10	4	4	140	9	21	180
Vegetables and Beef (Gerber)	1 jar	25	90	6	8	10	15	2	4	25	4	21	140
Vegetables and Beef (Gerber Chunky)	1 jar	20	35	4	4	8	10	2	6	451	4	15	120
Vegetables and Beef (Heinz)	1 jar	25	310	*	15	10	15	4	6	NA	3	18	120
Vegetable Beef Dinner (Beech-Nut Stage 3)	1 jar	15	380	6	6	15	10	4	4	90	4	20	130
Vegetable Chicken (Beech-Nut Stage 3)	1 jar	15	310	10	8	20	15	10	6	90	3	20	130

		% U.S. RDA											
Vegetables and Chicken (Gerber)	1 jar	15	100	10	4	4	10	6	4	21	3	17	110
Vegetables and Chicken (Gerber Chunky)	1 jar	25	50	6	6	6	15	2	4	499	3	16	120
Vegetables, Dumplings, and Beef (Heinz)	1 jar	20	50	*	10	10	10	2	6	NA	3	17	110
Vegetables, Egg Noodles, and Chicken (Heinz)	1 jar	25	75	*	15	15	15	10	4	NA	5	20	140
Vegetables, Egg Noodles, and Turkey (Heinz)	1 jar	20	60	*	10	10	4	10	2	NA	4	16	110
Vegetables and Ham (Gerber)	1 jar	20	80	6	10	8	8	2	2	30	4	20	140
Vegetables and Ham (Gerber Chunky)	1 jar	20	65	8	10	10	15	2	6	418	4	15	120
Vegetables and Ham (Heinz)	1 jar	30	60	2	15	15	6	4	2	NA	2	19	120
Vegetables and Lamb (Gerber)	1 jar	15	130	8	6	10	10	2	4	25	5	18	130
Vegetable Lamb Dinner (Beech-Nut Stage 3)	1 jar	15	250	15	8	10	15	4	6	60	4	21	140
Vegetables and Liver (Gerber)	1 jar	15	200	10	8	8	25	2	20	28	1	17	90
Vegetable Soup, Hearty (Beech-Nut Table Time)	6 oz	6	60	10	2	6	8	2	4	660	0	16	70

Baby Foods, Junior: Main Dishes	Amt.	Protein	A	C	B₁	B₂	Niacin	Calcium	Iron	Sodium (mg)	Fat (g)	Carbohydrate (g)	Calories
		% U.S. RDA											
Vegetable Stew w Chicken (Beech-Nut Table Time)	6 oz	10	170	15	4	15	15	8	8	510	6	21	160
Vegetables and Turkey (Gerber)	1 jar	15	100	10	4	6	10	4	2	32	3	19	90
Vegetables and Turkey (Gerber Chunky)	1 jar	20	35	6	4	8	10	6	6	474	4	16	120
Baby Foods, Junior: Meat													
Beef (Gerber)	1 jar	80	2	6	*	20	45	*	10	51	4	1	100
Beef and Beef Broth (Heinz)	1 jar	70	*	*	*	15	25	*	8	NA	8	0	130
Chicken (Gerber)	1 jar	80	2	4	2	20	45	8	6	39	9	0	140
Chicken and Chicken Broth (Heinz)	1 jar	70	*	*	4	15	40	12	6	NA	8	0	130
Chicken Sticks (Gerber)	1 jar	60	*	2	*	20	15	6	4	323	8	1	120
Ham (Gerber)	1 jar	80	2	6	15	25	35	*	6	39	6	1	120
Lamb (Gerber)	1 jar	80	*	2	*	25	35	*	10	52	4	1	100
Lamb and Lamb Broth (Heinz)	1 jar	70	*	*	4	15	20	*	10	NA	11	0	150
Meat Sticks (Gerber)	1 jar	60	*	2	8	20	15	4	6	325	7	1	110
Turkey (Gerber)	1 jar	80	2	6	2	30	45	4	6	49	8	0	130
Turkey Sticks (Gerber)	1 jar	50	*	2	*	20	15	8	4	331	9	1	120

Food	Serving					% U.S. RDA							
Veal (Gerber)	1 jar	80	2	6	*	25	50	*	6	54	4	0	100
Veal and Veal Broth (Heinz)	1 jar	70	2	4	4	20	40	*	6	NA	8	0	130
Baby Foods, Junior: Vegetables													
Carrots (Beech-Nut Stage 3)	1 jar	8	980	50	8	20	10	8	2	220	0	14	60
Carrots (Gerber)	1 jar	8	200	25	6	15	8	6	2	111	1	12	60
Carrots (Heinz)	1 jar	6	1300	15	8	8	4	6	2	NA	0	11	55
Corn, Creamed (Gerber)	1 jar	15	6	15	2	10	15	6	2	21	1	27	130
Corn, Creamed (Heinz)	1 jar	8	60	2	4	6	8	2	*	NA	2	37	160
Garden (Beech-Nut Stage 3)	1 jar	15	300	30	15	25	15	6	10	100	1	19	100
Green Beans (Beech-Nut Stage 3)	1 jar	10	70	40	8	35	6	15	15	NA	0	13	60
Green Beans, Creamed (Gerber)	1 jar	10	10	25	8	20	6	10	4	19	1	20	100
Green Beans, Creamed (Heinz)	1 jar	15	25	15	15	25	8	20	6	NA	3	12	90
Mixed (Beech-Nut Stage 3)	1 jar	10	390	8	10	8	10	4	4	75	0	20	90
Mixed (Gerber)	1 jar	10	200	8	10	6	15	4	4	77	1	18	90
Peas (Gerber)	1 jar	30	40	15	20	15	20	6	15	11	2	24	140
Peas, Creamed (Heinz)	1 jar	20	30	*	35	15	10	10	10	NA	4	21	140
Potatoes, Scalloped (Beech-Nut Stage 3)	1 jar	25	6	20	6	30	4	30	2	170	6	25	160

Baby Foods, Junior: Vegetables	Amt.	Protein	A	C	B$_1$	B$_2$	Niacin	Calcium	Iron	Sodium (mg)	Fat (g)	Carbohydrate (g)	Calories
			% U.S. RDA										
Squash (Gerber)	1 jar	8	200	40	6	10	10	8	2	4	1	13	70
Sweet Potatoes (Beech-Nut Stage 3)	1 jar	8	630	35	6	10	6	6	4	100	0	27	120
Sweet Potatoes (Gerber)	1 jar	10	200	60	8	10	10	4	2	51	1	31	140
Sweet Potatoes (Heinz)	1 jar	10	1420	25	15	10	8	4	6	NA	0	30	140
Bars													
Bar, Chocolate (Milk Break)	1 bar	10	4	0	4	10	2	15	2	75	13	22	230
Bar, Chocolate Mint (Milk Break)	1 bar	10	4	0	4	10	2	15	4	80	14	21	230
Bar, Peanut Butter (Milk Break)	1 bar	10	4	0	6	10	4	15	2	115	13	21	220
Bar, Natural Flavor (Milk Break)	1 bar	10	4	0	4	10	0	15	2	75	14	21	230
Breakfast Bar, Chocolate Chip (Carnation)	1 bar	10	35	45	20	2	25	2	25	180	11	20	200
Breakfast Bar, Chocolate Crunch (Carnation)	1 bar	10	35	45	20	2	25	2	25	145	10	20	190
Breakfast Bar, Honey Nut (Carnation)	1 bar	10	35	45	20	2	25	2	25	155	11	18	190
Breakfast Bar, Peanut Butter w Chocolate Chips (Carnation)	1 bar	10	35	45	20	2	25	2	25	170	11	20	200

Product	Serving	% U.S. RDA											
Breakfast Bar, Peanut Butter Crunch (Carnation)	1 bar	10	35	45	20	2	25	2	25	170	11	20	200
Diet Bar, Chocolate (Carnation Slender)	2 bars	25	25	25	25	25	25	25	25	285	14	26	270
Diet Bar, Chocolate Chip (Carnation Slender)	2 bars	25	25	25	25	25	25	25	25	315	14	26	270
Diet Bar, Chocolate Peanut Butter (Carnation Slender)	2 bars	25	25	25	25	25	25	25	25	285	15	24	270
Diet Bar, Vanilla (Carnation Slender)	2 bars	25	25	25	25	25	25	25	25	320	15	24	270
Diet Bar, All Flavors (Figurines)	2 bars	25	25	25	25	25	25	25	25	165–285	16	21	275
Granola Bar, Cinnamon (Nature Valley)	1 bar	4	*	*	4	2	*	2	4	80	4	17	110
Granola Bar, Coconut (Nature Valley)	1 bar	2	*	*	4	2	*	2	4	65	6	15	120
Granola Bar, Oats and Honey (Nature Valley)	1 bar	4	*	*	4	*	*	*	4	70	4	17	110
Granola Bar, Peanut (Nature Valley)	1 bar	4	*	*	4	*	2	*	4	85	5	16	120
Granola Bar, Peanut Butter (Nature Valley)	1 bar	4	*	*	2	*	2	*	4	80	6	15	120
Granola Bar, Roasted Almond (Nature Valley)	1 bar	4	*	*	4	2	*	*	4	85	5	16	120

Bars	Amt.	% U.S. RDA							Iron	Sodium (mg)	Fat (g)	Carbohydrate (g)	Calories
		Protein	A	C	B$_1$	B$_2$	Niacin	Calcium					
Granola Bar, Chewy, Apple (Nature Valley)	1 bar	2	*	*	2	*	2	*	4	70	5	20	130
Granola Bar, Chewy, Chocolate Chip (Nature Valley)	1 bar	2	*	*	2	*	*	*	4	80	7	19	150
Granola Bar, Chewy, Peanut Butter (Nature Valley)	1 bar	4	*	*	2	2	4	2	4	80	6	18	140
Granola Bar, Chewy, Raisin (Nature Valley)	1 bar	2	*	*	2	2	4	*	4	65	5	20	130
Granola & Fruit Bar, Apple (Nature Valley)	1 bar	2	*	*	2	*	*	*	4	150	5	25	150
Granola & Fruit Bar, Cherry (Nature Valley)	1 bar	2	*	*	2	*	*	*	4	165	5	24	150
Granola & Fruit Bar, Date (Nature Valley)	1 bar	2	*	*	2	*	*	2	4	140	5	26	160
Granola & Fruit Bar, Raspberry (Nature Valley)	1 bar	2	*	*	2	*	*	*	4	150	5	25	150
Granola Clusters, Almond (Nature Valley)	1 roll	4	*	*	4	4	*	2	4	100	4	27	150
Granola Clusters, Apple Cinnamon (Nature Valley)	1 roll	2	*	*	4	4	*	2	2	100	4	27	150

	Serving	% U.S. RDA											
Granola Clusters, Caramel (Nature Valley)	1 roll	2	*	*	4	2	*	2	2	95	3	28	150
Granola Clusters, Chocolate (Nature Valley)	1 roll	4	*	*	4	4	4	4	4	110	3	27	140
Granola Clusters, Chocolate Chip (Nature Valley)	1 roll	2	*	*	2	2	*	2	4	100	4	26	150
Granola Clusters, Raisin (Nature Valley)	1 roll	2	*	*	2	2	*	2	4	110	3	29	150
Biscuits													
Biscuits (Ballard Oven Ready)	2	4	0	0	10	6	6	0	6	355	1	20	100
Biscuits (1869 Brand Butter Tastin')	2	6	0	0	10	10	8	2	6	590	8	27	200
Biscuits (Hungry Jack Butter Tastin' Flaky)	2	4	0	0	10	6	8	0	6	550	9	23	180
Biscuits (Hungry Jack Flaky)	2	4	0	0	10	8	8	0	8	585	7	24	170
Biscuits (Pillsbury Country Style)	2	4	0	0	10	6	6	0	6	355	1	20	100
Biscuits (Pillsbury Good 'n Buttery Big Country)	2	6	0	0	15	8	10	0	6	650	8	27	190
Biscuits, Baking Powder (1869 Brand)	2	6	0	0	10	10	8	2	6	590	8	27	200
Biscuits, Baking Powder (Pillsbury Tenderflake)	2	2	0	0	6	4	4	0	4	355	5	14	110

| Biscuits | Amt. | % U.S. RDA | | | | | | | | Sodium (mg) | Fat (g) | Carbohydrate (g) | Calories |
		Protein	A	C	B₁	B₂	Niacin	Calcium	Iron				
Biscuits, Butter (Pillsbury)	2	4	0	0	10	6	6	0	6	355	1	20	100
Biscuits, Buttermilk (Ballard Oven Ready)	2	4	0	0	8	6	6	0	6	355	1	20	100
Biscuits, Buttermilk (1869 Brand)	2	6	0	0	10	10	8	2	6	590	8	27	200
Biscuits, Buttermilk (Hungry Jack Extra Rich)	2	4	0	0	8	4	4	0	4	345	3	19	110
Biscuits, Buttermilk (Hungry Jack Flaky)	2	4	0	0	10	6	8	0	6	590	7	25	170
Biscuits, Buttermilk (Hungry Jack Fluffy)	2	4	0	0	10	8	8	0	8	560	8	24	180
Biscuits, Buttermilk (Pillsbury)	2	4	0	0	10	6	6	0	6	355	1	20	100
Biscuits, Buttermilk (Pillsbury Big Country)	2	6	0	0	6	15	6	6	0	645	8	29	200
Biscuits, Buttermilk (Pillsbury Big Premium Heat 'n Eat)	2	6	0	0	10	20	8	2	8	605	15	32	280
Biscuits, Buttermilk (Pillsbury Extra Lights)	2	4	0	0	8	2	4	0	4	340	4	18	110
Biscuits, Buttermilk (Pillsbury Heat 'n Eat)	2	6	0	0	10	8	8	2	6	530	5	27	170
Biscuits, Buttermilk (Pillsbury Tenderflake)	2	2	0	0	6	4	4	0	4	335	5	14	110

		% U.S. RDA											
Biscuit Mix (Bisquick)	2 oz	6	*	*	20	15	10	8	6	700	8	38	240
Bread, Specialty													
Apple w Cinnamon (Pepperidge Farm)	2 sl	6	0	0	8	8	6	2	6	210	3	26	140
Bran w Diced Raisins (Pepperidge Farm)	2 sl	6	0	0	15	8	10	0	8	230	1	27	140
Brown, Canned (B & M)	½" sl	6	*	*	*	4	4	4	8	220	NA	18	80
Brown, Canned, w Raisins (B & M)	½" sl	6	*	*	*	4	4	4	8	220	NA	18	80
Buckwheat (Butter-Nut)	1 sl	4	*	*	8	4	6	2	4	150	2	12	80
Buckwheat (Weber's)	1 sl	4	*	*	8	4	6	2	4	150	2	12	80
Buttermilk (Butter-Nut)	1 sl	4	*	*	8	4	6	2	4	160	1	14	80
Buttermilk (Eddy's)	1 sl	4	*	*	8	4	.6	2	4	160	1	14	80
Buttermilk (Millbrook)	1 sl	4	*	*	8	4	6	2	4	160	1	14	80
Buttermilk (Sweetheart)	1 sl	4	*	*	8	4	6	2	4	160	1	14	80
Buttermilk (Weber's)	1 sl	4	*	*	8	4	6	2	4	160	1	14	80
Cinnamon (Pepperidge Farm)	2 sl	4	0	0	10	6	0	0	2	200	4	25	160
Cinnamon, Apple, and Walnut (Pepperidge Farm)	2 sl	6	0	0	10	8	8	2	10	200	5	26	160
Cinnamon-Raisin (Butter-Nut)	1 sl	4	*	*	2	*	*	2	2	140	2	14	80
Corn and Molasses (Pepperidge Farm)	2 sl	6	0	0	15	10	10	2	10	280	1	29	140

| Bread, Specialty | Amt. | % U.S. RDA | | | | | | | | Sodium (mg) | Fat (g) | Carbohydrate (g) | Calories |
		Protein	A	C	B₁	B₂	Niacin	Calcium	Iron				
Dark (Hollywood)	2 sl	8	0	0	15	15	10	10	10	325	2	25	140
Date-Walnut (Pepperidge Farm)	2 sl	6	0	0	8	4	6	2	6	220	5	23	150
Honey Bran (Pepperidge Farm) 1½ lb	2 sl	8	0	0	20	10	15	2	10	350	2	36	190
Honey Wheatberry (Pepperidge Farm)	2 sl	6	0	0	10	6	8	2	8	320	2	27	140
Honey Whole Grain (Butter-Nut)	1 sl	4	*	*	6	4	4	*	4	140	2	13	80
Honey Whole Grain (Eddy's)	1 sl	4	*	*	6	4	4	*	4	140	2	13	80
Honey Whole Grain (Millbrook)	1 sl	4	*	*	6	4	4	*	4	140	2	13	80
Honey Whole Grain (Sweetheart)	1 sl	4	*	*	6	4	4	*	4	140	2	13	80
Honey Whole Grain (Weber's)	1 sl	4	*	*	6	4	4	*	4	140	2	13	80
Multi Grain (Pepperidge Farm Very Thin Sliced)	2 sl	4	0	0	4	2	4	0	4	150	1	14	80
Oatmeal (Pepperidge Farm) 1½ lb	2 sl	6	0	0	15	6	8	4	8	340	2	25	140
Oatmeal (Pepperidge Farm Thin Sliced)	2 sl	6	0	0	10	6	6	2	6	370	3	25	140

Product	Serving											
				% U.S. RDA								
Onion (Pepperidge Farm Party Slices)	4 sl	4	0	6	4	4	2	2	100	1	11	60
Orange Raisin (Pepperidge Farm)	2 sl	4	0	15	8	8	2	10	160	3	27	150
Potato (Eddy's)	1 sl	4	*	8	4	6	2	4	170	1	14	70
Potato (Sweetheart)	1 sl	4	*	8	4	6	2	4	170	1	14	70
Pumpernickel (Pepperidge Farm Family)	2 sl	10	0	15	10	10	4	10	610	2	30	160
Pumpernickel (Pepperidge Farm Party Slices)	4 sl	4	0	6	4	4	2	4	200	1	12	70
Raisin w Cinnamon (Pepperidge Farm)	2 sl	6	0	10	8	10	2	6	190	3	28	150
Rye (Butter-Nut)	1 sl	4	*	8	8	8	*	6	220	1	13	70
Rye (Eddy's)	1 sl	4	*	8	8	8	*	6	220	1	13	70
Rye (Millbrook)	1 sl	4	*	8	8	8	*	6	220	1	13	70
Rye (Pepperidge Farm Family)	2 sl	10	0	20	10	10	4	10	490	2	31	170
Rye (Pepperidge Farm Party Slices)	4 sl	4	0	8	4	4	2	4	330	1	12	60
Rye (Pepperidge Farm Sandwich), 1½ lb	2 sl	8	0	15	10	15	2	10	450	4	32	190
Rye (Pepperidge Farm Very Thin Sliced)	2 sl	4	0	10	8	8	4	4	220	1	16	90
Rye (Sweetheart)	1 sl	4	*	8	8	8	*	6	220	1	13	70

Bread, Specialty	Amt.	% U.S. RDA								Sodium (mg)	Fat (g)	Carbohydrate (g)	Calories
		Protein	A	C	B₁	B₂	Niacin	Calcium	Iron				

Bread, Specialty	Amt.	Protein	A	C	B$_1$	B$_2$	Niacin	Calcium	Iron	Sodium (mg)	Fat (g)	Carbohydrate (g)	Calories
Rye, Dijon (Pepperidge Farm)	2 sl	6	0	0	6	10	10	4	10	340	2	18	110
Rye, Jewish (Pepperidge Farm)	2 sl	8	0	0	15	10	10	4	8	560	3	33	180
Rye, Seedless (Pepperidge Farm)	2 sl	10	0	0	20	10	10	4	8	500	2	31	160
Seven Grain (Home Pride)	2 sl	8	0	0	15	10	10	4	10	270	2	25	140
Wheat (Butter-Nut)	1 sl	4	*	*	8	4	4	*	4	180	1	14	70
Wheat (Eddy's)	1 sl	4	*	*	8	4	4	*	4	180	1	14	70
Wheat (Fresh Horizons)	2 sl	8	0	0	15	8	10	8	10	290	1	19	100
Wheat (Fresh & Natural)	2 sl	8	0	0	8	6	8	2	8	270	2	27	140
Wheat (Home Pride Butter Top)	2 sl	8	0	0	15	8	10	6	8	310	3	26	150
Wheat (Pepperidge Farm), 24-oz loaf	2 sl	10	0	0	15	8	10	2	10	390	3	35	190
Wheat (Pepperidge Farm Family), 32-oz loaf	2 sl	6	0	0	15	6	10	4	10	270	2	26	140
Wheat (Pepperidge Farm Sandwich)	2 sl	4	0	0	10	4	4	2	4	230	2	20	110
Wheat (Roman Meal)	2 sl	8	0	0	15	10	10	6	10	280	2	25	140
Wheat (Sweetheart)	1 sl	4	*	*	8	4	4	*	4	180	1	14	70

Food	Serving	% U.S. RDA										
Wheat (Weber's)	1 sl	4	*	*	8	4	*	4	180	1	14	70
Wheat (Wonder Family)	2 sl	8	0	*	15	10	10	10	300	2	27	150
Wheat, Cracked (Butter-Nut)	1 sl	4	*	*	4	2	*	2	180	1	13	70
Wheat, Cracked (Eddy's)	1 sl	4	*	*	4	2	*	2	180	1	13	70
Wheat, Cracked (Pepperidge Farm Thin Sliced)	2 sl	6	0	0	10	6	2	10	290	3	26	140
Wheat, Cracked (Sweetheart)	1 sl	4	*	*	4	2	*	2	180	1	13	70
Wheat, Cracked (Weber's)	1 sl	4	*	*	4	2	*	2	180	1	13	70
Wheat, Cracked (Wonder)	2 sl	8	0	0	10	8	2	10	300	2	27	150
Wheat, Honey (Home Pride)	2 sl	8	0	0	15	10	6	10	325	2	26	140
Wheat, Light, Fiber (Butter-Nut)	1 sl	4	*	*	8	4	2	4	175	0	11	50
Wheat, Light, Fiber (Millbrook)	1 sl	4	*	*	8	4	2	4	175	0	11	50
Wheat, Light, Fiber (Sweetheart)	1 sl	4	*	*	8	4	2	4	175	0	11	50
Wheat, Sprouted (Pepperidge Farm)	2 sl	8	0	0	10	8	2	10	220	3	23	140
Wheat, Whole, 100% (Home Pride)	2 sl	8	0	0	15	10	4	10	280	2	24	140
Wheat, Whole (Pepperidge Farm Thin Sliced)	2 sl	8	0	0	10	6	4	6	250	3	24	130

Bread, Specialty	Amt.	Protein	A	C	B₁	B₂	Niacin	Calcium	Iron	Sodium (mg)	Fat (g)	Carbohydrate (g)	Calories
						% U.S. RDA							
Wheat, Whole (Pepperidge Farm Very Thin Sliced)	2 sl	4	0	0	6	2	4	2	6	160	2	15	90
Wheat, Whole, 100% (Wonder)	2 sl	8	0	0	10	4	10	2	8	240	2	24	140
Wheatberry (Home Pride)	2 sl	8	0	0	15	8	10	6	10	300	2	25	140
Wheatberry, Honey (Home Pride)	2 sl	8	0	0	10	6	10	4	8	310	2	26	140
Wheat Germ (Pepperidge Farm Thin Sliced)	2 sl	8	0	0	10	10	10	4	10	280	1	25	130
Bread, White													
French (Pepperidge Farm Brown & Serve)	2 oz	8	0	0	20	15	10	4	8	360	2	26	140
French (Pepperidge Farm Twin)	2 oz	6	0	0	15	10	10	0	6	250	2	25	140
French (Wonder)	2 sl	8	0	0	15	8	10	6	8	340	2	27	150
French Style (Pepperidge Farm)	2 oz	8	0	0	20	10	15	4	6	320	2	28	150
Italian (Pepperidge Farm Brown & Serve)	2 oz	8	0	0	20	10	15	4	8	320	2	27	150
Low-Sodium (Wonder)	2 sl	8	0	0	15	8	10	4	8	6	2	27	140
Protein (Thomas' Protogen)	2 sl	10	*	*	8	4	6	4	6	188	.8	14.7	93.3
Sourdough (DiCarlo)	2 sl	8	0	0	15	8	10	6	8	300	1	27	140

Food	Serving	% U.S. RDA										
Vienna (Pepperidge Farm Thick Sliced)	2 sl	8	4	15	10	15	0	6	350	2	27	150
White (Butter-Nut)	1 sl	4	2	6	4	8	*	4	150	1	14	70
White (Eddy's)	1 sl	4	2	6	4	8	*	4	150	1	14	70
White (Fresh Horizons)	2 sl	10	8	10	10	15	0	8	285	1	19	100
White (Hillbilly)	2 sl	10	6	10	10	20	0	8	340	2	26	140
White (Hollywood Light)	2 sl	10	10	10	10	15	0	8	335	2	26	140
White (Home Pride Butter Top)	2 sl	10	8	10	10	15	0	8	300	3	26	150
White (Pepperidge Farm Enriched), 1½ lb	2 sl	8	2	10	10	25	0	8	350	3	34	190
White (Pepperidge Farm Large Family Enriched)	2 sl	6	4	10	10	15	0	6	350	3	27	150
White (Pepperidge Farm Sandwich Enriched)	2 sl	6	4	10	8	15	0	6	270	2	23	130
White (Pepperidge Farm Thin Sliced Enriched)	2 sl	6	4	10	10	15	0	6	270	3	25	150
White (Pepperidge Farm Very Thin Sliced Enriched)	2 sl	4	4	6	6	10	0	4	170	1	16	90
White (Pepperidge Farm Toasting Enriched)	2 sl	8	6	15	15	20	0	8	460	2	32	170
White (Sweetheart)	1 sl	4	2	6	4	8	*	4	150	1	14	70
White (Weber's)	1 sl	4	2	6	4	8	*	4	150	1	14	70

Bread, White	Amt.	Pro-tein	A	C	B$_1$	B$_2$	Nia-cin	Cal-cium	Iron	Sodium (mg)	Fat (g)	Carbohy-drate (g)	Calories
		<td colspan="8" align="center">% U.S. RDA</td>				
White (Wonder)	2 sl	8	0	0	15	8	10	6	8	305	2	27	140
White, Light, Fiber (Butter-Nut)	1 sl	4	*	*	8	4	6	2	4	175	0	11	50
White, Low Sodium (Butter-Nut)	1 sl	4	*	*	8	4	6	2	4	20	2	13	80
White, Low Sodium (Eddy's)	1 sl	4	*	*	8	4	6	2	4	20	2	13	80
White w Buttermilk (Wonder)	2 sl	8	0	0	15	10	10	8	10	340	2	27	150
White w Cracked Wheat (Pepperidge Farm)	2 sl	8	0	0	10	6	8	0	6	240	3	35	190
Bread Crumbs, Croutons, and Stuffing Mixes													
Bread Crumbs (Pepperidge Farm Premium)	1 oz	6	0	0	10	6	8	2	6	260	1	22	110
Bread Crumbs, Herb Seasoned (Pepperidge Farm Premium)	1 oz	6	0	0	10	6	8	2	6	260	1	22	110
Bread Crumbs, Seasoned (Contadina)	1 rounded tbsp	2	*	*	2	2	2	*	2	265	0–1	7	35
Bread Crumbs, Toasted (Old London Regular Style)	2 oz	10	*	*	15	8	8	6	8	NA	2	40	210
Corn Flake Crumbs (Kellogg's)	¼ c	4	25	25	25	25	25	*	10	285	0	25	110

Food	Serving												
						% U.S. RDA							
Cracker Meal (Nabisco)	1 c	15	*	*	60	35	35	2	25	NA	1	95	440
Croutons, Bacon and Cheese (Pepperidge Farm)	½ oz	4	0	0	4	4	6	2	4	130	3	8	70
Croutons, Bleu Cheese (Pepperidge Farm)	½ oz	4	0	0	4	4	4	2	2	170	4	7	70
Croutons, Cheddar and Romano Cheese (Pepperidge Farm)	½ oz	2	0	0	6	4	4	2	2	190	2	9	60
Croutons, Cheese and Garlic (Pepperidge Farm)	½ oz	2	0	0	4	4	4	2	2	190	3	9	70
Croutons, Dijon Mustard Rye and Cheese (Pepperidge Farm)	½ oz	4	0	0	4	4	4	2	2	150	4	7	70
Croutons, Onion and Garlic (Pepperidge Farm)	½ oz	2	0	0	6	4	4	0	2	160	3	9	70
Croutons, Seasoned (Pepperidge Farm)	½ oz	2	0	0	4	4	4	2	2	210	3	9	70
Croutons, Sour Cream & Chive (Pepperidge Farm)	½ oz	2	0	0	4	4	4	2	2	220	3	9	70
Stuffing (Kellogg's Croutettes)	½ c prep	4	6	*	6	8	6	2	6	350	9	14	150
Stuffing (Stove Top Americana New England) Prep w Butter	½ c prep	6	6	*	10	6	6	4	6	635	9	21	180
Stuffing (Stove Top Americana San Francisco) Prep w Butter	½ c prep	6	6	*	10	6	6	2	4	635	9	20	170

Bread Crumbs, Croutons, and Stuffing Mixes	Amt.	Protein	A	C	B₁	B₂	Niacin	Calcium	Iron	Sodium (mg)	Fat (g)	Carbohydrate (g)	Calories
		% U.S. RDA											
Stuffing, Beef (Stove Top) Prep w Butter	½ c prep	6	15	*	10	4	6	2	6	585	9	21	180
Stuffing, Chicken (Stove Top) Made w Butter	½ c prep	6	6	*	8	4	6	2	4	640	9	20	180
Stuffing, Chicken (Pepperidge Farm Pan Style)	1 oz	6	0	0	10	8	10	2	6	400	1	22	110
Stuffing, Corn Bread (Pepperidge Farm)	1 oz	4	0	0	10	6	8	2	6	530	1	22	110
Stuffing, Corn Bread (Stove Top) Prep w Butter	½ c prep	4	6	*	8	4	6	2	6	665	9	21	170
Stuffing, Cube (Pepperidge Farm)	1 oz	6	0	0	10	6	8	2	6	440	1	22	110
Stuffing, Cube, Unseasoned (Pepperidge Farm)	1 oz	4	0	0	10	6	6	2	4	510	2	22	110
Stuffing, Herb Seasoned (Pepperidge Farm)	1 oz	6	0	0	10	6	8	2	6	440	2	22	110
Stuffing, Pork (Stove Top) Made w Butter	½ c prep	6	8	*	10	6	6	4	6	620	9	20	170
Stuffing, Seasoned (Pepperidge Farm Pan Style)	1 oz	6	0	0	10	8	8	2	6	440	1	22	110
Stuffing, Turkey (Stove Top) Made w Butter	½ c prep	6	6	*	8	4	6	2	4	625	9	20	170

Food	Portion					% U.S. RDA								
Stuffing, w Rice (Stove Top) Made w Butter	1/2 c prep	180	23	8	505	6	0	2	6	2	10	*	6	4
Bread Mixes														
Applesauce Spice (Pillsbury)	1/12 loaf	150	28	3	155	4	0	6	4	4	8	4	0	2
Apricot Nut (Pillsbury)	1/12	160	27	4	150	6	0	4	4	6	8	0	6	4
Banana (Pillsbury)	1/12	150	27	4	150	4	0	4	4	6	8	0	0	2
Blueberry Nut (Pillsbury)	1/12	150	26	4	155	4	2	4	4	4	6	0	0	2
Carrot Nut (Pillsbury)	1/12	150	27	4	185	4	2	4	4	4	4	0	30	4
Cherry Nut (Pillsbury)	1/12	170	30	5	150	4	0	4	4	6	10	0	0	4
Corn (Ballard)	1/8 recipe	140	25	3	570	2	0	2	2	4	6	0	0	4
Corn (Dromedary)	2" sq	130	19	5	NA	2	6	2	2	4	8	*	2	4
Cranberry (Pillsbury)	1/12	160	10	3	155	2	0	4	6	4	6	0	0	2
Date (Pillsbury)	1/12	160	31	3	155	4	0	4	4	4	8	0	0	4
Nut (Pillsbury)	1/12	160	31	3	180	2	0	4	6	4	6	0	0	2
Rye (Pillsbury Poppin' Fresh)	1/2" slice	110	21	2	195	4	0	8	6	8	10	0	0	4
Wheat (Pillsbury Poppin' Fresh)	1/2" slice	110	20	2	195	4	0	6	8	6	10	0	0	6
White (Pillsbury Poppin' Fresh)	1/2" slice	110	21	2	195	4	0	6	8	8	10	0	0	4
Butter and Oils														
Butter	1 c	1630	1	184	2240	*	4	0	8	8	10	*	150	2

Butter and Oils	Amt.	Protein	A	C	B_1	B_2	Niacin	Calcium	Iron	Sodium (mg)	Fat (g)	Carbohydrate (g)	Calories
		% U.S. RDA											
Butter	1 tbsp	*	10	*	*	*	*	*	*	140	12	0-1	100
Butter, Whipped	1 c	2	100	*	*	*	*	2	*	1490	151	0-1	1080
Butter, Whipped	1 tbsp	*	6	*	*	*	*	*	*	89	8	0-1	70
Lard	1 c	*	*	*	*	*	*	*	*	0	205	0	1850
Margarine (Blue Bonnet)	1 tbsp	*	10	*	*	*	*	*	*	110	11	0	100
Margarine (Fleischmann's)	1 tbsp	*	10	*	*	*	*	*	*	110	11	0	100
Margarine (Imperial)	1 tbsp	*	10	*	*	*	*	*	*	NA	11	0	100
Margarine (Mazola)	1 tbsp	*	10	*	*	*	*	*	*	115	11	0	100
Margarine (Mrs. Filbert's Golden Quarters or Corn Oil Quarters)	1 tbsp	*	10	*	*	*	*	*	*	110	11	0	100
Margarine (Mrs. Filbert's Reduced Calorie)	1 tbsp	*	10	*	*	*	*	*	*	110	6	0	50
Margarine (Nucoa)	1 tbsp	*	10	*	*	*	*	*	*	165	11	0	100
Margarine, Soft (Blue Bonnet)	1 tbsp	*	10	*	*	*	*	*	*	110	11	0	100
Margarine, Soft (Fleischmann's)	1 tbsp	*	10	*	*	*	*	*	*	110	11	0	100
Margarine, Soft (Imperial)	1 tbsp	*	10	*	*	*	*	*	*	NA	11	0	100
Margarine, Soft (Mrs. Filbert's Golden or Corn Oil)	1 tbsp	*	10	*	*	*	*	*	*	110	11	0	100

Food	Serving	% U.S. RDA													
Margarine, Soft (Nucoa)	1 tbsp	*	10	*	*	*	*	*	*	*	*	155	10	0	90
Margarine, Soft, Unsalted (Mother's)	1 tbsp	*	10	*	*	*	*	*	*	*	*	NA	11	0	100
Margarine, Unsalted (Fleischmann's)	1 tbsp	*	10	*	*	*	*	*	*	*	*	1	11	0	100
Margarine, Unsalted (Fleischmann's Parve)	1 tbsp	*	10	*	*	*	*	*	*	*	*	0	11	0	100
Margarine, Unsalted (Mazola)	1 tbsp	*	10	*	*	*	*	*	*	*	*	0-1	11	0	100
Margarine, Unsalted (Mother's)	1 tbsp	*	10	*	*	*	*	*	*	*	*	NA	11	0	100
Margarine, Whipped (Blue Bonnet)	1 tbsp	*	10	*	*	*	*	*	*	*	*	70	7	0	70
Margarine, Whipped (Fleischmann's)	1 tbsp	*	10	*	*	*	*	*	*	*	*	70	7	0	70
Margarine, Whipped (Imperial)	1 tbsp	*	6	*	*	*	*	*	*	*	*	NA	5	0	50
Margarine, Imitation (Diet Blue Bonnet)	1 tbsp	*	10	*	*	*	*	*	*	*	*	110	6	0	50
Margarine, Imitation (Diet Fleischmann's)	1 tbsp	*	10	*	*	*	*	*	*	*	*	110	6	0	50
Margarine, Imitation (Diet Mazola)	1 tbsp	*	10	*	*	*	*	*	*	*	*	130	6	0	50
Oil, Corn (Mazola)	1 tbsp	*	*	*	*	*	*	*	*	*	*	0	14	0	120
Oil, Salad	1 c	*	*	*	*	*	*	*	*	*	*	0	218	0	1930

Butter and Oils	Amt.	Pro-tein	A	C	B₁	B₂	Nia-cin	Cal-cium	Iron	Sodium (mg)	Fat (g)	Carbohy-drate (g)	Calories
					% U.S. RDA								
Oil, Sunflower (Sunlite)	1 tbsp	*	*	*	*	*	*	*	*	NA	14	0	120
Oil, Vegetable (Wesson)	1 tbsp	*	*	*	*	*	*	*	*	NA	14	0	120
Oil for Popcorn (Orville Redenbacher Gourmet Buttery Flavor Popping Oil)	1 tbsp	*	*	*	*	*	*	*	*	NA	14	0	120
Shortening (Snowdrift)	1 tbsp	*	*	*	*	*	*	*	*	NA	12	0	110
Spread (Autumn)	1 tbsp	*	10	*	*	*	*	*	*	NA	8	0	80
Spread (Blue Bonnet)	1 tbsp	*	10	*	*	*	*	*	*	110	8	0	80
Spread (Fleischmann's)	1 tbsp	*	10	*	*	*	*	*	*	110	8	0	80
Spread (Imperial)	1 tbsp	*	10	*	*	*	*	*	*	NA	7	0	70
Spread (Imperial Light)	1 tbsp	*	10	*	*	*	*	*	*	NA	8	0	80
Spread (Mrs. Filbert's Family)	1 tbsp	*	10	*	*	*	*	*	*	85	7	0	70
Spread (Mrs. Filbert's Spread 25)	1 tbsp	*	10	*	*	*	*	*	*	105	8	0	80
Spread (Promise)	1 tbsp	*	10	*	*	*	*	*	*	NA	10	0	90
Spread, Soft (Imperial Light)	1 tbsp	*	10	*	*	*	*	*	*	NA	7	0	60
Spread, Soft (Promise)	1 tbsp	*	10	*	*	*	*	*	*	NA	10	0	90
Vegetable Coating (Mazola No Stick)	.7 gm (2-second spray)	*	*	*	*	*	*	*	*	NA	1	0	6

Cakes		% U.S. RDA											
Angel Food (Dolly Madison)	1/6	2	*	*	2	6	4	4	2	150	5	17	120
Apple-Walnut w Cream Cheese Icing (Pepperidge Farm Old Fashioned)	1⅜ oz	2	0	2	0	2	0	2	2	140	7	18	150
Boston Cream (Pepperidge Farm Cake Supreme)	2⅞ oz	4	0	0	0	4	0	2	4	190	14	39	290
Butter Pound (Pepperidge Farm Old Fashioned)	1 oz	2	0	0	0	2	0	0	0	150	7	16	130
Butterscotch Pecan Layer (Pepperidge Farm)	1⅝ oz	2	0	0	0	4	0	2	2	110	7	23	160
Carrot w Cream Cheese Icing (Pepperidge Farm Old Fashioned)	1⅜ oz	0	15	2	0	2	0	0	2	150	8	17	140
Chocolate (Pepperidge Farm Cake Supreme)	2⅞ oz	4	0	0	0	4	2	2	6	140	17	37	310
Chocolate Fudge Layer (Pepperidge Farm)	1⅝ oz	2	0	0	0	2	0	0	4	140	10	23	180
Chocolate Mint Layer (Pepperidge Farm)	1⅝ oz	2	0	0	0	2	0	2	6	140	9	22	170
Coconut Layer (Pepperidge Farm)	1⅝ oz	0	0	0	0	2	0	0	2	120	9	25	180
Devil's Food Layer (Pepperidge Farm)	1⅝ oz	2	0	0	0	2	0	0	2	135	9	24	180

Cakes	Amt.	Protein	A	C	B₁	B₂	Niacin	Calcium	Iron	Sodium (mg)	Fat (g)	Carbohydrate (g)	Calories
							% U.S. RDA						
German Chocolate Layer (Pepperidge Farm)	1⅜ oz	2	0	0	0	2	0	2	2	170	10	23	180
Golden Layer (Pepperidge Farm)	1⅜ oz	2	0	0	0	2	0	0	2	115	9	24	180
Lemon Coconut (Pepperidge Farm Cake Supreme)	3 oz	2	0	4	2	4	0	2	2	220	13	38	280
Pineapple Cream (Pepperidge Farm Cake Supreme)	2 oz	2	0	10	0	2	0	0	4	145	8	27	180
Pound (Dolly Madison)	⅙	6	*	*	10	6	6	4	6	290	8	33	220
Strawberry Cream (Pepperidge Farm Cake Supreme)	2 oz	0	0	4	0	2	0	0	2	145	8	27	190
Vanilla Layer (Pepperidge Farm)	1⅜ oz	0	0	0	0	2	0	0	0	120	8	25	190
Walnut (Pepperidge Farm Cake Supreme)	2½ oz	2	0	0	0	2	0	2	4	200	17	33	300
Cake Mixes													
Angel Food, Chocolate (Betty Crocker)	1/12 pkg	4	*	*	*	4	*	*	4	300	0	35	150
Angel Food, Confetti (Betty Crocker)	1/12 pkg	4	*	*	*	4	*	6	*	255	0	36	160

Food	Serving	% U.S. RDA											
Angel Food, Lemon Custard (Betty Crocker)	½ pkg	4	*	*	*	4	*	6	*	260	0	35	150
Angel Food, Raspberry (Pillsbury)	½ pkg	4	0	0	2	2	2	2	0	300	0	32	140
Angel Food, Strawberry (Betty Crocker)	½ pkg	4	*	*	4	4	*	6	*	260	0	35	150
Angel Food, Traditional White (Betty Crocker)	½ pkg	4	*	*	*	4	*	4	*	165	0	31	140
Angel Food, White (Betty Crocker)	½ pkg	4	*	*	*	4	*	6	*	260	0	35	150
Angel Food, White (Pillsbury)	½ cake	4	0	0	4	4	0	2	2	345	0	33	140
Apple Cinnamon (Betty Crocker SuperMoist)	½ pkg	4	*	6	6	4	4	6	4	275	11	36	260
Applesauce Raisin (Betty Crocker Snackin' Cake)	⅑ pkg	2	*	6	6	4	4	4	2	250	4	33	180
Applesauce Spice (Pillsbury Plus)	½ cake	4	2	8	6	6	2	4	4	300	11	36	250
Banana (Betty Crocker SuperMoist)	½ pkg	4	*	6	6	6	4	6	4	255	11	36	260
Banana (Pillsbury Plus)	½ cake	4	2	8	6	6	8	4	4	290	11	36	250
Banana Walnut (Betty Crocker Snackin' Cake)	⅑ pkg	2	*	6	6	4	4	4	2	260	6	31	190
Bundt, Boston Cream (Pillsbury Bundt)	1/16 cake	4	2	6	6	6	4	4	4	305	10	43	270

75

Cake Mixes	Amt.	% U.S. RDA								Sodium (mg)	Fat (g)	Carbohy-drate (g)	Calories
		Pro-tein	A	C	B₁	B₂	Nia-cin	Cal-cium	Iron				
Bundt, Chocolate Macaroon (Pillsbury Bundt)	⅟₁₆ cake	4	4	0	6	2	6	0	4	305	11	37	250
Bundt, Fudge (Pillsbury Bundt Tunnel of Fudge)	⅟₁₆ cake	4	2	0	6	6	2	2	4	315	12	37	270
Bundt, Fudge Nut Crown (Pillsbury Bundt)	⅟₁₆ cake	4	4	0	4	4	2	2	6	290	9	31	220
Bundt, Lemon (Pillsbury Bundt Tunnel of Lemon)	⅟₁₆ cake	4	2	0	6	4	4	4	4	295	9	45	270
Bundt, Lemon Blueberry (Pillsbury Bundt)	⅟₁₆ cake	4	4	0	6	6	2	4	6	270	8	28	200
Bundt, Marble Supreme (Pillsbury Bundt)	⅟₁₆ cake	4	4	0	6	6	4	2	4	265	9	38	250
Bundt, Pound (Pillsbury Bundt)	⅟₁₆ cake	4	4	0	8	8	4	2	4	260	9	33	230
Butter Brickle (Betty Crocker SuperMoist)	⅟₁₂ pkg	4	*	*	6	6	4	6	6	275	11	38	260
Butter Pecan (Betty Crocker Snackin' Cake)	⅙ pkg	2	*	*	8	4	4	6	2	250	6	31	190
Butter Pecan (Betty Crocker SuperMoist)	⅟₁₂ pkg	4	*	*	6	4	4	4	4	250	11	35	250
Butter Recipe (Pillsbury Plus)	⅟₁₂ pkg	4	6	0	8	6	4	4	4	345	9	36	240
Butter Recipe Yellow (Betty Crocker SuperMoist)	⅟₁₂ pkg	4	6	*	6	4	4	6	2	350	11	37	260

Item	Serving										
		% U.S. RDA									
Carrot (Betty Crocker SuperMoist)	1/12 pkg	4	*	6	4	4	4	255	12	34	260
Carrot Nut (Betty Crocker Snackin' Cake)	1/9 pkg	4	8	8	4	8	4	240	6	30	180
Carrot w Cream Cheese Frosting (Betty Crocker Stir 'n Frost)	1/6 pkg	2	*	6	4	6	4	215	6	43	230
Carrot 'n Spice (Pillsbury Plus)	1/12 cake	4	25	6	6	4	4	330	11	36	260
Cheesecake (Jell-O)	1/8 cake	15	8	8	15	2	2	365	14	38	300
Cherry Chip (Betty Crocker SuperMoist)	1/12 pkg	4	*	6	4	*	2	265	3	36	180
Chocolate Chip (Betty Crocker SuperMoist)	1/12 pkg	4	*	6	2	*	2	230	4	35	190
Chocolate Chip w Chocolate Frosting (Betty Crocker Stir 'n Frost)	1/6 pkg	2	2	6	4	4	4	205	6	41	230
Chocolate Chocolate Chip (Betty Crocker SuperMoist)	1/12 pkg	4	*	6	2	6	6	425	12	33	250
Chocolate Chocolate Chip w Chocolate Chocolate Chip Frosting (Betty Crocker Stir 'n Frost)	1/6 pkg	2	2	4	2	2	6	260	6	41	230
Chocolate Fudge (Betty Crocker SuperMoist)	1/12 pkg	6	*	6	4	6	6	450	11	35	250

Cake Mixes	Amt.	% U.S. RDA Protein	A	C	B_1	B_2	Niacin	Calcium	Iron	Sodium (mg)	Fat (g)	Carbohydrate (g)	Calories
Chocolate Fudge Chip (Betty Crocker Snackin' Cake)	1/9 pkg	4	*	*	6	4	4	6	6	205	6	32	190
Chocolate Fudge w Vanilla Frosting (Betty Crocker Stir 'n Frost)	1/6 pkg	4	2	*	8	4	4	2	10	275	5	43	230
Chocolate Mint (Pillsbury Plus)	1/12 cake	4	2	0	4	6	6	10	6	340	12	35	260
Coconut Pecan (Betty Crocker Snackin' Cake)	1/9 pkg	2	*	*	8	4	4	6	2	255	7	30	190
Coffee Cake, Apple Cinnamon (Pillsbury)	1/8 cake	4	2	0	10	8	6	6	6	155	7	40	240
Coffee Cake, Butter Pecan (Pillsbury)	1/8 cake	6	8	0	10	8	4	4	4	335	15	39	310
Coffee Cake, Cinnamon Streusel (Pillsbury)	1/8 cake	4	2	0	8	6	4	4	6	225	8	41	250
Coffee Cake, Sour Cream (Pillsbury)	1/8 cake	6	4	0	8	8	4	4	4	235	12	35	270
Dark Chocolate (Pillsbury Plus)	1/12 cake	4	2	0	4	6	4	10	8	440	12	35	260
Devil's Food (Betty Crocker SuperMoist)	1/12 pkg	6	*	*	6	6	4	2	10	425	13	35	270
Devil's Food (Pillsbury Plus)	1/12 cake	4	2	0	2	4	4	10	6	405	11	35	250

				% U.S. RDA							
Devil's Food w Chocolate Frosting (Betty Crocker Stir 'n Frost) 1/6 pkg	4	2	*	6	4	4	2	8	260	6	41	230
Fudge Marble (Pillsbury Plus) 1/12 cake	4	2	0	8	6	4	4	6	300	12	36	270
Fudge Peanut Butter Chip (Betty Crocker Snackin' Cake) 1/9 pkg	4	*	*	8	6	6	6	6	250	7	32	200
German Black Forest (Betty Crocker Classics) 1/12 pkg	4	*	*	4	4	2	6	2	325	7	28	180
German Chocolate (Betty Crocker SuperMoist) 1/12 pkg	6	*	*	6	4	4	6	4	420	11	36	260
German Chocolate (Pillsbury Plus) 1/12 cake	4	2	0	4	4	4	4	2	340	11	36	250
German Chocolate Coconut Pecan (Betty Crocker Snackin' Cake) 1/9 pkg	2	*	*	6	2	4	6	2	255	5	32	180
Gingerbread (Betty Crocker Classics) 1/9 pkg	4	*	*	8	6	4	2	10	325	7	35	210
Gingerbread (Dromedary) 2" sq	2	*	*	4	4	4	2	6	NA	2	20	100
Gingerbread (Pillsbury) 3" sq	2	0	0	10	10	6	4	10	310	4	36	190
Golden Chocolate Chip (Betty Crocker Snackin' Cake) 1/9 pkg	2	*	*	6	4	4	6	4	255	5	34	190
Lemon (Betty Crocker SuperMoist) 1/12 pkg	4	*	*	6	4	4	4	4	260	11	36	260

Cake Mixes	Amt.	% U.S. RDA								Sodium (mg)	Fat (g)	Carbohydrate (g)	Calories
		Protein	A	C	B$_1$	B$_2$	Niacin	Calcium	Iron				
Lemon (Pillsbury Plus)	1/12 cake	4	2	0	10	6	4	4	4	310	11	36	260
Lemon Chiffon (Betty Crocker)	1/12 pkg	6	*	*	6	8	2	2	4	190	4	35	190
Marble (Betty Crocker SuperMoist)	1/12 pkg	4	*	*	6	6	4	4	6	255	11	36	260
Milk Chocolate (Betty Crocker SuperMoist)	1/12 pkg	6	*	*	6	6	4	4	6	290	11	35	250
Mint Fudge Chip (Betty Crocker Snackin' Cake)	1/9 pkg	2	*	*	6	4	4	6	4	210	6	32	190
Oats 'n Brown Sugar (Pillsbury Plus)	1/12 cake	4	2	0	6	6	4	4	6	305	12	35	260
Orange (Betty Crocker SuperMoist)	1/12 pkg	4	*	*	6	4	4	6	4	280	11	36	260
Pineapple Upside-Down (Betty Crocker Classics)	1/9 pkg	2	4	*	4	4	2	4	2	215	10	43	270
Pound, Golden (Betty Crocker Classics)	1/12 pkg	4	*	*	4	4	2	2	2	155	9	27	200
Pound (Dromedary)	3/4" sl	4	2	*	6	4	2	2	2	NA	9	29	210
Pudding, Chocolate (Betty Crocker Classics)	1/9 pkg	4	2	*	4	4	2	4	6	255	5	45	230
Pudding, Lemon (Betty Crocker Classics)	1/9 pkg	4	2	*	4	4	2	4	2	270	5	45	230

Product	Serving	% U.S. RDA										
Sour Cream Chocolate (Betty Crocker SuperMoist)	¹⁄₁₂ pkg	6	*	*	6	4	4	6	6	430	11	36	260
Sour Cream White (Betty Crocker SuperMoist)	¹⁄₁₂ pkg	4	*	*	6	4	4	4	*	2	260	3	36	180
Spice (Betty Crocker SuperMoist)	¹⁄₁₂ pkg	4	*	*	6	6	4	6	6	275	11	37	260
Spice w Vanilla Frosting (Betty Crocker Stir 'n Frost)	⅙ pkg	4	2	*	8	6	6	2	4	315	9	48	280
Strawberry (Betty Crocker SuperMoist)	¹⁄₁₂ pkg	4	*	*	6	4	4	4	4	260	11	36	260
Strawberry (Pillsbury Plus)	¹⁄₁₂ cake	2	2	0	8	6	4	4	4	300	11	37	260
Streusel, Banana (Pillsbury Streusel Swirl)	¹⁄₁₆ cake	4	2	0	8	6	4	4	6	200	11	38	260
Streusel, Rich Butter (Pillsbury Streusel Swirl)	¹⁄₁₆ cake	4	2	0	8	6	4	2	6	235	11	38	260
Streusel, Cinnamon (Betty Crocker Stir 'n Streusel)	⅙ pkg	4	*	*	8	4	6	*	4	230	7	42	240
Streusel, Cinnamon (Pillsbury Streusel Swirl)	¹⁄₁₆ cake	4	2	0	6	6	4	4	6	200	11	38	260
Streusel, Dutch Apple (Pillsbury Streusel Swirl)	¹⁄₁₆ cake	4	2	0	6	6	4	2	6	200	11	38	260
Streusel, Fudge Marble (Pillsbury Streusel Swirl)	¹⁄₁₆ cake	4	2	0	6	6	4	2	6	200	11	38	260

Cake Mixes	Amt.	Pro-tein	A	C	B₁	B₂	Nia-cin	Cal-cium	Iron	Sodium (mg)	Fat (g)	Carbohy-drate (g)	Calories
					% U.S. RDA								
Streusel, German Chocolate (Betty Crocker Stir 'n Streusel)	⅙ pkg	4	*	*	8	4	6	2	6	245	7	42	240
Streusel, German Chocolate (Pillsbury Streusel Swirl)	1/16 cake	4	2	0	4	4	2	4	4	290	11	36	260
Streusel, Lemon (Pillsbury Streusel Swirl)	1/16 cake	4	2	0	6	6	4	6	4	335	11	39	270
Streusel, Pecan and Brown Sugar (Pillsbury Streusel Swirl)	1/16 cake	4	2	0	6	4	4	2	6	200	11	37	260
White (Betty Crocker SuperMoist)	1/12 pkg	4	*	*	10	8	4	6	6	245	10	37	250
White (Pillsbury Plus)	1/12 cake	4	0	0	2	2	2	2	0	295	10	35	240
Yellow (Betty Crocker SuperMoist)	1/12 pkg	4	*	*	6	4	4	6	4	270	12	36	260
Yellow (Pillsbury Plus)	1/12 cake	4	2	0	8	6	6	4	4	300	12	36	260
Yellow w Chocolate Frosting (Betty Crocker Stir 'n Frost)	⅙ pkg	2	2	*	6	4	4	2	4	215	8	37	230
Snack Cakes													
Chip Flips (Hostess)	1	4	0	0	6	6	4	2	6	165	16	47	330
Choco-Diles (Hostess)	1	2	0	0	4	4	0	2	4	280	11	35	240

Product	Serving					% U.S. RDA						
Coffee Cake (Drake's)	1 pc	220	32	9	220	6	2	6	4	8	*	6
Crumb Cakes (Hostess)	1	130	22	4	95	4	2	2	4	4	0	2
Cupcake, Chocolate (Dolly Madison)	1	170	29	5	290	4	*	4	4	2	*	2
Cup Cakes, Chocolate (Hostess)	1	170	29	6	250	4	2	2	4	4	0	2
Cup Cakes, Orange (Hostess)	1	150	28	5	175	2	2	2	4	4	0	2
Dessert Cups (Hostess)	1	60	14	0	120	2	2	2	2	4	0	2
Devil Dogs (Drake's)	1 pc	170	22	8	165	4	*	2	4	2	*	2
Ding Dongs / Big Wheels	1	170	21	9	130	2	2	2	2	0	0	2
Fruit Loaf (Hostess)	1	400	77	9	520	10	4	8	8	15	0	6
Funny Bones (Drake's)	1 pc	160	18	9	130	4	2	2	4	2	*	4
Ho Hos (Hostess)	1	120	17	6	90	2	2	0	2	0	0	2
Hostess O's	1	240	33	11	265	2	4	4	2	2	0	4
Lil' Angels (Hostess)	1	90	14	2	95	2	2	0	2	2	0	2
Peanut Putters, Filled (Hostess)	1	360	46	15	240	8	4	10	10	8	0	8
Peanut Putters, Unfilled (Hostess)	1	410	43	21	240	6	4	18	10	6	0	10
Ring Ding Jr. (Drake's)	1 pc	160	20	9	120	4	*	*	2	*	*	2
Sno Balls	1	150	28	4	170	2	2	2	2	2	0	2
Suzy Q's, Banana (Hostess)	1	240	38	9	195	4	4	4	6	6	0	4

Snack Cakes	Amt.	Protein	A	C	B₁	B₂	Niacin	Calcium	Iron	Sodium (mg)	Fat (g)	Carbohydrate (g)	Calories
		% U.S. RDA											
Suzy Q's, Chocolate (Hostess)	1	2	0	0	4	4	2	2	4	300	10	37	240
Tiger Tail	1	2	0	0	4	4	2	2	4	240	6	38	210
Twinkies (Hostess)	1	2	0	0	4	4	2	2	2	150	5	26	160
Yankee Doodles (Drake's)	1 pc	2	*	*	*	2	2	*	2	130	5	15	110
Candy													
Almond Joy, Bar	1.6 oz	2	*	*	*	4	*	2	2	90	12	26	220
Caramello, Bar	2 oz	6	*	*	2	8	*	10	2	110	13	37	280
Chocolate, Bar (Cadbury Dairy Milk)	2 oz	6	2	*	2	10	2	14	8	90	16	34	300
Chocolate, Bar (Hershey's)	1.45 oz	4	*	*	2	6	*	8	4	35	13	23	220
Chocolate w Almond, Bar (Cadbury)	2 oz	8	2	*	2	14	2	14	4	80	18	31	310
Chocolate w Almonds, Bar (Hershey's)	1.45 oz	6	*	*	*	10	*	8	2	35	14	22	230
Chocolate w Brazil Nuts, Bar (Cadbury Brazil Nut)	2 oz	8	*	*	4	10	2	14	4	80	18	32	310
Chocolate w Fruit and Nuts, Bar (Cadbury)	2 oz	8	2	*	2	10	4	12	6	80	16	33	300
Chocolate w Hazelnuts, Bar (Cadbury Whole Hazels)	2 oz	8	*	*	2	12	2	14	4	90	17	32	310

Food	Serving	% U.S. RDA											Calories
Chocolate Coated Bridge Mix (Deran)	1 oz	2	*	*	*	2	*	2	*	25	5	20	130
Chocolate Malted Milk Balls (Deran)	1 oz	2	*	*	*	4	2	4	2	70	6	20	140
Golden Almond, Bar (Hershey's)	1 oz	4	*	*	*	6	6	6	4	20	11	12	160
Kisses (Hershey's)	1 oz (6 pcs)	2	*	*	*	4	6	4	2	25	9	16	150
Kit Kat, Bar	1.5 oz	4	*	*	*	6	6	6	2	45	11	25	210
Krackel, Bar	1.45 oz	4	*	*	*	6	8	6	2	60	12	25	220
Marshmallows (Campfire)	2 lg or 24 mini	*	*	*	*	*	*	*	*	10	0	10	40
Milk Chocolate Covered Raisins (Deran)	1 oz	2	*	*	*	2	2	2	*	35	4	20	120
Mounds, Bar	1.65 oz	2	*	*	*	2	*	2	4	90	12	28	230
Mr. Goodbar, Bar	1.65 oz	10	*	*	4	6	10	6	6	20	15	23	250
Peanut Clusters (Deran)	1 oz	8	*	*	2	2	10	2	2	15	9	13	150
Power House, Bar	2.2 oz	8	*	*	2	6	12	4	4	210	11	42	290
Reese's Peanut Butter Cups (Plain or Crunchy)	1.6 oz (2 pcs)	10	*	*	*	4	10	4	2	145	14	23	240
Reese's Peanut Butter Chips	¼ c	15	*	*	8	8	20	6	4	90	13	19	230
Reese's Pieces	1 oz (35 pcs)	6	*	*	4	4	8	4	2	45	6	17	140
Rolo	1 oz (5 pcs)	2	*	*	4	8	*	8	2	65	6	19	140
Rum Wafers (Deran)	1 oz	*	*	*	*	*	*	*	2	15	7	20	150

Candy	Amt.	Protein	A	C	B₁	B₂	Niacin	Calcium	Iron	Sodium (mg)	Fat (g)	Carbohydrate (g)	Calories
							% U.S. RDA						
Special Dark, Bar (Hershey's)	1.45 oz	4	*	*	*	2	*	*	8	2	12	26	220
Whatchamacallit, Bar	1.4 oz	6	*	*	*	6	6	6	*	100	12	22	210
York Mint	1.5 oz	*	*	*	*	*	*	*	2	15	5	33	180
Cereal, Cold													
All-Bran	⅓ c	6	25	25	25	25	25	2	25	320	1	22	70
Alpha-Bits	1 oz	2	25	NA	25	25	25	*	10	195	1	24	110
Apple Jacks	1 c	2	25	25	25	25	25	*	25	125	0	26	110
Body Buddies, Brown Sugar and Honey	1 c	2	25	25	25	25	25	10	45	290	0–1	24	110
Body Buddies, Natural Fruit Flavor	1 c	2	25	25	25	25	25	10	45	285	1	24	110
BooBerry	1 c	2	25	25	25	25	25	2	25	210	1	24	110
Bran Buds	⅓ c	4	25	25	25	25	25	2	25	175	1	22	70
Bran Chex	⅔ c	4	*	25	25	4	25	*	25	300	0	23	90
Bran Flakes, 40% (Kellogg's)	⅔ c	4	25	*	25	25	25	*	45	220	0	23	90
Bran Flakes, 40% (Post)	1 oz	4	25	NA	25	25	25	*	25	225	1	23	90
Bran Flakes, 40% (Ralston)	¾ c	4	25	25	25	25	25	*	25	285	0	20	90
BucWheats	¾ c	2	45	45	45	45	45	6	45	235	1	24	110

Cereal	Serving												
				% U.S. RDA									
C-3PO's	3/4 c	4	25	25	25	25	25	*	10	160	0	24	110
Cheerios	1¼ c	6	25	25	25	25	25	4	25	330	2	20	110
Cheerios, Honey Nut	3/4 c	4	25	25	25	25	25	2	25	255	1	23	110
Cinnamon Toast Crunch	2/3 c	2	25	25	25	25	25	4	25	225	3	23	120
Cocoa Krispies	3/4 c	2	25	25	25	25	25	*	10	195	0	25	110
Cocoa Puffs	1 c	2	*	25	25	25	25	*	25	205	1	25	110
Cookie-Crisp, Chocolate Chip or Vanilla Wafer	1 c	2	25	25	25	25	25	*	25	200	1	25	110
Corn Chex	1 c	2	*	25	25	2	25	*	10	310	0	25	110
Corn Flakes (General Mills Country)	1 c	4	25	25	25	25	25	*	45	310	0–1	25	110
Corn Flakes (Kellogg's)	1 c	4	25	25	35	35	35	*	10	285	0	25	110
Corn Flakes (Post Toasties)	1 oz	2	25	NA	25	25	25	*	2	305	1	24	110
Corn Flakes (Ralston)	1 c	2	25	25	25	*	25	*	10	270	0	25	110
Corn Total	1 c	4	100	100	100	100	100	4	100	310	1	24	110
Count Chocula	1 c	2	25	25	25	25	25	2	25	205	1	24	110
Cracklin' Oat Bran	½ c	4	25	25	25	25	25	2	10	190	4	20	120
Crispix	3/4 c	2	25	25	25	25	25	*	10	230	0	24	110
Crispy Oatmeal & Raisin Chex	3/4 c	4	*	2	25	4	25	*	25	240	1	31	140
Crispy Rice (Ralston)	1 c	2	25	25	25	*	25	*	10	205	0	25	110
Crispy Wheats 'n Raisins	3/4 c	2	25	*	25	25	25	4	25	185	1	23	110

Cereal, Cold	Amt.	Pro-tein	A	C	B₁	B₂	Nia-cin	Cal-cium	Iron	Sodium (mg)	Fat (g)	Carbohy-drate (g)	Calories
					% U.S. RDA								
C.W. Post	1 oz	2	25	NA	25	25	25	*	25	55	4	20	130
C.W. Post w Raisins	1 oz	2	25	NA	25	25	25	*	25	50	4	21	120
Donkey Kong	1 c	2	25	25	25	25	25	*	25	130	1	25	110
Donkey Kong Junior	1 c	2	25	25	25	25	25	*	25	120	1	25	110
E.T.	¾ c	4	25	25	25	25	25	*	25	170	5	19	130
FrankenBerry	1 c	2	25	25	25	25	25	2	25	205	1	24	110
Froot Loops	1 c	2	25	100	25	25	25	*	25	135	1	-25	110
Frosted Flakes (Kellogg's)	¾ c	2	25	25	25	25	25	*	10	190	0	26	110
Frosted Flakes, Banana (Kellogg's)	⅔ c	2	25	25	25	25	25	*	10	180	1	25	110
Frosted Krispies	¾ c	2	25	25	25	25	25	*	10	200	0	25	110
Frosted Mini-Wheats, Sugar Frosted or Apple Flavored	4 biscuits (1 oz)	4	25	25	25	25	25	*	10	0–10	0	24	110
Fruit & Fibre, Apples and Cinnamon	1 oz	4	25	NA	25	25	25	*	25	195	1	22	90
Fruit & Fibre, Dates, Raisins, and Walnuts	1 oz	4	25	NA	25	25	25	*	25	170	1	21	90
Fruitful Bran	¾ c	4	25	*	25	25	25	*	45	240	0	27	110
Fruit Rings (Ralston)	1 c	2	25	25	25	25	25	*	25	NA	1	26	110
Golden Grahams	¾ c	2	25	25	25	25	25	*	25	285	1	24	110

Cereal	Serving				% U.S. RDA						
Granola, Cinnamon and Raisins (Nature Valley)	1/3 c	4	*	*	6	*	*	6	35	5	19	130
Granola, Coconut and Honey (Nature Valley)	1/3 c	4	*	*	6	*	*	6	35	7	18	150
Granola, Fruit and Nut (Nature Valley)	1/3 c	4	*	*	6	2	2	4	35	5	19	130
Granola, Toasted Oat Mixture (Nature Valley)	1/3 c	4	*	*	6	2	2	6	35	5	19	130
Grape-Nuts	1 oz	6	25	NA	25	25	*	4	195	1	23	100
Grape-Nuts, Raisin	1 oz	4	25	NA	25	25	*	4	160	1	22	100
Grape-Nuts Flakes	1 oz	4	25	NA	25	25	*	25	195	1	23	100
Honey & Nut Corn Flakes (Kellogg's)	3/4 c	2	25	25	25	25	*	10	190	1	24	110
Honey Nut Crunch, Raisin Bran (Post)	1 oz	4	25	NA	25	25	*	20	150	1	23	90
Honey Smacks	3/4 c	2	25	25	25	25	*	10	70	0	25	110
Honeycomb	1 oz	2	25	NA	25	25	*	10	195	1	25	110
Honeycomb, Strawberry	1 oz	2	25	NA	25	25	*	10	160	2	25	120
Kaboom	1 c	4	45	45	45	45	4	45	370	1	23	110
Kix	1 1/2 c	4	25	25	25	25	4	45	315	1	24	110
Lucky Charms	1 c	4	25	25	25	25	2	25	185	1	24	110
Marshmallow Krispies	1 1/4 c	4	25	25	25	25	*	10	285	0	33	140
Most	1/2 c	6	100	100	100	100	100	100	30	0	22	100

Cereal, Cold	Amt.	Protein	A	C	B_1	B_2	Niacin	Calcium	Iron	Sodium (mg)	Fat (g)	Carbohydrate (g)	Calories
							% U.S. RDA						
Natural (Heartland, All Varieties)	¼ c	4	*	*	6	2	*	*	6	NA	6	18	130
Nutri-Grain, Corn	½ c	4	25	25	25	25	25	*	4	185	1	24	110
Nutri-Grain, Wheat	⅔ c	4	25	25	25	25	25	*	6	195	0	24	110
Nutri-Grain, Wheat and Raisins	⅔ c	4	25	*	25	25	25	*	6	165	0	33	140
Oat Flakes, Fortified (Post)	1 oz	10	25	NA	25	25	25	2	45	275	1	20	100
Pac-Man	1 c	2	25	25	25	25	25	2	25	195	0-1	25	110
Pebbles, Cocoa	1 oz	*	25	NA	25	25	25	*	10	165	2	25	110
Pebbles, Fruity	1 oz	*	25	NA	25	25	25	*	10	160	2	25	110
Product 19	¾ c	4	100	100	100	100	100	*	100	320	0	24	110
Raisin Bran (Kellogg's)	¾ c	4	25	*	25	25	25	*	45	205	1	30	110
Raisin Bran (Post)	1 oz	4	25	NA	25	25	25	*	25	170	1	22	90
Raisin Bran (Ralston)	¾ c	4	25	2	25	25	25	2	25	315	0	30	120
Raisins, Rice & Rye	¾ c	4	*	*	25	25	25	*	25	235	0	31	140
Rice Chex	1⅛ c	2	*	25	25	*	25	*	10	280	0	25	110
Rice Krispies	1 c	2	25	25	25	25	25	*	10	285	0	25	110
Smurf-Berry Crunch	1 oz	2	25	NA	25	25	25	*	25	65	1	25	110
Strawberry Krispies	¾ c	2	25	25	25	25	25	*	10	200	0	25	110
Special K	1 c	10	25	25	35	35	35	*	25	220	0	20	110

		% U.S. RDA											
Strawberry Shortcake	1 c	2	25	25	25	25	25	*	25	190	1	25	110
Sugar Corn Pops	1 c	2	25	25	25	25	25	*	10	95	0	26	110
Sugar Frosted Flakes (Ralston)	¾ c	2	25	25	25	25	25	*	10	180	0	26	110
Sugar Frosted Rice (Ralston)	1 c	2	25	25	25	25	25	*	10	150	1	26	110
Super Sugar Crisp	1 oz	2	25	NA	25	25	25	*	10	25	0	26	110
Tasteeos	1¼ c	6	25	25	25	25	25	*	25	210	1	22	110
Total	1 c	4	100	100	100	100	100	4	100	375	1	23	110
Trix	1 c	2	25	25	25	25	25	*	25	170	0-1	25	110
Wheat Chex	⅔ c	4	*	25	4	25	*	*	25	200	0	23	100
Wheat & Raisin Chex	¾ c	4	*	2	4	25	*	*	30	215	1	31	130
Wheaties	1 c	4	25	25	25	25	4	4	25	370	1	23	110
Cereal, Hot													
Farina (Pillsbury)	⅔ c cooked	2	0	0	8	4	4	0	4	265	0-1	17	80
Grits, Hominy Quick (Albers)	¼ c dry	6	*	*	10	6	8	*	6	NA	0	33	150
Oatmeal, Instant (Harvest Brand)	1 pkt	6	*	*	15	*	*	*	6	220	2	18	110
Oatmeal, Instant w Apples and Cinnamon (Harvest Brand)	1 pkt	6	*	*	10	*	*	*	6	230	2	26	140
Oatmeal, Instant w Cinnamon and Spice (Harvest Brand)	1 pkt	6	*	*	10	2	*	*	6	300	2	35	180

Cereal, Hot	Amt.	Protein	A	C	B$_1$	B$_2$	Niacin	Calcium	Iron	Sodium (mg)	Fat (g)	Carbohydrate (g)	Calories
		% U.S. RDA											
Oatmeal, Instant w Maple and Brown Sugar (Harvest Brand)	1 pkt	6	*	*	10	*	*	*	8	290	2	32	170
Oatmeal, Instant w Peaches and Cream (Harvest Brand)	1 pkt	4	*	*	10	*	*	*	4	200	2	27	140
Oats (3-Minute Brand Old-Fashioned)	1 oz	6	*	*	10	*	*	*	6	0	2	18	110
Oats (3-Minute Brand Quick)	1 oz	6	*	*	10	*	*	*	6	*	2	18	110
Oats, Regular and Quick (Ralston)	⅓ c uncooked	8	*	*	15	2	*	*	6	5	2	18	110
Ralston, Instant and Regular	¼ c uncooked	6	*	*	10	2	6	*	6	5	1	20	90
Cheese													
American, Process (Borden)	1 oz	15	4	*	*	6	*	20	*	445	9	1	110
American, Process (Kraft Deluxe)	1 oz	10	4	*	*	6	*	15	*	425	9	1	110
American, Process, Slices (Kraft Deluxe)	1 oz	15	6	*	*	6	*	15	*	465	9	1	110
American, Cheese Food (Borden)	1 oz	10	4	*	*	6	*	15	*	490	7	3	90

		% U.S. RDA											
American, Sharp, Process (Kraft Old English)	1 oz	10	4	*	*	6	*	15	*	405	9	1	110
American, Sharp, Process, Slices (Kraft Old English)	1 oz	10	4	*	*	6	*	15	*	395	9	1	110
American Flavor Process Cheese Product, Slices (Lite-line)	1 oz	15	*	*	*	2	*	20	*	410	2	1	50
American Flavor Process Cheese Product (Lite-line Reduced Sodium)	1 oz	15	4	*	*	4	*	20	*	90	4	2	70
American Flavor Process Cheese Product (Lite-line Sodium Lite)	1 oz	15	4	*	*	4	*	20	*	200	4	2	70
Blue	1 oz	15	8	*	*	10	2	8	*	NA	9	1	110
Blue (Kraft)	1 oz	10	2	*	*	4	*	15	*	395	8	1	100
Brick (Kraft)	1 oz	15	6	*	*	6	*	20	*	205	9	1	110
Camembert, Domestic, 4-oz pkg (3 wedges)	1 wedge	15	8	*	2	15	2	4	2	NA	10	1	110
Caraway (Kraft)	1 oz	15	6	*	*	6	*	20	*	195	8	1	100
Cheddar, Domestic	1 oz	15	8	*	*	8	*	20	2	198	9	1	110
Cheddar, Domestic, Shredded	1 c	60	30	*	2	30	*	80	6	791	37	3	450
Cheddar, Mild (Kraft)	1 oz	15	6	*	*	6	*	20	*	180	9	1	110
Cheddar, Mild, Imitation (Kraft Golden Image)	1 oz	15	4	*	*	6	*	20	*	170	9	1	110

Cheese	Amt.	% U.S. RDA								Sodium (mg)	Fat (g)	Carbohydrate (g)	Calories
		Protein	A	C	B₁	B₂	Niacin	Calcium	Iron				
Cheddar, Sharp (Kraft)	1 oz	15	4	*	*	6	*	20	*	175	9	1	110
Cheese Spread, Process (Velveeta)	1 oz	10	4	*	*	8	*	15	*	430	6	2	80
Cheese Spread, Process, Slices (Velveeta)	1 oz	10	6	*	*	6	*	15	*	400	6	2	90
Cheese Spread, Process, Jalapeno (Kraft)	1 oz	10	4	*	*	6	*	15	*	420	6	2	80
Cheese Spread, Process, Pimento (Velveeta)	1 oz	10	4	*	*	8	*	15	*	450	6	2	80
Colby (Kraft)	1 oz	15	4	*	*	6	*	15	*	175	9	1	110
Colby, Imitation (Kraft Golden Image)	1 oz	15	4	*	*	6	*	15	*	140	9	1	110
Colby Flavor Process Cheese Product (Lite-line)	1 oz	15	2	*	*	2	*	20	*	470	2	1	50
Cottage, Creamed, Packed	1 c	70	8	*	4	35	*	25	4	561	10	7	260
Cottage, Uncreamed, Packed	1 c	80	*	*	4	35	*	20	4	580	1	6	170
Cottage, 4% Milkfat (Borden)	½ c	30	4	*	*	10	*	6	*	465	5	4	120
Cottage, 4% Milkfat (Meadow Gold)	½ c	30	4	*	*	10	*	6	*	NA	5	4	120
Cottage, 2% Milkfat (Meadow Gold Viva Lowfat)	½ c	30	*	*	*	10	*	6	*	NA	2	4	100

94

		% U.S. RDA											
Cottage, Lowfat (Lite-line)	½ c	30	*	*	*	10	*	6	*	375	2	4	90
Cream Cheese (Kraft Philadelphia Brand)	1 oz	4	6	*	*	2	*	2	*	85	10	1	100
Cream Cheese w Chives (Kraft Philadelphia Brand)	1 oz	4	6	*	*	2	*	2	*	115	10	1	100
Cream Cheese w Pimentos (Kraft Philadelphia Brand)	1 oz	4	6	*	*	2	*	2	*	115	10	1	100
Cream Cheese, Whipped (Kraft Philadelphia Brand)	1 oz	4	6	*	*	2	*	2	*	110	10	1	100
Cream Cheese, Whipped, w Bacon and Horseradish (Kraft Philadelphia Brand)	1 oz	4	8	*	*	2	*	2	*	130	9	1	90
Cream Cheese, Whipped, w Blue Cheese (Kraft Philadelphia Brand)	1 oz	6	10	*	*	4	*	6	*	145	9	2	100
Cream Cheese, Whipped, w Chives (Kraft Philadelphia Brand)	1 oz	4	6	*	*	2	*	2	*	145	8	1	90
Cream Cheese, Whipped, w Onions (Kraft Philadelphia Brand)	1 oz	4	10	*	*	2	*	4	*	160	8	2	90
Cream Cheese, Whipped, w Pimentos (Kraft Philadelphia Brand)	1 oz	4	10	4	*	4	*	4	*	140	8	2	90

Cheese	Amt.	% U.S. RDA								Sodium (mg)	Fat (g)	Carbohydrate (g)	Calories
		Protein	A	C	B₁	B₂	Niacin	Calcium	Iron				
Cream Cheese, Whipped, w Smoked Salmon (Kraft Philadelphia Brand)	1 oz	4	6	*	*	2	*	2	*	90	9	1	100
Edam (Kraft)	1 oz	10	2	2	*	4	*	15	*	275	8	1	100
Gouda (Kraft)	1 oz	10	2	*	*	4	*	15	*	230	8	1	100
Limburger	1 oz	15	6	*	2	8	*	15	2	NA	8	1	100
Limburger (Mohawk Valley Little Gem Size)	1 oz	15	8	*	*	8	*	15	*	225	8	0	100
Monterey Jack (Kraft)	1 oz	15	6	*	*	4	*	20	*	195	9	0	110
Monterey Jack Flavor Process Cheese Product (Lite-line)	1 oz	15	2	*	*	2	*	20	*	470	2	1	50
Mozzarella, Low Moisture Part Skim (Kraft)	1 oz	20	4	*	*	4	*	20	*	190	5	1	80
Muenster (Kraft)	1 oz	15	6	*	*	6	*	15	*	170	8	1	100
Muenster Flavor Process Cheese Product (Lite-line)	1 oz	15	2	*	*	2	*	20	*	470	2	1	50
Neufchatel (Kraft)	1 oz	6	6	*	*	2	*	2	*	110	7	1	80
Parmesan, Grated	1 oz	25	8	*	*	15	*	40	*	247	9	1	130
Parmesan, Grated (Kraft)	1 oz	25	4	*	*	6	*	40	*	425	9	1	130
Parmesan, Natural (Kraft)	1 oz	20	2	*	*	4	*	30	*	455	7	1	110

		% U.S. RDA										
Pimento Cheese, Process (Kraft Deluxe)	1 oz	10	4	*	*	6	*	15	320	9	1	110
Provolone (Kraft)	1 oz	15	2	*	*	4	*	15	250	7	1	90
Romano, Grated (Kraft)	1 oz	25	4	*	*	6	*	35	405	9	1	130
Romano, Natural (Kraft Casino)	1 oz	20	4	*	*	4	*	25	340	7	1	100
Roquefort	1 oz	15	8	*	*	10	2	8	NA	9	1	110
Scamorze, Low Moisture Part Skim (Kraft)	1 oz	15	4	*	*	6	*	20	150	5	1	80
Sharp Cheddar Flavor Process Cheese Product (Lite-line)	1 oz	15	2	*	*	2	*	20	445	2	1	50
Snack Mate Process Cheese Spread, All Flavors (Nabisco)	1 oz	10	4	*	*	8	*	10	NA	6	2	80
Swiss, Domestic	1 oz	15	6	*	*	6	2	25	201	8	1	110
Swiss, Process	1 oz	15	6	*	*	6	2	25	331	8	1	100
Swiss, Aged (Kraft)	1 oz	15	4	*	*	4	*	25	75	8	0	100
Swiss, Chunk (Kraft)	1 oz	20	6	*	*	4	*	30	40	8	1	110
Swiss, Process (Borden)	1 oz	15	4	*	*	4	*	35	355	8	1	100
Swiss, Slices (Kraft)	1 oz	20	6	*	*	4	*	30	105	8	1	110
Swiss Flavor Process Cheese Product (Lite-line)	1 oz	15	*	*	*	2	*	20	330	2	1	50
Substitute, Cheese Food, Process (Lite-line)	1 oz	10	4	*	*	6	*	15	450	7	2	90

Chocolate, Baking	Amt.	Pro-tein	A	C	B$_1$	B$_2$	Nia-cin	Cal-cium	Iron	Sodium (mg)	Fat (g)	Carbohy-drate (g)	Calories
					% U.S. RDA								
Chocolate, Baking (Hershey's)	1 oz	*	*	*	*	8	2	2	10	1	16	7	190
Chocolate Chips, Milk (Hershey's)	¼ c	4	*	*	2	6	*	8	2	55	11	27	220
Chocolate Chips, Semi-Sweet (Borden)	1 oz	2	*	*	*	*	*	*	4	5	7	20	150
Chocolate Chips, Semi-Sweet (Hershey's)	¼ c	4	*	*	*	2	*	*	8	5	12	26	220
Chocolate Chips, Semi-Sweet, Mini (Hershey's)	¼ c	4	*	*	*	2	*	*	8	5	12	26	220
Cocoa													
Cocoa (Hershey's)	⅓ c	*	*	*	*	8	2	4	25	5	4	13	120
Mix (Hershey's)	1 oz	6	*	*	*	6	*	10	4	145	2	21	120
Mix, Instant (Hershey's) Prep w Milk	3 tbsp	15	6	2	4	25	*	30	4	160	10	29	240
Mix, Instant (Ovaltine 50 Calorie)	1 pkt	2	10	10	10	10	10	10	10	NA	2	8	50
Mix, Instant (Ovaltine Hot 'n Rich)	1 pkt	2	10	10	10	10	10	10	10	NA	3	22	120
Mix, Instant (Superman)	1 env	NA	NA	NA	NA	NA	NA	10	*	210	2	12	70
Mix, Instant, Chocolate Marshmallow (Alba)	1 env	NA	NA	NA	NA	NA	NA	30	*	180	0	10	60

Food	Serving				% U.S. RDA							
Mix, Instant, Chocolate w Mini-Marshmallows (Carnation)	1 oz	4	*	*	*	8	*	6	*	115	1	23	110
Mix, Instant, Milk Chocolate (Alba)	1 env	NA	NA	NA	NA	NA	*	30	*	180	0	9	60
Mix, Instant, Milk Chocolate (Carnation)	1 oz	6	*	*	*	10	*	8	*	115	1	23	110
Mix, Instant, Mocha (Alba)	1 env	NA	NA	NA	NA	NA	*	30	*	180	0	10	60
Mix, Instant, Rich Chocolate (Carnation)	1 oz	4	*	*	*	8	*	6	*	115	1	23	110
Mix, Instant, Rich Chocolate (Carnation 70 Calorie)	1 pkt	6	*	*	*	8	*	10	*	125	0	15	70
Mix, Instant, Sugar Free (Carnation)	1 pkt	8	*	*	2	10	*	10	4	160	0-1	8	50
Mix, Instant, Sugar Free (Ovaltine)	1 pkt	2	10	10	10	10	10	10	10	NA	1	7	40
Mix, Instant, Sugar Free Mint (Ovaltine)	1 pkt	2	10	10	10	10	10	10	10	NA	1	7	40
Coconut													
Coconut, Fresh, Meat Only	2"x2"x½" pc	4	*	2	*	2	*	*	4	10	16	4	160
Coconut, Fresh, Shredded or Grated	1 c packed	10	*	6	4	4	2	2	10	30	46	12	450
Coconut, Dried, Unsweetened	1 oz	4	*	*	2	*	*	*	4	NA	18	7	190

Coffee	Amt.	Protein	A	C	B$_1$	B$_2$	Niacin	Calcium	Iron	Sodium (mg)	Fat (g)	Carbohydrate (g)	Calories
		% U.S. RDA											
Instant (Kava)	1 tsp	*	*	*	*	*	2	*	*	0-5	0	1	2
Café Amaretto, Instant (General Foods International Coffees)	6 fl oz	*	*	*	*	*	4	*	*	30	2	7	50
Café Francais, Instant (General Foods International Coffee)	6 fl oz	*	*	*	*	*	2	*	*	30	3	7	60
Café Vienna, Instant (General Foods International Coffee)	6 fl oz	*	*	*	*	*	2	*	*	95	2	10	60
Irish Mocha Mint, Instant (General Foods International Coffee)	6 fl oz	*	*	*	*	*	*	*	*	25	3	7	50
Orange Cappuccino, Instant (General Foods International Coffees)	6 fl oz	*	*	*	*	*	*	*	*	100	2	10	60
Suisse Mocha, Instant (General Foods International Coffee)	6 fl oz	*	*	*	*	*	*	*	*	25	3	7	60
Coffeelike Instant Beverage (Postum)	6 fl oz	*	*	*	*	*	4	*	*	5	0	3	12
Condiments													
Garden Mix (Vlasic Hot & Spicy)	1 oz	*	2	6	*	*	*	*	2	380	0	1	4

Food	Portion	% U.S. RDA							Sodium (mg)			Calories
Mustard (French's Bold 'n Spicy)	1 tbsp	*	*	*	*	*	*	*	145	1	1	16
Mustard, Brown (Heinz)	1 tsp	*	NA	NA	NA	NA	*	*	58	.4	.5	8
Mustard, Mild or Pourable (Heinz)	1 tsp	*	NA	NA	NA	NA	*	*	71	.2	.5	5
Mustard (French's Medford)	1 tbsp	*	*	*	*	*	*	*	240	1	1	16
Mustard, Prepared Yellow (French's)	1 tbsp	*	*	*	*	*	*	*	180	1	1	10
Mustard w Horseradish (French's)	1 tbsp	*	*	*	*	*	*	*	265	1	1	16
Mustard w Onion (French's)	1 tbsp	*	*	*	*	*	*	*	190	1	5	25
Olives, Green, Medium	4	*	*	*	*	*	*	2	360	2	0–1	20
Olives, Ripe	3 sm or 2 lg	*	*	*	*	2	*	2	82	2	0–1	18
Onions, Cocktail, Lightly Spiced (Vlasic)	1 oz	*	*	*	*	*	*	*	365	0	1	4
Onions, Spiced (Heinz)	1 oz	0	NA	NA	NA	NA	*	*	600	0	0	2
Onions, Sweet (Heinz)	1 oz	0	NA	NA	NA	NA	*	*	165	0	9	40
Pepperoncini (Vlasic Mild Greek)	1 oz	*	*	*	*	*	*	2	450	0	1	4
Peppers, Hot Banana (Heinz)	1 oz	0	NA	NA	NA	NA	2	2	305	0	1	6
Peppers, Rings or Slices (Heinz)	1 oz	0	NA	NA	NA	NA	2	2	305	0	1	4
Peppers, Hot Banana Rings (Vlasic)	1 oz	*	15	*	*	*	*	2	465	0	1	4

Condiments	Amt.	Protein	A	C	B₁	B₂	Niacin	Calcium	Iron	Sodium (mg)	Fat (g)	Carbohydrate (g)	Calories
								% U.S. RDA					
Peppers, Sweet (Heinz Mementos)	1 oz	0	NA	NA	NA	NA	NA	2	*	320	0	1	6
Picalilli (Heinz)	1 oz	0	NA	NA	NA	NA	NA	*	*	145	0	7	30
Pickles, Bread and Butter (Heinz Slices)	1 oz	0	NA	NA	NA	NA	NA	*	*	170	0	6	25
Pickles, Bread and Butter (Vlasic Deli Chunks)	1 oz	*	*	*	*	*	*	*	*	120	0	6	25
Pickles, Bread and Butter (Vlasic Old Fashioned Chunks)	1 oz	*	*	*	*	*	*	*	*	120	0	6	25
Pickles, Bread and Butter, Sweet (Vlasic Butter Chips)	1 oz	*	*	*	*	*	*	*	*	155	0	6	27
Pickles, Bread and Butter, Sweet (Vlasic Butter Stix)	1 oz	*	*	*	*	*	*	*	*	110	0	5	18
Pickles, Dill	1 (3¾" × 1¼")	*	2	6	*	*	*	2	4	928	0	2	8
Pickles, Dill (Vlasic Half the Salt Hamburger Chips)	1 oz	*	*	*	*	*	*	*	*	175	0	1	2
Pickles, Dill (Vlasic Kosher Baby)	1 oz	*	*	*	*	*	*	*	2	210	0	1	4
Pickles, Dill (Vlasic Kosher Crunchy)	1 oz	*	*	*	*	*	*	*	2	210	0	1	4

Food	Amount	% U.S. RDA										
Pickles, Kosher Crunchy Dill (Vlasic Half the Salt)	1 oz	*	*	*	*	*	*	*	125	0	1	4
Pickles, Dill (Vlasic Kosher Deli Dills)	1 oz	*	*	*	*	*	*	*	290	1	1	4
Pickles, Dill (Vlasic No Garlic)	1 oz	*	*	*	*	*	2	*	210	0	1	4
Pickles, Dill (Vlasic Original)	1 oz	*	*	*	*	*	*	*	375	0	1	2
Pickles, Dill, Gherkins (Vlasic Kosher)	1 oz	*	*	*	*	*	2	*	210	0	1	4
Pickles, Dill, Sliced	1 c	2	4	15	2	*	4	8	221	0	4	18
Pickles, Dill, Spears (Vlasic Kosher)	1 oz	*	*	*	*	*	*	*	175	0	1	4
Pickles, Dill, Spears (Vlasic Kosher Half the Salt)	1 oz	*	*	*	*	*	*	*	120	0	1	4
Pickle Relish, Dill (Vlasic)	1 oz	*	*	*	*	*	*	*	415	0	1	2
Pickle Relish, Hamburg (Vlasic)	1 oz	*	2	*	*	*	*	*	255	0	9	40
Pickle Relish, Hamburger (Heinz)	1 oz	0	NA	NA	NA	NA	NA	NA	325	0	7	30
Pickle Relish, Hot Dog (Heinz)	1 oz	0	NA	NA	NA	NA	2	NA	200	0	8	35
Pickle Relish, Hot Dog (Vlasic)	1 oz	*	*	2	*	*	*	2	255	1	8	40
Pickle Relish, India (Heinz)	1 oz	0	NA	NA	NA	NA	NA	NA	215	0	9	35

| Condiments | Amt. | % U.S. RDA | | | | | | | | Sodium (mg) | Fat (g) | Carbohy-drate (g) | Calories |
		Pro-tein	A	C	B₁	B₂	Nia-cin	Cal-cium	Iron				
Pickle Relish, Sweet	1 tbsp.	*	*	2	*	*	*	*	*	107	0	5	12
Pickle Relish, Sweet (Heinz)	1 oz	0	NA	NA	NA	NA	NA	*	*	205	0	9	35
Pickle Relish, Sweet (Vlasic)	1 oz	*	*	*	*	*	*	*	*	220	0	8	30
Pickles, Sweet (Heinz)	1 oz	0	NA	NA	NA	NA	NA	*	*	210	0	8	35
Pickles, Sweet (Heinz Cucumber Slices)	1 oz	0	NA	NA	NA	NA	NA	*	*	195	0	5	20
Pickles, Sweet (Heinz Cucumber Stix)	1 oz	0	NA	NA	NA	NA	NA	*	*	145	0	6	25
Pickles, Sweet (Heinz Mixed)	1 oz	0	NA	NA	NA	NA	NA	*	*	200	0	9	40
Pickles, Sweet (Heinz Salad Cubes)	1 oz	0	NA	NA	NA	NA	NA	*	*	270	0	7	30
Pickles, Sweet (Heinz Slices)	1 oz	0	NA	NA	NA	NA	NA	*	*	205	0	8	35
Pickles, Sweet Butter (Vlasic Half the Salt Chips)	1 oz	*	*	*	*	*	*	*	*	80	0	7	30
Pickles, Sweet, Gherkin	1 (2½" × ¾")	*	*	2	*	*	*	*	2	NA	0	6	22
Pickles, Sweet, Gherkin (Heinz)	1 oz	0	NA	NA	NA	NA	NA	*	*	210	0	8	35
Soy Sauce	1 tbsp	2	*	*	*	2	*	2	4	1320	0–1	2	12

Food	Serving	% U.S. RDA											
Tartar Sauce (Hellmann's/ Best Foods)	1 tbsp	*	*	*	*	*	*	*	*	185	8	0	70
Cookies													
Almond Supreme (Pepperidge Farm)	2	4	0	0	2	2	*	2	4	45	10	13	140
Almond Windmill (Nabisco)	3	2	*	*	6	4	4	4	4	NA	5	21	140
Animal Crackers (Barnum's Animals)	11	2	*	*	4	6	4	*	4	NA	4	21	130
Animal Crackers (Ralston)	15 (1 oz)	2	*	*	2	6	4	*	4	30	3	22	130
Apple Crisp (Nabisco)	3	2	*	*	8	6	6	*	4	NA	6	21	150
Apple Nut Bar (Pepperidge Farm)	1	2	0	0	0	2	0	0	2	90	5	33	170
Applesauce Raisin, Iced (Nabisco Almost Home)	2	2	*	*	4	2	2	2	4	NA	8	17	140
Apricot-Raspberry (Pepperidge Farm)	3	2	0	0	0	0	0	0	0	80	6	23	150
Arrowroot Biscuit (Nabisco National)	6	2	*	*	6	4	4	2	*	NA	4	21	130
Biscos Peanut Creme Patties (Nabisco)	4	4	*	*	*	2	6	*	2	NA	7	15	140
Blueberry (Pepperidge Farm)	3	2	0	0	2	2	2	2	0	80	6	27	170
Blueberry Bar (Pepperidge Farm)	1	2	0	0	0	0	0	0	2	90	3	36	170

105

Cookies	Amt.	% U.S. RDA								Sodium (mg)	Fat (g)	Carbohy-drate (g)	Calories
		Pro-tein	A	C	B₁	B₂	Nia-cin	Cal-cium	Iron				

Cookies	Amt.	Pro-tein	A	C	B$_1$	B$_2$	Nia-cin	Cal-cium	Iron	Sodium (mg)	Fat (g)	Carbohy-drate (g)	Calories
Bordeaux (Pepperidge Farm)	3	0	0	0	0	0	0	0	0	70	5	16	110
Brown Edge Sandwich (Nabisco)	2	2	*	*	4	6	4	*	6	NA	8	20	160
Brown Edge Wafers (Nabisco)	5	2	*	*	6	2	4	*	2	NA	6	21	140
Brownie Chocolate Nut (Pepperidge Farm)	3	2	0	0	0	0	0	0	4	80	10	19	170
Brownie Nut Bar (Pepperidge Farm)	1	2	0	2	0	2	0	0	4	100	7	30	190
Brussels (Pepperidge Farm)	3	2	0	0	2	0	0	0	2	95	8	20	160
Brussels Mint (Pepperidge Farm)	3	2	0	0	2	0	0	0	2	120	10	25	200
Butter Flavored (Nabisco)	6	2	*	*	6	4	4	*	2	NA	5	21	140
Butter (Pepperidge Farm)	3	2	0	0	0	0	0	0	2	55	6	14	110
Cappucino (Pepperidge Farm)	3	0	0	0	0	0	0	0	0	210	60	9	160
Capri (Pepperidge Farm)	2	2	0	0	0	0	0	0	2	90	9	20	160
Champagne (Pepperidge Farm)	3	0	0	0	0	0	0	0	2	55	5	12	95
Chessmen Assortment (Pepperidge Farm)	3	2	0	0	0	0	0	0	2	80	6	18	130

		% U.S. RDA										
Chips Ahoy! (Nabisco)	3	2	*	*	4	4	4	4	NA	7	21	160
Chocolate Chip (Nabisco Cookie Little)	20	2	*	*	4	4	4	4	NA	6	20	140
Chocolate Chip (Pepperidge Farm)	3	2	0	0	0	0	0	0	90	8	20	150
Chocolate Chip, Real (Nabisco Almost Home)	2	2	*	*	4	2	2	*	NA	5	20	130
Chocolate Chip Macaroon Bar (Pepperidge Farm)	1	2	0	2	2	2	0	2	80	11	28	210
Chocolate Chip Snaps (Nabisco)	6	2	*	*	4	4	2	*	NA	4	20	120
Chocolate Chocolate Chip (Nabisco)	3	2	*	*	2	4	2	*	NA	7	22	160
Chocolate Chocolate Chip (Pepperidge Farm)	3	2	0	0	0	0	0	0	74	9	19	160
Chocolate Chunk Pecan (Pepperidge Farm)	2	2	0	0	0	2	2	0	50	7	15	130
Chocolate and Peanut Bars (Nabisco Ideal)	2	4	*	*	6	4	6	*	NA	10	20	190
Chocolate Snaps (Nabisco)	8	2	*	*	2	4	4	*	NA	4	22	130
Chocolate Wafers (Nabisco Famous)	5	2	*	*	2	4	4	*	NA	4	23	140
Cinnamon Chip (Pepperidge Farm)	3	2	0	0	0	2	0	2	80	7	21	150

| Cookies | Amt. | % U.S. RDA | | | | | | | | Sodium (mg) | Fat (g) | Carbohydrate (g) | Calories |
		Protein	A	C	B_1	B_2	Niacin	Calcium	Iron				
Cinnamon Raisin, Old Fashioned (Nabisco Almost Home)	2	2	*	*	4	2	2	*	4	NA	7	18	140
Cinnamon Treats (Nabisco)	.9 oz	2	*	*	*	4	4	*	4	NA	2	20	110
Coconut Bars (Nabisco Bakers Bonus)	3	2	*	*	*	2	2	*	2	NA	6	16	130
Coconut Chocolate Chip (Nabisco)	2	2	*	*	4	2	2	2	4	NA	8	18	150
Coconut Macaroon Soft Cakes (Nabisco)	2	2	*	*	*	2	*	*	4	NA	10	23	190
Coconut Macaroon Bar (Pepperidge Farm)	1	2	0	0	0	2	0	0	4	80	11	28	210
Creme Sandwich (Nabisco Baronet)	3	2	*	*	6	4	4	*	2	NA	7	24	160
Creme Sandwich (Nabisco Cameo)	2	2	*	*	4	4	2	*	2	NA	5	21	140
Creme Sandwich (Nabisco Mayfair)	2	2	*	*	2	4	4	*	2	NA	6	18	130
Creme Sandwich (Nabisco Mayfair Crown)	3	2	*	*	*	4	4	*	8	NA	7	24	160
Creme Sandwich (Nabisco Mayfair Tea Rose)	3	2	*	*	4	6	6	*	4	NA	7	23	160

		% U.S. RDA										
Creme Sandwich (Nabisco Oreo Swiss)	3	2	*	*	4	4	4	*	2	NA	7	22	150
Creme Sandwich, Fudge (Nabisco)	3	2	*	*	2	4	4	*	4	NA	7	23	160
Creme Sandwich, Fudge (Nabisco Gaiety)	3	2	*	*	2	4	2	*	4	NA	7	21	160
Creme Sandwich, Fudge 'n Chocolate (Nabisco Almost Home)	1	2	*	*	2	2	2	2	4	NA	6	20	140
Creme Sandwich, Mixed (Nabisco Cookie Break)	3	2	*	*	4	4	4	*	4	NA	7	22	160
Creme Sandwich, Peanut Butter (Nabisco Almost Home)	1	4	*	*	4	2	6	2	2	NA	6	20	140
Creme Sandwich, Vanilla (Nabisco Cookie Break)	3	2	*	*	4	4	4	*	4	NA	6	22	150
Creme Wafer Sticks (Nabisco)	3	*	*	*	*	2	2	*	2	NA	7	19	140
Date Nut Granola (Pepperidge Farm)	3	2	0	0	2	0	0	0	4	95	9	20	160
Date Nut Bar (Pepperidge Farm)	1	2	0	2	2	2	0	0	4	90	7	30	190
Date Pecan (Pepperidge Farm)	3	2	0	0	2	0	0	0	2	60	8	22	160
Fig Bars, Whole Wheat (Nabisco Fig Wheats)	2	2	*	*	2	2	2	4	4	NA	2	23	120

Cookies	Amt.	Pro-tein	A	C	B$_1$	B$_2$	Nia-cin	Cal-cium	Iron	Sodium (mg)	Fat (g)	Carbohy-drate (g)	Calories
		% U.S. RDA											
Fig Newtons (Nabisco)	2	2	*	*	2	2	2	2	4	NA	2	22	120
Fruit Sticks, All Flavors (Nabisco Almost Home)	1	*	*	*	2	*	*	*	2	NA	2	14	70
Fudge and Butterscotch Chips (Nabisco Bakers Bonus Double Chips)	2	2	*	*	4	4	4	2	2	NA	7	22	160
Fudge Chocolate Chip (Nabisco Almost Home)	2	2	*	*	4	2	2	*	4	NA	5	20	130
Geneva (Pepperidge Farm)	3	2	0	0	0	0	0	0	4	65	10	19	170
Gingerman (Pepperidge Farm)	3	0	0	0	0	0	0	0	2	75	4	15	100
Ginger Snaps, Old Fashion (Nabisco)	4	2	*	*	2	4	4	2	8	NA	3	22	120
Graham Crackers (Nabisco Honey Maid)	4	2	*	*	2	4	6	*	4	NA	3	22	120
Graham Crackers (Nabisco)	4	2	*	*	2	4	6	*	4	NA	3	21	120
Graham Crackers (Rokeach)	8	2	*	*	2	4	2	*	4	NA	3	21	120
Graham Crackers, Sugar Honey (Ralston)	8 (1 oz)	2	*	*	6	4	4	*	2	140	3	22	120
Grahams, Chocolate (Nabisco)	3	2	*	*	6	4	4	*	6	NA	8	21	170

					% U.S. RDA							
Grahams, Fancy Dip (Nabisco)	2	2	*	2	2	2	*	4	NA	6	16	130
Grahams, Party (Nabisco)	3	2	*	4	2	2	2	2	NA	7	18	140
Hazelnut (Pepperidge Farm)	3	2	0	0	0	0	0	2	110	9	22	170
Heyday (Nabisco)	1	2	*	*	2	4	*	*	NA	7	13	120
Irish Oatmeal (Pepperidge Farm)	3	2	0	2	0	0	0	2	120	7	20	140
Kettle (Nabisco)	4	2	*	6	4	4	*	4	NA	5	21	140
Lemon Nut Crunch (Pepperidge Farm)	3	2	0	2	0	0	0	4	75	10	19	170
Lido (Pepperidge Farm)	2	2	0	0	0	0	0	2	85	11	21	190
Lorna Doone (Nabisco)	4	2	*	6	6	4	*	4	NA	8	20	160
Mallomars (Nabisco)	2	*	*	*	2	*	*	2	NA	5	17	120
Malted Milk Peanut Butter Sandwich (Nabisco)	4	4	*	10	4	8	2	4	NA	7	18	150
Marseilles Assortment (Pepperidge Farm)	2	2	0	0	0	0	0	2	50	5	12	90
Marshmallow Puffs (Nabisco)	2	2	*	2	4	2	2	2	NA	6	28	170
Marshmallow Twirls (Nabisco)	1	*	*	2	4	*	2	2	NA	5	20	130
Milano (Pepperidge Farm)	3	2	0	0	0	0	0	0	80	10	21	180
Mint Milano (Pepperidge Farm)	3	2	0	0	0	0	0	2	105	13	25	230

Cookies	Amt.	Protein	A	C	B₁	B₂	Niacin	Calcium	Iron	Sodium (mg)	Fat (g)	Carbohydrate (g)	Calories
					% U.S. RDA								
Molasses (Nabisco Pantry)	2	2	*	*	8	4	4	*	8	NA	4	19	120
Molasses Crisps (Pepperidge Farm)	3	0	0	0	0	0	0	2	2	75	5	12	100
Mystic Mint (Nabisco)	2	2	*	*	2	2	2	*	4	NA	9	22	180
Nassau (Pepperidge Farm)	2	2	0	0	0	0	4	0	2	90	10	18	170
Nilla Wafers (Nabisco)	7	2	*	*	4	4	4	*	2	NA	4	21	130
Nutter Butter (Nabisco)	2	4	*	*	6	4	4	*	2	NA	6	18	140
Nutter Butter, Chocolate	3	4	*	*	4	4	6	*	2	NA	8	22	170
Oatmeal (Drake's)	3	4	*	*	6	4	2	*	4	200	7	29	190
Oatmeal (Nabisco Bakers Bonus)	2	2	*	*	4	4	4	*	4	NA	6	24	160
Oatmeal (Nabisco Cookie Little)	20	2	*	*	4	2	2	*	2	NA	5	20	130
Oatmeal Creme (Nabisco Almost Home)	1	2	*	*	4	2	2	2	4	NA	5	21	140
Oatmeal, Iced (Nabisco Almost Home)	2	2	*	*	4	2	2	*	4	NA	5	19	130
Oatmeal Raisin (Nabisco Almost Home)	2	2	*	*	4	2	2	*	4	NA	5	20	130
Oatmeal Raisin (Pepperidge Farm)	3	2	0	0	2	0	0	0	4	170	8	23	170
Orange (Pepperidge Farm)	3	2	0	0	2	2	2	0	2	65	6	27	170

Product				% U.S. RDA								
Orange Milano (Pepperidge Farm)	3	2	0	0	0	0	0	2	105	13	25	230
Oreo (Nabisco)	3	*	*	*	2	2	*	4	NA	7	22	150
Oreo Double Stuf (Nabisco)	2	*	*	*	2	2	*	2	NA	7	18	140
Orleans (Pepperidge Farm)	3	0	0	0	0	0	0	2	30	6	11	90
Orleans Sandwich (Pepperidge Farm)	3	2	0	0	0	0	0	2	60	12	21	180
Peanut Brittle Cookies (Nabisco)	3	4	6	*	6	8	2	4	NA	7	19	150
Peanut Butter (Nabisco Almost Home)	2	4	4	*	2	8	2	2	NA	7	16	140
Peanut Butter Chip (Pepperidge Farm)	3	2	0	0	0	2	0	2	135	9	19	160
Peanut Butter Fudge (Nabisco)	3	4	4	*	4	4	*	4	NA	7	20	150
Peanut Butter Fudge (Nabisco Almost Home)	2	4	4	*	2	8	2	2	NA	7	16	140
Peanut Butter Sugar Wafer (Nabisco Biscos)	3	4	6	*	4	8	*	2	NA	7	17	140
Pecan Shortbread (Nabisco)	2	2	6	*	4	4	*	2	NA	10	17	160
Piccolo Rolled Wafers (Nabisco)	6	2	2	*	2	2	*	0	NA	4	20	130
Pirouettes, Original (Pepperidge Farm)	3	0	0	0	0	0	0	0	55	7	13	110

Cookies	Amt.	Protein	A	C	B_1	B_2	Niacin	Calcium	Iron	Sodium (mg)	Fat (g)	Carbohydrate (g)	Calories
		% U.S. RDA											
Pirouettes, Chocolate Laced (Pepperidge Farm)	3 0	0	0	0	0	0	0	0	2	45	7	13	110
Raisin Bran (Pepperidge Farm)	3	2	0	0	2	0	2	0	2	80	8	20	160
Raisin Fruit Biscuit (Nabisco)	2	2	*	*	6	2	2	*	4	NA	2	24	120
Seville Assortment (Pepperidge Farm)	2	2	0	0	0	0	0	0	2	50	6	14	110
Shortbread (Pepperidge Farm)	2	0	0	0	0	0	0	0	0	85	8	17	150
Shortcake (Nabisco Melt Away)	2	2	*	*	2	2	2	*	*	NA	7	16	140
Social Tea Biscuit (Nabisco)	6	2	*	*	6	4	4	*	4	NA	4	21	130
Southport Assortment (Pepperidge Farm)	2	2	0	0	0	0	0	0	4	70	9	18	150
Spiced Wafers (Nabisco)	4	2	*	*	2	4	4	*	4	NA	3	24	130
Strawberry (Pepperidge Farm)	3	2	0	0	0	0	0	0	2	70	7	23	150
Striped Shortbread (Nabisco)	3	2	*	*	2	4	4	*	2	NA	7	19	150
Sugar (Pepperidge Farm)	3	2	0	0	0	0	0	0	2	115	8	20	150

Item	Serving					% U.S. RDA					
Sugar Rings (Nabisco Bakers Bonus)	2	140	21	5	NA	4	*	4	6	*	2
Sugar Wafers (Nabisco Biscos)	8	150	21	7	NA	2	*	4	2	*	2
Tahiti (Pepperidge Farm)	2	170	17	11	50	2	0	0	0	*	2
Tea Time Biscuit (Nabisco Mayfair)	4	100	15	3	NA	2	*	4	4	*	2
Twiddle Sticks (Nabisco)	3	160	21	8	NA	2	*	2	2	*	*
Waffle Cremes (Nabisco Biscos)	3	130	18	6	NA	2	*	2	2	*	*
Cookie Mixes											
Brownie, Fudge (Betty Crocker Family Size)	1/24 pkg	130	21	5	95	4	*	2	2	*	2
Brownie, Fudge (Betty Crocker Regular Size)	1/16 pkg	150	22	6	100	4	*	2	2	*	2
Brownie, Fudge (Pillsbury)	1 2" sq	150	23	6	95	2	0	2	0	0	2
Brownie, Fudge (Pillsbury Family Size)	1 2" sq	150	22	7	90	2	0	0	0	0	2
Brownie, Supreme Fudge (Betty Crocker)	1/24 pkg	120	25	2	90	4	*	2	*	*	*
Brownie, Supreme Golden (Betty Crocker Family Size)	1/24 pkg	130	19	5	105	2	*	2	*	*	2
Brownie, Walnut (Betty Crocker Family Size)	1/24 pkg	130	19	6	85	4	*	2	2	*	2

Cookie Mixes	Amt.	% U.S. RDA								Sodium (mg)	Fat (g)	Carbohydrate (g)	Calories
		Protein	A	C	B₁	B₂	Niacin	Calcium	Iron				
Brownie, Walnut (Betty Crocker Regular Size)	1/16 pkg	2	*	*	2	2	2	*	4	100	7	22	160
Brownie, Walnut (Pillsbury Family Size)	1 2" sq	2	0	0	4	2	2	0	4	95	7	23	160
Chocolate Chip (Betty Crocker Big Batch)	1/18 (2 cookies)	2	2	*	2	2	*	*	2	95	6	16	120
Chocolate Chip (Pillsbury)	3 cookies	2	0	0	4	4	4	0	6	125	8	23	170
Coconut Macaroon (Betty Crocker Classics)	1/24 pkg	2	*	*	*	*	*	2	*	15	4	10	80
Date Bar (Betty Crocker Classics)	1/32 pkg	*	*	*	*	*	*	*	*	35	2	9	60
Double Chocolate (Pillsbury)	3 cookies	2	0	0	4	4	2	0	2	160	6	23	150
Fudge, Brown Sugar and Oatmeal (Pillsbury Fudge Jumbles)	1 bar	0	0	0	0	0	0	0	2	60	4	15	100
Fudge, Chocolate Chip and Oatmeal (Pillsbury Fudge Jumbles)	1 bar	0	0	0	0	0	0	0	0	60	4	14	100
Fudge, Coconut and Oatmeal (Pillsbury Fudge Jumbles)	1 bar	0	0	0	0	0	0	0	2	60	5	14	100
Fudge, Peanut Butter and Oatmeal (Pillsbury Fudge Jumbles)	1 bar	2	0	0	2	2	2	0	2	55	4	14	100

					% U.S. RDA							
Oatmeal (Betty Crocker Big Batch)	1/18 (2 cookies)	2	2	*	4	*	*	2	100	6	17	130
Peanut Butter (Pillsbury)	3 cookies	4	0	0	4	6	0	2	190	7	20	150
Sugar (Betty Crocker Big Batch)	1/18 (2 cookies)	2	2	*	4	2	*	2	95	5	18	120
Sugar (Pillsbury)	3 cookies	2	0	0	6	4	0	2	170	8	23	170
Vienna Dream Bar (Betty Crocker Classics)	1/14 pkg	*	*	*	2	*	*	*	65	5	10	90
Crackers												
Bacon 'n Dip (Nabisco)	17	2	*	*	10	6	2	4	NA	8	16	150
Buttery Flavored Sesame Snack (Nabisco)	1 oz	4	*	*	10	6	2	4	NA	8	17	150
Cheddar Snacks (Ralston)	18 (1 oz)	4	*	*	6	4	2	4	320	5	20	130
Cheddar Triangles (Nabisco)	1 oz	4	*	*	6	6	4	2	NA	8	16	150
Cheddar 'n Sesame (Nabisco Country)	1 oz	4	*	*	10	6	2	4	NA	8	16	150
Cheese Nips (Nabisco)	1 oz	4	*	*	10	8	2	4	NA	6	18	140
Cheese Peanut Butter Sandwich (Nabisco)	1 oz	4	*	*	10	6	4	4	NA	6	17	140
Cheese Sandwich (Nabisco)	4	4	*	*	8	4	4	4	NA	6	13	110
Cheese Snacks (Ralston)	25 (1 oz)	4	*	*	6	4	2	4	330	7	18	140
Cheese Tid-Bit (Nabisco)	1 oz	2	*	*	8	6	4	4	NA	9	16	150
Chicken in a Biskit (Nabisco)	1 oz	2	*	*	6	4	*	4	NA	9	16	150

| Crackers | Amt. | % U.S. RDA | | | | | | | | Sodium (mg) | Fat (g) | Carbohy-drate (g) | Calories |
		Protein	A	C	B_1	B_2	Niacin	Calcium	Iron				
Chippers (Nabisco)	1 oz	2	*	*	10	6	6	2	4	NA	8	17	150
Cracked Wheat (Pepperidge Farm)	4	2	0	0	2	0	2	0	2	200	4	14	110
Crown Pilot (Nabisco)	1 oz	4	*	*	10	8	8	*	6	NA	4	26	150
Dip in a Chip (Nabisco)	1 oz	2	*	*	8	6	4	2	4	NA	8	16	150
Dixies (Nabisco)	1 oz	2	*	*	8	6	4	*	4	NA	7	17	140
English Water Biscuits (Pepperidge Farm)	4	2	0	0	2	0	2	0	2	90	1	13	70
Escort (Nabisco)	1 oz	2	*	*	8	6	6	*	4	NA	8	18	150
French Onion (Nabisco)	1 oz	2	*	*	8	6	6	4	4	NA	7	18	150
Goldfish, Cheddar Cheese (Pepperidge Farm)	45	4	0	0	4	2	2	2	2	180	6	18	140
Goldfish, Parmesan Cheese (Pepperidge Farm)	45	4	0	0	4	2	2	2	2	250	6	18	140
Goldfish, Pizza Flavored (Pepperidge Farm)	45	4	0	0	4	2	2	0	2	180	7	18	140
Goldfish, Pretzel (Pepperidge Farm)	40	4	0	0	4	4	4	0	2	160	3	21	120
Goldfish, Salted (Pepperidge Farm)	45	2	0	0	4	2	2	0	0	180	7	18	140
Hearty Wheat (Pepperidge Farm)	4	4	0	0	2	2	2	0	2	180	4	13	100

Product	Serving				% U.S. RDA								Calories
Holland Rusk	2	4	*	4	4	4	*	2	NA	2	15	80
Meal Mates (Nabisco)	1 oz	4	*	15	8	6	6	4	NA	5	19	130
Melba Toast (Old London)	3 sl	2	*	4	2	2	*	2	NA	0	10	50
Melba Toast, Bacon (Old London Bacon Rounds)	5	2	*	4	2	2	*	2	NA	2	9	60
Melba Toast, Cheese (Old London Cheese Rounds)	5	2	*	4	2	2	*	2	NA	2	9	60
Melba Toast, Garlic (Old London Garlic Rounds)	5	2	*	4	2	2	*	2	NA	1	9	50
Melba Toast, Onion (Old London Onion Rounds)	5	2	*	4	2	2	*	2	NA	1	9	50
Melba Toast, Pumpernickel (Old London)	3	2	*	4	2	2	*	2	NA	0	10	50
Melba Toast, Rye (Old London)	3	2	*	4	2	2	*	2	NA	0	10	50
Melba Toast, Salty Rye (Old London Salty-Rye Rounds)	5	2	*	4	2	2	*	2	NA	1	9	50
Melba Toast, Sesame (Old London Sesame Rounds)	5	2	*	4	2	2	2	4	NA	2	8	60
Melba Toast, Unsalted (Old London)	3	2	*	4	2	2	*	2	5	0	10	50
Melba Toast, Whole Grain (Old London)	3	2	*	4	2	2	*	2	NA	1	10	60
Milk Crackers (Nabisco Royal Lunch)	2	2	*	8	4	4	4	4	NA	4	16	110

Crackers	Amt.	Pro-tein	A	C	B₁	B₂	Nia-cin	Cal-cium	Iron	Sodium (mg)	Fat (g)	Carbohy-drate (g)	Calories
		% U.S. RDA											
Oyster (Ralston)	65 (1 oz)	4	*	*	2	6	4	*	4	380	3	20	120
Rich & Crisp (Ralston)	9 (1 oz)	2	*	*	8	6	6	*	4	200	7	19	140
Ritz (Nabisco)	9	2	*	*	6	6	6	4	4	NA	8	18	150
Rye Snacks (Ralston)	15 (1 oz)	4	*	*	6	4	2	*	4	235	6	20	130
RyKrisp, Natural	2	2	*	*	2	*	*	*	2	110	0	10	50
RyKrisp, Seasoned	2	2	*	*	2	*	*	*	2	220	1	10	50
RyKrisp, Sesame	2	2	*	*	2	*	*	*	2	220	2	11	50
Saltine (Nabisco Premium)	10	4	*	*	8	8	8	4	6	NA	4	20	120
Saltine, Unsalted Tops (Nabisco Premium)	10	4	*	*	8	8	8	4	6	NA	4	20	120
Saltine (Ralston)	10 (1 oz)	4	*	*	8	6	4	*	4	400	3	21	120
Saltine, Kosher (Rokeach)	10	2	*	*	8	6	6	*	4	NA	3	20	120
Sea Rounds (Nabisco)	2 (1 oz)	2	*	*	15	10	8	2	6	NA	2	15	90
Sesame (Pepperidge Farm)	4	4	0	0	2	2	2	0	2	105	3	11	80
Sesame Wheats! (Nabisco)	1 oz	4	*	*	8	4	6	4	6	NA	9	16	150
Snack (Rokeach)	9	2	*	*	8	6	6	2	4	NA	5	19	130
Snackers (Ralston)	8 (1 oz)	2	*	*	2	6	4	*	2	210	7	18	140
Snacks Ahoy (Nabisco)	1 oz	2	*	*	6	4	4	*	2	NA	7	17	140
Snack Sticks, Cheese (Pepperidge Farm)	8	4	0	0	2	0	0	2	2	350	6	18	140

Food	Amount				% U.S. RDA					Sodium (mg)	Calories
		Protein	Vit. A	Vit. C	Thiamine	Riboflavin	Niacin	Calcium	Iron		
Snack Sticks, Original (Pepperidge Farm)	8	2	0	2	0	0	2	5	20	320	130
Snack Sticks, Pumpernickel (Pepperidge Farm)	8	4	0	2	2	0	2	5	20	380	130
Snack Sticks, Rye (Pepperidge Farm)	8	2	0	2	2	0	2	4	20	390	130
Snack Sticks, Sesame (Pepperidge Farm)	8	4	0	2	0	0	2	6	18	350	130
Sociables (Nabisco)	1 oz	4	*	10	6	4	6	7	18	NA	150
Soup and Oyster (Nabisco Dandy)	1 oz	4	*	6	6	*	6	3	20	NA	120
Soup and Oyster (Nabisco Oysterettes)	1 oz	4	*	6	6	*	6	3	20	NA	120
Swiss Cheese Naturally Flavored (Nabisco)	1 oz	4	*	10	6	4	6	8	17	NA	150
Thins, Bacon Flavored (Nabisco)	14	2	*	10	6	4	6	8	17	NA	150
Thins, Butter Flavored (Pepperidge Farm)	4	2	0	2	0	0	2	3	10	100	80
Thins, Gold Fish, Cheese (Pepperidge Farm)	4	2	0	2	2	2	2	3	8	105	70
Thins, Goldfish, Salted (Pepperidge Farm)	4	2	0	2	2	2	2	3	8	100	60
Thins, Goldfish, Wheat (Pepperidge Farm)	4	4	0	2	2	0	2	3	8	105	60

Crackers	Amt.	Protein	A	C	B₁	B₂	Niacin	Calcium	Iron	Sodium (mg)	Fat (g)	Carbohydrate (g)	Calories
						% U.S. RDA							
Thins, Vegetable (Nabisco)	1 oz	2	*	*	8	6	6	4	4	NA	8	17	150
Thins, Wheat (Nabisco)	1 oz	2	*	*	6	4	6	*	4	NA	6	19	140
Triscuit (Nabisco)	7	4	*	*	4	2	6	*	4	NA	5	21	140
Twigs (Nabisco)	1 oz	4	*	*	10	6	6	6	6	NA	7	16	140
Uneeda Biscuit (Nabisco)	6	4	*	*	8	8	8	*	8	NA	4	22	130
Unsalted Top (Ralston)	10 (1 oz)	4	*	*	8	6	4	*	4	205	3	21	120
Waverly Wafers (Nabisco)	8	2	*	*	8	6	6	4	4	NA	6	21	140
Wheat Snacks (Ralston)	15 (1 oz)	2	*	*	6	4	4	*	4	200	6	19	130
Wheatsworth (Nabisco)	9	4	*	*	10	6	6	2	6	NA	6	16	130
Zwieback (Nabisco)	4	2	*	*	6	8	4	*	4	NA	3	21	120
Cream													
Regular and Whipped	1 oz	6	8	*	*	4	*	2	*	71	11	1	110
Half and Half	1 c	15	25	4	4	25	*	25	*	111	29	11	320
	1 tbsp	2	2	*	*	2	*	2	*	7	2	1	20
Light, Coffee or Table	1 c	15	40	4	4	20	*	25	*	103	50	10	510
	1 tbsp	*	2	*	*	2	*	2	*	6	3	1	30
Sour Cream	1 c	15	40	4	4	20	*	25	*	331	48	1	485
	1 tbsp	*	2	*	*	*	*	*	*	6	3	1	25

		% U.S. RDA									
Sour Cream, Imitation	1 c	15	2	4	20	*	30	235	45	15	440
	1 tbsp	*	*	*	*	*	2	NA	NA	NA	20
Sour Cream, Imitation (Pet)	1 tbsp	*	*	*	*	*	*	NA	2	1	25
Whipping, Heavy	1 c	70	4	4	15	*	20	76	90	8	840
	1 tbsp	4	*	*	2	*	2	5	6	0-1	60
Whipping, Light	1 c	60	4	4	15	*	20	86	75	9	720
	1 tbsp	4	*	*	2	*	2	5	5	0-1	45
Creamers, Nondairy											
Coffee-mate	1 pkt (3 g)	*	*	*	*	*	*	5	1	1.6	17
	1 tsp	*	*	*	*	*	*	4	1	1.1	11
	1 fl oz	*	*	*	*	*	*	9	2	2.6	27
Cremora	1 tsp	*	*	*	*	*	*	5	1	1	12
Eggs											
Large, Whole	1	10	*	2	8	6	2	61	6	0-1	80
Large, White Only	1	*	*	*	6	*	*	48	0	0-1	18
Large, Yolk Only	1	10	*	2	4	4	2	26	5	0-1	60
Large, Fried	1	15	*	4	8	6	2	169	NA	NA	100
Large, Scrambled w Milk and Table Fat	1	15	*	4	10	6	6	NA	8	1	110
Egg Substitute (Morningstar Farms Scramblers)	¼ c	NA	NA	15	30	2	4	150	3	2	60

Entrees, Canned	Amt.	Pro-tein	A	C	B$_1$	B$_2$	Nia-cin	Cal-cium	Iron	Sodium (mg)	Fat (g)	Carbohy-drate (g)	Calories
		% U.S. RDA											
Beef Goulash (Heinz)	7½ oz	NA	NA	NA	NA	NA	NA	*	10	920	11	22	240
Chicken & Dumplings (Swanson)	7½ oz	20	10	*	*	6	10	2	4	965	12	19	220
Chicken a la King (Swanson)	5¼ oz	20	*	*	2	8	10	4	4	695	12	9	180
Chili con Carne (Heinz)	7¾ oz	NA	NA	NA	NA	NA	NA	6	20	1000	21	27	350
Chili con Carne (Old El Paso)	1 c	41	0	*	*	20	16	7	51	906.9	21.4	12.3	349
Chili w Beans, Hot (Heinz)	7¾ oz	NA	NA	NA	NA	NA	NA	10	15	1140	16	30	330
Chili w Beans (Old El Paso)	1 c	25	0	*	4	13	9	9	30	1037.4	27.6	27.2	423
Chili Mac (Heinz)	7½ oz	NA	NA	NA	NA	NA	NA	6	10	860	12	26	250
Stew, Beef (Heinz)	7½ oz.	NA	NA	NA	NA	NA	NA	2	10	1245	9	19	210
Stew, Chicken (Swanson)	7⅝ oz	20	110	8	*	4	15	2	4	960	7	16	170
Stew, Chicken, w Dumplings (Heinz)	7½ oz	NA	NA	NA	NA	NA	NA	4	6	850	9	22	210
Tamales (Old El Paso)	2 tamales	8	*	*	*	7	8	3	18	377.8	11.9	16.5	192
Entrees, Frozen													
Asparagus w Mornay Sauce in Pastry (Pepperidge Farm Vegetables in Pastry)	1	8	10	20	10	10	8	2	10	250	17	18	250

Food	Serving				% U.S. RDA							
Beef w Barbecue Sauce in Pastry (Pepperidge Farm Deli's)	1	30	6	4	15	20	2	20	640	11	28	270
Beef Burgundy w Rice, Carrots (Green Giant)	9 oz	30	30	10	4	10	2	10	855	8	33	280
Beef Chop Suey w Rice (Stouffer's)	12 oz	25	6	*	8	10	*	10	2040	10	48	355
Beef Chow Mein w Rice, Vegetables (Green Giant)	10 oz	20	4	20	2	10	4	8	1050	6	33	240
Beef, Creamed Chipped (Stouffer's)	5½ oz	20	*	*	6	10	10	6	900	16	10	235
Beef Enchilada (Swanson)	11¼ oz	25	20	10	10	10	15	15	1220	23	49	470
Beef Enchilada (Swanson Hungry-Man)	16 oz	35	35	15	20	15	20	35	2010	35	65	660
Beef, Oriental, in Sauce w Vegetables and Rice (Stouffer's Lean Cuisine)	8⅝ oz	30	20	4	8	20	2	10	1150	8	32	280
Beef Ribs, Boneless, w BBQ Sauce, Corn on the Cob (Green Giant)	1 pkg	40	50	30	6	35	4	20	1440	13	40	390
Beef, Sliced (Swanson Hungry-Man)	12¼ oz	80	*	20	10	45	2	25	1045	8	24	330
Beef, Sliced, w Bacon Sauce in Pastry (Pepperidge Farm Deli's)	1	25	2	2	15	20	2	15	570	11	26	260

Entrees, Frozen	Amt.	Pro-tein	A	C	B₁	B₂	Nia-cin	Cal-cium	Iron	Sodium (mg)	Fat (g)	Carbohy-drate (g)	Calories
		% U.S. RDA											
Beef, Sliced, and Gravy (Swanson)	8 oz	35	*	6	4	10	20	*	15	805	7	18	200
Beef Stroganoff w Noodles (Green Giant)	9 oz	35	2	10	15	25	20	8	20	820	16	35	380
Beef Stroganoff w Parsley Noodles (Stouffer's)	9¾ oz	30	4	*	20	15	25	4	20	1300	20	31	390
Beef Teriyaki w Rice and Vegetables (Stouffer's)	10 oz	40	*	*	8	20	20	2	25	1450	11	41	365
Beef and Pork Cannelloni w Mornay Sauce (Stouffer's Lean Cuisine)	9⅝ oz	30	50	*	10	20	10	20	8	950	10	24	260
Broccoli w Cheese in Pastry (Pepperidge Farm Vegetables in Pastry)	1	6	6	30	10	10	6	6	10	460	17	19	250
Cabbage Rolls, Stuffed, w Beef, Tomato Sauce (Green Giant)	½ pkg	10	10	10	*	4	10	4	6	800	12	19	220
Cauliflower and Cheese Sauce in Pastry (Pepperidge Farm Vegetables in Pastry)	1	6	2	30	10	10	8	4	10	470	13	20	220
Cheese Cannelloni w Tomato Sauce (Stouffer's Lean Cuisine)	9⅛ oz	35	25	10	6	15	6	30	4	900	10	24	270

126

		% U.S. RDA											
Cheese Soufflé (Stouffer's)	6 oz	25	15	15	10	25	2	30	8	1360	26	14	355
Chicken w BBQ Sauce, Corn on the Cob (Green Giant)	1 pkg	45	15	30	6	10	50	4	10	885	5	45	350
Chicken w Broccoli, Rice, Cheese Sauce (Green Giant)	9½ oz	40	10	50	4	15	20	20	6	915	14	26	330
Chicken Cacciatore w Spaghetti (Stouffer's)	11¼ oz	35	15	*	10	15	25	4	10	1135	11	29	310
Chicken Chow Mein w/o Noodles (Stouffer's)	8 oz	20	6	*	8	10	15	4	10	1115	6	10	145
Chicken Chow Mein w Rice, Vegetables (Green Giant)	9 oz	25	4	8	10	6	15	4	4	1075	5	29	220
Chicken Chow Mein w Rice (Stouffer's Lean Cuisine)	11¼ oz	25	8	20	6	8	15	2	4	1200	5	36	250
Chicken, Creamed (Stouffer's)	6½ oz	30	8	*	8	8	20	6	8	680	22	6	300
Chicken Divan (Stouffer's)	8½ oz	30	35	15	10	15	20	20	6	830	22	14	335
Chicken Fillets Cacciatore (Buitoni)	11 oz	19	20	*	15	15	20	4	15	1120	3	40	260
Chicken Fillets Marsala (Buitoni)	11 oz	19	30	*	15	10	10	4	50	1410	3	40	260
Chicken, Fried (Swanson)	7¼ oz	40	*	8	10	10	35	4	15	1075	21	30	390

Entrees, Frozen	Amt.	Protein	A	C	B₁	B₂	Niacin	Calcium	Iron	Sodium (mg)	Fat (g)	Carbohydrate (g)	Calories
		% U.S. RDA											
Chicken, Fried, Breast Portions (Swanson Hungry-Man)	11¾ oz	60	*	10	20	20	70	10	20	1710	37	51	670
Chicken, Fried, Dark Portions (Swanson Hungry-Man)	11 oz	60	*	10	15	30	45	4	20	1340	36	46	640
Chicken, Glazed, w Vegetable Rice (Stouffer's Lean Cuisine)	8½ oz	40	2	4	8	8	50	*	4	810	8	23	270
Chicken w Herb Butter, Stuffed Potato (Green Giant)	1 pkg	45	10	30	6	10	60	6	8	965	22	30	430
Chicken a la King w Biscuits (Green Giant)	9 oz	30	10	20	25	20	20	10	10	1545	15	40	370
Chicken a la King w Rice (Stouffer's)	9½ oz	30	4	*	6	10	25	10	8	900	11	38	330
Chicken Nibbles (Swanson)	5 oz	25	*	2	10	6	15	2	10	865	25	31	400
Chicken Nibbles (Swanson Plump and Juicy)	3¼ oz	25	*	*	6	8	15	*	10	645	21	16	300
Chicken and Noodles, Escalloped (Stouffer's)	5¾ oz	20	*	*	10	10	10	6	8	720	15	16	250
Chicken w Noodles, Vegetables (Green Giant)	9 oz	35	6	8	20	25	30	15	15	940	16	38	390

		% U.S. RDA										
Chicken Paprikash w Egg Noodles (Stouffer's)	10½ oz	45	10	*	15	15	30	6	20	1325	15	32	385
Chicken w Pea Pods, Sauce, Rice, Vegetables (Green Giant)	10 oz	25	4	15	4	8	10	4	6	995	12	32	300
Chicken and Vegetables w Vermicelli (Stouffer's Lean Cuisine)	12¾ oz	35	25	40	10	10	20	10	6	1325	7	28	260
Chili con Carne w Beans (Stouffer's)	8¾ oz	30	30	*	10	20	15	10	20	1265	10	26	270
Corn Soufflé (Stouffer's)	4 oz	6	15	*	6	8	2	4	4	510	7	19	155
Crepes, Chicken, w Mushroom Sauce (Stouffer's)	8½ oz	45	8	*	10	25	25	15	8	1040	22	19	390
Crepes, Ham and Asparagus (Stouffer's)	6¼ oz	25	10	*	25	20	10	20	6	840	20	21	325
Crepes, Ham and Swiss Cheese w Cream Sauce (Stouffer's)	7½ oz	35	50	*	15	30	15	45	10	905	25	23	410
Crepes, Spinach w Cheddar Cheese Sauce (Stouffer's)	9½ oz	25	50	*	10	40	6	30	25	995	25	30	415
Eggs, Scrambled, Canadian Bacon, and Cheese in Pastry (Pepperidge Farm Deli's)	1	15	8	2	20	15	15	10	10	670	17	24	290
Eggplant Parmigiana (Buitoni)	12 oz	17	8	8	10	50	30	30	10	1160	26	33	430

129

Entrees, Frozen	Amt.	Protein	A	C	B₁	B₂	Niacin	Calcium	Iron	Sodium (mg)	Fat (g)	Carbohydrate (g)	Calories
						% U.S. RDA							
Enchilada Sonora Style (Green Giant)	12 oz	50	70	50	6	40	25	60	35	1245	42	48	700
Filet of Fish Divan (Stouffer's Lean Cuisine)	12⅜ oz	45	15	50	10	15	10	15	6	780	10	16	270
Filet of Fish Florentine (Stouffer's Lean Cuisine)	9 oz	40	15	*	10	15	10	15	6	810	9	13	240
Green Bean Mushroom Casserole (Stouffer's)	4¾ oz	6	10	*	4	10	2	10	4	675	9	12	150
Green Beans w Mushroom Sauce in Pastry (Pepperidge Farm Vegetables in Pastry)	1	8	2	10	8	6	6	4	8	250	19	20	270
Green Pepper Steak w Rice (Stouffer's)	10½ oz	35	8	*	4	15	25	2	15	1500	13	35	350
Green Peppers, Stuffed (Green Giant)	½ pkg	15	6	35	2	6	6	2	6	785	11	15	200
Green Peppers, Stuffed, w Beef in Tomato Sauce (Stouffer's)	7¾ oz	15	10	*	10	8	20	4	10	960	11	18	225
Lobster Newburg (Stouffer's)	6½ oz	20	20	*	2	20	4	10	6	700	29	9	350
Meatballs w Brown Gravy (Swanson)	8½ oz	25	*	8	4	8	25	4	15	885	17	20	280

Food	Serving				% U.S. RDA								
Meatballs, Swedish, w Parsley Noodles (Stouffer's)	11 oz	35	10	*	15	20	25	8	25	1620	27	33	475
Meatballs, Sweet and Sour, w Rice, Vegetables (Green Giant)	9.4 oz	20	6	10	4	6	15	4	10	820	10	57	370
Meat Loaf w Tomato Sauce (Swanson)	9 oz	30	6	15	10	10	20	6	10	1020	16	30	310
Mushrooms Dijon in Pastry (Pepperidge Farm Vegetables in Pastry)	1	4	2	2	10	10	8	2	15	420	16	19	230
Omelet, Western Style, in Pastry (Pepperidge Farm Deli's)	1	15	2	2	20	15	15	4	10	590	18	27	300
Oriental Garden Vegetables in Szechwan Spiced Sauce, in Pastry (Pepperidge Farm Vegetables in Pastry)	1	6	6	6	8	4	15	2	8	300	15	19	230
Pie, Beef (Stouffer's)	10 oz	30	15	*	10	20	15	4	15	1600	36	38	550
Pie, Chicken (Stouffer's)	10 oz	30	15	*	15	10	20	8	10	1530	28	40	500
Pie, Turkey (Stouffer's)	10 oz	30	15	*	15	10	15	15	8	1735	26	35	460
Pot Pie, Beef (Swanson)	8 oz	25	25	4	20	15	20	2	15	810	22	40	420
Pot Pie, Beef (Swanson Chunky)	10 oz	35	50	8	25	20	25	2	20	935	30	57	580
Pot Pie, Beef (Swanson Hungry-Man)	16 oz	50	60	10	40	30	35	2	30	1565	37	65	700

131

Entres, Frozen	Amt.	Protein	A	C	B₁	B₂	Niacin	Calcium	Iron	Sodium (mg)	Fat (g)	Carbohydrate (g)	Calories
						% U.S. RDA							
Pot Pie, Chicken (Swanson)	8 oz	25	40	4	20	15	20	2	10	850	24	39	420
Pot Pie, Chicken (Swanson Chunky)	10 oz	35	60	*	25	20	30	4	15	850	30	56	570
Pot Pie, Chicken (Swanson Hungry-Man)	16 oz	60	80	*	30	25	40	6	25	1680	41	64	730
Pot Pie, Steak Burger (Swanson Hungry-Man)	16 oz	45	45	*	20	35	40	2	35	1460	49	65	830
Pot Pie, Turkey (Swanson)	8 oz	25	35	4	20	20	15	2	10	890	25	40	430
Pot Pie, Turkey (Swanson Chunky)	10 oz	30	70	4	20	15	20	2	10	975	31	48	540
Pot Pie, Turkey (Swanson Hungry-Man)	16 oz	50	70	8	30	25	35	4	20	1730	42	63	750
Ratatouille (Stouffer's)	5 oz	*	10	35	4	4	4	2	4	1320	3	9	60
Ratatouille w Cheese in Pastry (Pepperidge Farm Vegetables in Pastry)	1	8	6	2	8	8	10	8	8	400	16	18	230
Roast Beef Hash (Stouffer's)	5¾ oz	25	*	*	4	10	15	*	10	760	16	11	265
Salisbury Steak (Swanson)	5½ oz	35	*	4	6	8	15	4	15	635	24	20	370
Salisbury Steak (Swanson Hungry-Man)	11¾ oz	60	*	8	8	25	50	10	40	1330	36	30	570
Salisbury Steak (Swanson Main Course)	10 oz	50	6	2	8	25	30	4	25	1435	29	16	430

					% U.S. RDA								
Salisbury Steak w Creole Sauce (Green Giant)	9 oz	50	6	15	8	15	35	2	25	910	26	11	410
Salisbury Steak w Gravy (Green Giant)	½ pkg	20	15	8	4	6	10	2	10	1095	19	11	280
Salisbury Steak w Italian Style Sauce and Vegetables (Stouffer's Lean Cuisine)	9½ oz	40	15	10	10	15	25	10	15	800	13	14	270
Salisbury Steak w Mashed Potatoes (Green Giant)	11 oz	30	20	10	4	15	25	10	15	1515	29	27	450
Salisbury Steak w Onion Gravy (Stouffer's)	6 oz	30	*	*	6	10	25	2	15	1150	15	5	250
Sausage and Peppers (Buitoni)	10½ oz	23	20	4	80	50	25	*	35	1745	19	49	460
Scallops, Oriental, and Vegetables w Rice (Stouffer's Lean Cuisine)	11 oz	25	15	15	*	6	8	4	4	1200	3	32	220
Scallops and Shrimp Mariner w Rice (Stouffer's)	10¼ oz	35	8	*	8	10	8	100	40	1120	16	40	400
Short Ribs of Beef, Boneless, w Vegetable Gravy (Stouffer's)	5¾ oz	45	*	*	4	15	25	2	45	560	25	2	350
Shrimp Marinara (Buitoni)	11 oz	24	20	8	20	15	20	6	20	1795	2	24	210
Spinach Almondine in Pastry (Pepperidge Farm Vegetables in Pastry)	1	8	35	0	10	10	6	8	10	330	18	19	260

Entrees, Frozen	Amt.	Pro-tein	A	C	B₁	B₂	Nia-cin	Cal-cium	Iron	Sodium (mg)	Fat (g)	Carbohy-drate (g)	Calories
		% U.S. RDA											
Spinach Soufflé (Stouffer's)	4 oz	8	15	*	8	8	2	8	8	600	7	12	135
Steak and Green Peppers (Swanson Main Course)	8½ oz	35	8	50	4	15	20	4	20	1105	7	11	200
Steak w Green Peppers, Sauce, Rice, Vegetables (Green Giant)	9 oz	30	6	35	4	10	20	2	10	1170	5	32	250
Stew, Beef (Green Giant)	9 oz	30	40	10	8	8	20	2	15	275	3	20	180
Stew, Beef (Stouffer's)	10 oz	30	25	*	10	15	20	2	15	1675	17	16	310
Stew, Meatball (Stouffer's Lean Cuisine)	10 oz	35	20	6	10	25	25	4	10	1250	7	21	240
Stir Fry Beef Teriyaki (Green Giant)	10 oz	30	20	25	6	15	15	2	10	780	11	36	320
Stir Fry Cashew Chicken (Green Giant)	10 oz	30	6	15	4	15	20	2	10	965	13	37	340
Stir Fry Chicken and Garden Vegetables (Green Giant)	10 oz	25	35	20	10	15	35	4	10	705	7	29	250
Stir Fry Shrimp Fried Rice (Green Giant)	10 oz	20	15	20	4	10	10	6	6	1130	5	49	300
Stir Fry Sweet and Sour Chicken (Green Giant)	10 oz	20	45	25	4	8	30	4	6	585	6	47	300
Stir Fry Szechwan Beef (Green Giant)	10 oz	35	70	35	15	15	20	6	20	590	11	26	290

Food	Serving	% U.S. RDA											
Swiss Steak w Gravy, Stuffed Potato (Green Giant)	1 pkg	35	20	20	10	6	30	6	15	1235	13	37	350
Tuna Noodle Casserole (Stouffer's)	5¾ oz	15	2	*	10	10	15	10	6	670	9	18	200
Turkey (Swanson)	8¾ oz	30	*	10	8	8	40	2	8	1070	7	27	230
Turkey (Swanson Hungry-Man)	13¼ oz	60	*	10	15	20	60	4	15	1645	11	39	370
Turkey, Breast Slices w White and Wild Rice Stuffing (Green Giant)	9 oz	30	10	8	8	8	35	4	8	1225	28	34	460
Turkey Casserole w Gravy and Dressing (Stouffer's)	9¾ oz	35	8	4	10	10	25	8	10	1125	18	29	370
Turkey, Ham, and Cheese in Pastry (Pepperidge Farm Deli's)	1	30	0	4	20	15	25	8	10	770	13	23	270
Turkey Tetrazzini (Stouffer's)	6 oz	15	*	*	10	10	10	8	8	620	14	17	240
Veal Patty Pomodoro (Buitoni)	10½ oz	23	10	*	30	20	25	4	25	1590	5	53	350
Vegetables, Mexican Style Picante, in Pastry (Pepperidge Farm Vegetables in Pastry)	1	6	10	15	8	8	10	6	6	470	14	21	220
Welsh Rarebit (Stouffer's)	5 oz	10	20	*	6	15	*	40	2	660	29	17	355
Zucchini Provencal in Pastry (Pepperidge Farm Vegetables in Pastry)	1	4	8	8	10	8	8	2	20	290	13	21	210

Entrees, Mixes	Amt.	Pro-tein	A	C	B_1	B_2	Nia-cin	Cal-cium	Iron	Sodium (mg)	Fat (g)	Carbohy-drate (g)	Calories
		% U.S. RDA											
Beef Noodle (Hamburger Helper)	⅕ prep	40	*	*	20	20	25	2	20	970	15	25	320
Beef Romanoff (Hamburger Helper)	⅕ pkg (w ⅕ lb grd beef)	40	*	*	20	15	25	6	15	1095	16	28	340
Burger 'n Cheese Dinner (Creamette Hamburger Mate)	⅕ prep	45	*	*	40	20	25	10	20	NA	10	32	310
Cheeseburger Macaroni (Hamburger Helper)	⅕ prep	40	4	*	20	20	25	6	15	1025	18	28	360
Chili Tomato (Hamburger Helper)	⅕ prep	40	4	*	20	15	25	2	15	1310	14	32	330
Country Dumplings, Noodles, and Tuna (Tuna Helper)	⅕ prep	25	*	*	20	10	30	4	10	1020	6	31	230
Creamy Noodles and Tuna (Tuna Helper)	⅕ prep	25	6	*	20	10	30	2	10	880	11	31	280
Hamburger Hash (Hamburger Helper)	⅕ prep	35	*	2	4	10	25	2	15	920	15	24	300
Hamburger Pizza Dish (Hamburger Helper)	⅕ prep	40	10	2	20	15	30	2	20	960	14	33	340
Hamburger Stew (Hamburger Helper)	⅕ prep	35	10	*	4	10	20	2	15	945	14	23	290
Noodles, Cheese Sauce, and Tuna (Tuna Helper)	⅕ prep	25	*	*	15	10	30	4	8	745	7	28	230

Food	Serving	% U.S. RDA										Calories
Potatoes au Gratin (Hamburger Helper)	1/5 prep	35	*	6	6	25	4	10	890	15	27	320
Potato Stroganoff (Hamburger Helper)	1/5 prep	35	*	4	10	25	2	10	965	15	27	320
Rice Oriental (Hamburger Helper)	1/5 prep	35	*	15	10	25	2	20	1085	14	35	340
Tamale Pie (Hamburger Helper)	1/5 prep	40	10	20	15	25	2	15	910	16	37	370
Tuna Tetrazzini (Tuna Helper)	1/5 prep	30	4	15	10	25	6	6	840	11	26	260

Fast Food

Arby's

Food	Serving	% U.S. RDA										Calories
Arby's Sub (No Dressing)	1	30	4	20	20	15	20	25	1354	16	37	484
Beef 'n Cheddar Sandwich	1	45	4	45	25	20	25	10	1745	21	46	484
Chicken Breast Sandwich	1	40	*	15	15	50	10	20	1323	28	55	584
French Dip	1	35	*	10	15	25	6	25	1111	12	47	386
French Fries	2.5 oz	3	*	*	*	3	*	*	39	12	26	216
Ham 'n Cheese Sandwich	1	45	4	45	25	20	25	10	1745	21	46	484
Potato Cakes	2 cakes	2	30	*	*	4	*	2	476	9	24	190
Roast Beef Sandwich, Deluxe	1	40	*	20	20	25	10	35	1288	23	43	486
Roast Beef Sandwich, Junior	1	20	*	10	10	15	4	10	530	9	21	220
Roast Beef Sandwich, Regular	1	35	*	20	20	25	8	20	880	15	32	350

Fast Food	Amt.	% U.S. RDA								Sodium (mg)	Fat (g)	Carbohy- drate (g)	Calories
		Pro- tein	A	C	B₁	B₂	Nia- cin	Cal- cium	Iron				
Roast Beef Sandwich, Super	1	45	*	*	35	25	35	10	30	1420	28	61	620
Sauce, Arby's	1 oz	NA	140	2	*	*	*	6	*	1255	9	24	34
Sauce, Horsey	1 oz	*	*	*	*	*	*	*	*	NA	5.5	2.5	120
Turnover, Apple	1	4	*	*	2	2	2	2	4	240	21	30	310
Turnover, Blueberry	1	4	2	2	2	2	2	*	2	255	20	30	340
Turnover, Cherry	1	4	*	2	2	2	2	2	4	254	20	32	320
Arthur Treacher's Fish & Chips													
Chicken	2 pcs	40	*	2	4	8	55	*	4	495	16	17	370
Chicken Sandwich	1	25	*	30	10	10	40	6	8	708	12	44	410
Chips	1 svg	6	*	10	10	2	10	*	2	393	12	35	280
Chowder	1 svg	7	6	2	4	8	2	6	*	835	3	11	110
Cole Slaw	1 svg	2	4	90	2	*	2	2	*	266	8	11	120
Fish	2 pcs	30	*	2	6	4	10	*	2	450	13	25	360
Fish Sandwich	1	25	*	2	15	10	20	8	8	836	15	40	444
Krunch Pup	1	8	*	6	2	2	6	*	2	446	26	12	200
Lemon Luvs	1	4	*	2	10	4	8	*	4	314	16	35	280
Shrimp	7 pcs	20	*	2	4	2	8	6	4	538	21	27	380

Burger King

							% U.S. RDA							
Apple Pie	1 pie	4	*	*	*	*	2	*	*	2	335	12	32	240
Bacon Double Cheeseburger	1	50	8	*	20	25	35	25	25	985	35	36	600	
Cheeseburger	1	30	*	2	8	10	10	4	15	730	17	30	350	
Cheeseburger, Double	1	50	*	*	10	15	20	8	15	990	31	32	530	
Chicken Sandwich	1	40	4	2	20	15	50	6	10	775	42	52	690	
French Fries, Regular	1 svg	4	*	4	4	*	4	*	2	230	11	25	210	
Hamburger	1	25	*	*	10	10	10	*	15	525	13	29	290	
Onion Rings, Regular	1 svg	4	*	*	4	*	*	8	2	450	16	29	270	
Shake, Chocolate	10 oz	10	*	*	8	15	*	25	*	280	10	57	340	
Shake, Vanilla	10 oz	10	*	*	10	20	*	30	*	320	11	52	340	
Veal Parmigiana	1	45	20	10	25	30	35	30	25	1130	25	65	600	
Whaler	1	35	*	*	15	10	10	8	15	745	24	57	540	
Whaler w Cheese	1	40	4	*	15	15	10	20	15	885	28	58	590	
Whopper	1	40	*	*	4	15	20	4	15	990	36	50	630	
Whopper w Cheese	1	50	*	*	8	20	15	15	15	1435	45	52	740	
Whopper, Double Beef	1	70	*	*	6	25	30	2	25	1080	52	52	850	
Whopper, Double Beef w Cheese	1	80	*	*	6	25	30	15	20	1535	60	54	950	
Whopper Junior	1	25	*	15	15	10	15	*	10	560	20	31	370	
Whopper Junior w Cheese	1	30	*	15	15	10	15	8	10	785	25	32	420	

Carl's Jr.

| Fast Food | Amt. | % U.S. RDA | | | | | | | | Sodium (mg) | Fat (g) | Carbohy-drate (g) | Calories |
		Pro-tein	A	C	B₁	B₂	Nia-cin	Cal-cium	Iron				
Bacon	2 strips	8	*	*	*	2	2	4	*	220	6	0	70
California Roast Beef Sandwich	1	50	8	10	30	25	35	20	30	505	7	34	300
Carrot Cake	1 piece	6	4	*	4	4	4	4	8	375	18	44	350
Charbroiler Chicken Sandwich	1	40	2	4	8	25	100	10	12	1380	14	55	450
Charbroiler Steak	1	40	2	*	4	8	20	*	15	215	17	0	230
Charbroiler Steak Sandwich	1	60	8	4	60	30	30	10	25	700	33	54	630
Cheese Sandwich, American	1	8	2	*	*	4	*	10	*	120	6	1	70
Cheese Sandwich, Swiss	1	8	2	*	*	4	*	10	*	125	5	1	70
Chicken Breasts	2	85	0	0	4	15	70	2	8	600	4	0	200
Crispirito	1	50	4	0	20	20	25	25	15	1050	40	55	670
Eggs, Scrambled	1 svg	25	2	*	4	15	2	4	8	110	12	1	150
English Muffin w Butter and Jelly	1	6	2	*	15	6	10	15	10	245	9	34	228
Famous Star Hamburger	1	50	10	4	40	25	25	10	25	705	32	38	530
Fillet of Fish Sandwich	1	40	6	4	40	20	25	25	15	790	27	61	570
French Fries, Regular	1 svg	4	*	10	6	8	2	8	2	460	15	25	250
Garlic Bread	1 svg	4	0	0	6	4	4	2	10	260	5	18	130
Ground Beef	1 svg	85	0	0	8	20	45	2	30	130	40	0	520

		% U.S. RDA											
Happy Star Hamburger	1	45	4	*	30	15	30	8	20	670	13	33	330
Hashed Brown Potatoes	2	4	*	*	4	6	10	*	4	260	19	26	280
Hot Cakes w Syrup and Butter	1 svg	10	*	*	25	15	10	20	15	530	15	80	480
Hot Chocolate	1 svg	6	4	4	245	8	*	10	4	120	2	20	110
Old Time Star Hamburger	1	50	8	*	40	30	35	6	30	625	20	45	450
Omelette, Bacon 'n Cheese	1	45	6	*	6	25	8	25	10	660	28	2	290
Omelette, California	1	40	6	*	4	25	6	30	15	550	24	3	310
Omelette, Cheese	1	35	6	*	2	25	4	25	10	440	22	2	280
Onion Rings	1 svg	8	2	*	8	2	8	2	10	75	17	39	330
Onion Ring Garnish	1 svg	3	1	*	3	1	3	1	3	25	6	13	110
Potato, Baked	1	12	NA	43	NA	NA	NA	NA	13	6	.2	33	167
Potatoes, Wedge Cut	1 svg	6	0	34	8	0	15	2	6	8	13	32	252
Salad, Regular	1	15	80	45	10	15	25	10	15	695	4	33	210
Salad Dressing, Bleu Cheese	2 oz	2	*	*	*	*	*	2	*	230	16	2	160
Salad Dressing, Low-Cal Italian	2 oz	*	*	*	*	*	*	*	*	360	10	0	80
Salad, Dressing, Thousand Island	2 oz	*	*	*	*	*	*	*	*	320	24	8	240
Sausage	1 patty	15	*	*	10	4	6	*	2	235	9	0	110
Shake, Regular	1	30	*	*	8	35	6	60	6	350	8	90	490
Sunrise Sandwich w Bacon	1	35	6	*	20	20	15	20	15	780	24	28	410

Fast Food	Amt.	Pro-tein	A	C	B₁	B₂	Nia-cin	Cal-cium	Iron	Sodium (mg)	Fat (g)	Carbohy-drate (g)	Calories
		% U.S. RDA											
Sunrise Sandwich w Sausage	1	40	2	*	25	25	15	20	15	790	27	28	450
Super Star Hamburger	1	100	10	*	45	35	45	10	35	785	50	38	780
Sweet Roll w Butter	1	10	4	*	20	15	15	8	15	450	18	57	420
Tartar Sauce	¾ oz	*	*	NA	NA	NA	NA	*	*	NA	NA	NA	39
Top Sirloin Steak	1 svg	80	0	0	6	15	35	0	25	85	7	0	210
Trout w Lemon Garlic Butter	1 svg	50	0	0	4	10	40	15	6	190	11	0	200
Turnover, Apple	1	6	*	*	4	6	10	*	15	470	23	45	400
Western Bacon Cheese-burger	1	80	4	0	25	25	50	20	25	1330	40	42	670
Zucchini	1 svg	5	2	5	13	7	9	4	9	516	19	32	311
Dairy Queen/Brazier													
Banana Split	1 svg	15	15	25	10	30	2	25	10	150	11	103	540
Buster Bar	1	20	2	*	8	10	10	10	6	175	29	41	460
Chicken Sandwich	1 svg	2	*	15	4	*	4	*	2	870	41	46	670
Cone, Large	1	20	8	*	8	30	*	25	8	115	10	57	340
Cone, Regular	1	10	4	*	4	20	*	15	4	80	7	38	240
Cone, Small	1	6	2	*	2	10	*	10	2	45	4	22	140
Cone, Dipped, Chocolate, Large	1	20	8	*	8	30	*	25	8	145	24	64	510

		% U.S. RDA											
Cone, Dipped, Chocolate, Regular	1	10	4	*	4	20	*	15	4	100	16	42	340
Cone, Dipped, Chocolate, Small	1	6	2	*	2	10	*	10	2	55	9	25	190
Dilly Bar	1	6	2	*	2	10	*	10	2	50	13	21	210
Double Delight	1	20	6	*	10	20	2	20	8	150	20	69	490
DQ Sandwich	1	6	*	*	2	4	2	6	*	40	4	24	140
Fish Sandwich	1 svg	30	*	*	10	15	15	6	4	875	17	41	400
Fish Sandwich w Cheese	1 svg	35	2	*	10	15	15	15	2	1035	21	39	440
Float	1	10	4	*	4	15	*	20	6	85	7	82	410
Freeze	1	20	8	*	10	30	*	30	10	180	12	89	500
French Fries	1 svg	4	*	25	6	2	6	*	6	115	10	25	200
French Fries, Large	1 svg	6	*	4	6	*	2	2	4	185	16	40	320
Hamburger, Double	1	60	2	*	30	20	45	10	35	660	28	33	530
Hamburger, Double w Cheese	1	70	8	*	30	25	45	35	35	980	37	34	650
Hamburger, Single	1	30	2	*	20	10	25	10	20	630	16	33	360
Hamburger, Single w Cheese	1	35	4	*	20	10	25	20	20	790	20	33	410
Hamburger, Triple	1	80	4	*	40	30	70	10	50	690	45	33	710
Hamburger, Triple w Cheese	1	90	8	*	40	35	70	35	50	1010	50	34	820
Hot Dog	1	15	*	*	8	8	15	8	8	830	16	21	280

Fast Food	Amt.	Pro-tein	A	C	B₁	B₂	Nia-cin	Cal-cium	Iron	Sodium (mg)	Fat (g)	Carbohy-drate (g)	Calories
						% U.S. RDA							
Hot Dog w Cheese	1	20	2	*	8	10	15	15	8	990	21	21	330
Hot Dog w Chili	1	20	*	*	10	15	20	8	10	985	20	23	320
Hot Dog, Super	1	25	*	*	15	15	25	15	15	1365	27	44	520
Hot Dog, Super, w Cheese	1	35	2	*	15	15	25	25	8	1605	34	45	580
Hot Dog, Super, w Chili	1	30	*	*	15	25	30	15	15	1595	32	47	570
Hot Fudge Brownie Delight	1	20	6	*	8	20	*	20	10	225	25	85	600
Malt, Chocolate, Large	1	45	20	*	25	70	6	70	30	360	25	187	1060
Malt, Chocolate, Regular	1	30	15	*	20	50	4	45	25	260	18	134	760
Malt, Chocolate, Small	1	20	10	*	10	35	2	35	15	180	13	91	520
Mr. Misty Float	1	10	4	*	4	15	*	20	4	95	7	74	390
Mr. Misty Freeze	1	20	8	*	8	30	*	30	8	140	12	91	500
Mr. Misty Kiss	1	*	*	*	*	*	*	*	*	0-10	0	17	70
Mr. Misty, Large	1	*	*	*	*	*	*	*	*	0-10	0	84	340
Mr. Misty, Regular	1	*	*	*	*	*	*	*	*	0-10	0	63	250
Mr. Misty, Small	1	*	*	*	*	*	*	*	*	0-10	0	48	190
Onion Rings	1 svg	45	*	*	20	20	50	10	25	140	16	31	280
Parfait	1	15	8	6	6	25	*	25	8	140	8	76	430
Peanut Buster Parfait	1	35	6	*	10	25	10	25	10	250	34	94	740
Shake, Chocolate, Large	1	45	20	*	20	60	4	70	20	360	26	168	990

							% U.S. RDA						
Shake, Chocolate, Regular	1	30	15	*	15	45	2	45	15	260	19	120	710
Shake, Chocolate, Small	1	20	10	*	10	35	*	35	10	180	13	82	490
Strawberry Shortcake	1	15	8	20	15	30	*	25	10	215	11	100	540
Sundae, Chocolate, Large	1	15	8	*	6	25	*	25	8	165	10	78	440
Sundae, Chocolate, Regular	1	10	4	*	4	20	*	20	6	120	8	56	310
Sundae, Chocolate, Small	1	6	2	*	2	10	*	10	2	75	4	33	190
Hardee's													
Bacon Cheeseburger	1	53	16	5	3	23	32	15	35	1074	42	42	686
Bacon & Egg Biscuit	1	20	3	3	7	10	9	14	16	823	26	30	405
Biscuit	1	7	*	*	23	14	4	15	14	650	13	35	275
Biscuit w Egg	1	17	15	*	26	23	4	18	20	819	22	35	383
Cheeseburger	1	26	15	*	34	19	27	5	15	789	17	28	335
Chicken Fillet	1	41	22	22	34	37	47	8	27	360	26	42	510
Cookie, Big	1	4	0	4	*	4	*	2	6	258	15	33	278
Fisherman Fillet	1	38	6	0	12	17	17	14	12	1013	20	47	469
French Fries, Large	1 svg	7	0	26	7	3	8	2	7	192	20	44	381
French Fries, Small	1 svg	5	0	16	4	*	5	*	4	121	13	28	239
Ham Biscuit	1	19	2	*	40	25	9	18	17	1414	17	37	349
Ham Biscuit w Egg	1	28	17	*	43	34	9	21	24	1584	25	37	458
Ham and Cheese Sandwich, Hot	1	NA	NA	NA	NA	NA	NA	NA	NA	1067	15	37	376

Fast Food	Amt.	% U.S. RDA								Sodium (mg)	Fat (g)	Carbohy-drate (g)	Calories
		Pro-tein	A	C	B_1	B_2	Nia-cin	Cal-cium	Iron				
Hamburger	1	25	*	*	36	34	32	2	20	682	13	29	305
Hashrounds	1 svg	4	*	6	6	*	8	*	6	310	13	20	200
Hot Dog	1	17	0	0	19	13	21	4	14	744	22	26	346
Milk Shake	1	17	0	0	13	45	3	45	3	NA	10	63	391
Mushroom 'n Swiss Hamburger	1	49	4	0	16	39	30	11	23	1051	23	43	512
Roast Beef Sandwich	1	31	11	5	62	11	18	5	35	1030	17	36	376
Roast Beef Sandwich, Big	1	42	13	12	68	13	26	7	44	1770	19	33	418
Sausage Biscuit	1	15	*	*	23	13	14	14	15	864	26	34	413
Sausage Biscuit w Egg	1	25	15	*	27	21	14	17	22	1033	35	34	521
Steak Biscuit	1	21	*	*	22	25	16	12	25	803	22	40	419
Steak Biscuit w Egg	1	30	15	*	26	33	16	15	32	973	31	41	527
Turkey Club Sandwich	1	38	16	8	21	16	45	4	12	1185	22	32	426
Turnover, Apple	1	4	*	*	2	2	2	*	5	NA	14	37	282
McDonald's													
Big Mac	1	39	10	3	25	21	32	15	22	1010	33	40	563
Biscuit, Plain	1	NA	NA	NA	NA	NA	NA	NA	NA	786	18	NA	312
Biscuit, Buttered	1	NA	NA	NA	NA	NA	NA	NA	NA	830	23	NA	342
Biscuit w Bacon, Egg, and Cheese	1	NA	NA	NA	NA	NA	NA	NA	NA	1269	31	NA	509

Item	Serving				% U.S. RDA								
Biscuit w Sausage	1	NA	NA	NA	NA	NA	NA	NA	NA	1209	30	NA	522
Biscuit w Sausage and Egg	1	NA	NA	NA	NA	NA	NA	NA	NA	1301	39	NA	612
Cheeseburger	1	23	6	2	16	13	18	13	13	767	14	29	307
Chicken McNuggets	1 svg	31	NA	3	8	9	42	*	5	525	19	15	314
Cone	1	6	NA	NA	3	21	2	18	*	109	5	30	185
Cookies, Chocolaty Chip	2½ oz (69 g)	6	4	*	8	12	8	2	8	313	16	44	342
Cookies, McDonaldland	2½ oz (67 g)	6	NA	*	15	13	14	*	8	358	10	48	308
Egg McMuffin	1	28	11	NA	31	26	18	22	16	884	14	31	330
Eggs, Scrambled	1 svg	29	13	2	5	27	*	6	14	205	13	2	180
English Muffin w Butter	1	7	3	*	18	28	13	11	8	318	5	29	186
Filet-o-Fish	1	22	3	NA	17	11	13	9	9	781	25	37	432
Fries, Regular	1 svg	4	NA	20	8	*	11	*	3	109	11	26	220
Hamburger	1	19	*	2	16	10	19	5	12	520	9	29	255
Hash Brown Potatoes	1 svg	2	NA	6	4	NA	4	*	2	325	7	14	125
Hotcakes w Butter and Syrup	1 svg	12	5	7	17	21	11	10	12	1070	10	93	500
Pie, Apple	1 pie	2	NA	NA	*	*	*	*	3	398	14	29	253
Pie, Cherry	1 pie	3	2	NA	*	*	*	*	3	427	13	32	260
Quarter Pounder	1	37	2	NA	21	16	32	6	22	735	21	32	424
Quarter Pounder w Cheese	1	46	13	4	20	21	36	21	23	1236	30	32	524
Sauce, Barbeque (for McNuggets)	1 svg	*	NA	NA	NA	NA	NA	NA	NA	309	0–1	13	60

147

Fast Food	Amt.	Pro-tein	A	C	B₁	B₂	Nia-cin	Cal-cium	Iron	Sodium (mg)	Fat (g)	Carbohy-drate (g)	Calories
		% U.S. RDA											
Sauce, Honey (for McNuggets)	1 svg	*	NA	NA	NA	NA	NA	NA	NA	0-3	0-1	12	50
Sauce, Hot Mustard (for McNuggets)	1 svg	*	NA	NA	NA	NA	NA	NA	NA	259	2	10	63
Sauce, Sweet and Sour (for McNuggets)	1 svg	*	NA	NA	NA	NA	NA	NA	NA	186	0-1	15	64
Sausage	1 svg	19	NA	NA	18	6	10	*	4	615	18	0-1	206
Sausage McMuffin	1	NA	NA	NA	NA	NA	NA	NA	NA	942	24	NA	417
Sausage McMuffin w Egg	1	NA	NA	NA	NA	NA	NA	NA	NA	1044	30	NA	507
Shake, Chocolate	1	22	7	NA	7	25	2	32	4	300	9	65	383
Shake, Strawberry	1	20	7	6	7	25	*	32	*	207	8	62	362
Shake, Vanilla	1	20	7	5	7	41	*	32	*	201	8	59	352
Sundae, Caramel	1	11	5	6	4	18	5	20	*	195	10	52	328
Sundae, Hot Fudge	1	10	4	4	4	18	5	21	3	175	10	46	310
Sundae, Strawberry	1	10	5	4	4	17	5	17	2	96	8	46	289
Fish													
Anchovies, Pickled, Canned	5	8	*	*	*	2	6	4	4	NA	2	0	35
Bass, Striped, Oven-fried	3 oz	40	*	*	6	2	8	2	4	NA	8	6	170
Bluefish, Baked or Broiled w Butter or Margarine	3 oz	50	*	*	6	4	8	2	4	88	4	0	140

Food	Serving	% U.S. RDA											Calories
Bluefish, Fried	3 oz	45	2	*	6	6	8	2	4	124	9	4	140
Clams, Canned, Drained, Chopped or Minced	1 c	60	4	*	2	10	8	8	35	NA	4	3	160
Clams, Canned, Minced (Snow's)	6½ oz	45	*	*	*	8	6	4	15	920	1	4	100
Clams, Raw, Cherry-stones or Little Necks, Meat Only	4–5	15	2	10	4	6	4	4	30	25	2	1	60
Clam Juice (Doxsee)	8 fl oz	*	*	*	4	*	2	*	*	570	0	4	20
Clam Juice (Snow's)	3 fl oz	2	*	*	*	*	2	*	2	470	0	2	14
Cod, Broiled w Butter or Margarine	3 oz	60	4	*	4	6	15	2	4	94	5	0	140
Crabmeat, Canned, Drained	3 oz	35	20	*	4	4	8	4	4	850	2	1	90
Crabmeat, Steamed	3 oz	35	35	10	4	4	10	4	4	NA	2	1	80
Flounder, Baked w Butter or Margarine	3 oz	60	*	4	4	4	10	2	6	201	7	0	170
Gefilte, Jelled (Rokeach)	1 pc	10	4	*	*	4	2	4	2	835	1	4	60
Gefilte, Jellied (Mother's Old World)	1 pc	10	2	10	*	6	2	2	2	NA	1	7	70
Gefilte, in Jellied Broth (Rokeach Old Vienna)	1 pc	10	*	4	*	*	2	4	*	NA	1	8	70
Gefilte, in Jellied Broth, Low Sodium (Rokeach)	1 pc	10	5	*	*	*	*	2	2	15	2	3	50
Gefilte, in Jellied Broth, Unsalted (Mother's)	1 pc	10	4	*	*	*	*	2	2	10	1	2	45

Fish	Amt.	Protein	A	C	B₁	B₂	Niacin	Calcium	Iron	Sodium (mg)	Fat (g)	Carbohydrate (g)	Calories
								% U.S. RDA					
Gefilte, in Liquid Broth (Mother's Old Fashioned)	1 pc	10	2	8	*	6	2	4	2	NA	1	7	70
Gefilte, in Natural Liquid Broth (Rokeach)	1 pc	6	*	2	*	4	*	4	*	NA	1	4	50
Haddock, Pan-fried or Oven-fried	3 oz	35	*	4	2	4	15	4	6	150	6	5	140
Halibut, Broiled w Butter or Margarine	3 oz	50	10	*	2	4	35	2	4	114	6	0	150
Herring, Canned, Smoked, Kippered	4⅜" × 1¾" × ¼" fillet	20	*	*	*	6	6	2	4	NA	6	0	80
Lobster, Northern, Cooked	3 oz	35	*	*	6	4	6	6	4	179	2	0-1	80
Mackerel, Atlantic, Broiled w Butter or Margarine	3 oz	40	8	*	8	15	35	*	6	NA	14	0	200
Ocean Perch, Atlantic, Fried	3 oz	35	*	*	6	6	8	2	6	130	12	6	190
Oysters, Eastern, Raw, Meat Only	1 c (13–19 med or 19–31 standard)	45	15	*	25	25	30	25	70	175	4	8	160
Oysters, Pacific, Raw, Meat Only	1 c (4–6 med)	60	15	*	20	25	15	20	100	NA	6	16	220
Rockfish, Oven-steamed	3 oz	35	10	2	2	6	35	2	4	58	2	2	90
Roe, Herring, Canned	3 oz	40	*	4	6	40	6	2	6	NA	3	0-1	100

Food	Serving												
		% U.S. RDA											
Salmon, Pink, Canned (Del Monte)	½ c	45	*	0	*	10	35	20	4	660	7	0	160
Salmon, Red. Canned (Del Monte)	½ c	50	4	0	*	10	30	25	4	660	9	0	180
Salmon, Steak, Broiled or Baked w Butter or Margarine	3 oz	50	2	*	10	2	40	10	6	99	6	0	160
Salmon, Smoked	1 oz	15	*	*	*	4	4	*	2	NA	3	0	50
Sardines in Mustard Sauce (Underwood)	1 can (3¾ oz)	40	6	*	*	8	10	25	6	850	17	NA	230
Sardines in Soya Bean Oil (Underwood)	1 can (3¾ oz)	40	6	*	*	8	10	25	6	800	34	NA	380
Sardines in Tomato Sauce (Del Monte)	½ c	40	6	8	*	20	15	30	20	540	12	45	360
Sardines in Tomato Sauce (Underwood)	1 can (3¾ oz)	40	6	2	*	8	10	25	6	850	17	1	230
Scallops, Frozen, Breaded	1 (15–20 per lb)	10	*	*	*	2	*	2	4	NA	2	3	50
Shrimp, Canned	3 oz	45	2	*	*	2	8	10	15	NA	1	1	100
Shrimp, French-fried	3 oz	40	*	2	2	4	10	6	10	158	9	9	190
Swordfish, Broiled w Butter or Margarine	3 oz	50	35	*	2	2	45	2	6	NA	6	0	140
Tuna, Chunk, Light, in Oil (Chicken of the Sea)	1 c	100	*	2	2	8	100	*	10	NA	42	0	550
Tuna, Chunk, Light, in Water (Chicken of the Sea)	1 c	100	*	2	2	8	100	*	10	NA	2	0	200

Fish	Amt.	Pro-tein	A	C	B₁	B₂	Nia-cin	Cal-cium	Iron	Sodium (mg)	Fat (g)	Carbohy-drate (g)	Calories
		% U.S. RDA											
Tuna, Chunk, White, in Oil (Chicken of the Sea)	1 c	100	*	*	2	6	100	*	4	NA	35	0	500
Tuna, Chunk, White, in Water (Chicken of the Sea Dietetic Pack, Low Sodium)	1 c	100	*	*	4	4	110	*	4	95	6	0	220
Tuna, Solid, Light, in Oil (Chicken of the Sea)	1 c	100	*	*	4	8	110	*	8	NA	30	0	460
Tuna, Solid, Light, in Water (Chicken of the Sea)	1 c	110	*	*	4	6	120	*	4	NA	4	0	240
Tuna, Solid, White, in Oil (Chicken of the Sea)	1 c	110	*	*	4	8	110	*	6	NA	28	0	450
Tuna, in Water	3 oz	50	*	*	*	6	60	*	8	744	1	0	110
Tuna Salad (The Spreadables)	1.9 oz (¼ can)	15	*	*	*	*	15	*	2	270	7	3	100
Whitefish and Pike, Jelled (Mother's)	1 pc	10	2	2	*	4	2	2	2	NA	1	4	60
Whitefish and Pike, in Jelled Broth (Rokeach)	1 pc	10	2	8	*	4	2	4	*	NA	1	4	60
Flour													
Cornmeal, White (Albers)	1 oz	2	*	*	8	4	6	*	4	NA	0	22	100

		2	4	*	8	4	6	*	4	NA	0	22	100
Cornmeal, Yellow (Albers)	1 oz	2	4	*	8	4	6	*	4	NA	0	22	100
Flour, High Protein (Gold Medal Better for Bread)	4 oz	20	*	*	45	25	30	2	25	0-5	1	83	400
Flour, Rye, Medium (Pillsbury's Best)	1 c	20	0	0	20	8	15	2	15	0-5	2	83	400
Flour, Rye and Wheat (Pillsbury's Best Bohemian Style)	1 c	15	0	0	20	10	15	2	20	0-5	1	86	400
Flour, White (Ballard All Purpose)	1 c	15	0	0	45	25	30	0	25	0-5	1	87	400
Flour, White (Drifted Snow)	4 oz	15	*	*	45	25	30	2	25	0-5	1	87	400
Flour, White (Gold Medal All Purpose)	4 oz	15	*	*	45	25	30	2	25	0-5	1	87	400
Flour, White Gold Medal Self-Rising	4 oz	15	*	*	45	25	30	20	25	1520	1	83	380
Flour, White (Gold Medal Unbleached)	4 oz	15	*	*	45	25	30	2	25	0-5	1	87	400
Flour, White (Pillsbury's Best All Purpose)	1 c	15	0	0	45	25	30	0	25	0-5	1	87	400
Flour, White (Pillsbury's Best Bread)	1 c	20	0	0	45	25	30	0	25	0-5	2	83	400
Flour, White (Pillsbury's Best Self-Rising Unbleached or Bleached)	1 c	15	0	0	45	25	30	30	25	1290	1	84	380
Flour, White (Pillsbury's Best Unbleached)	1 c	15	0	0	45	25	30	0	25	0-5	1	86	400

% U.S. RDA

Flour	Amt.	Protein	A	C	B_1	B_2	Niacin	Calcium	Iron	Sodium (mg)	Fat (g)	Carbohydrate (g)	Calories
		% U.S. RDA											
Flour, White (Red Band Plain)	4 oz	15	*	*	45	25	30	4	25	0-5	1	87	400
Flour, White (Red Band Self-Rising)	4 oz	15	*	*	45	25	30	20	25	1520	1	83	380
Flour, White (Red Band Unbleached)	4 oz	15	*	*	45	25	20	2	25	0-5	1	87	400
Flour, White (Red Star Self-Rising)	4 oz	15	*	*	45	25	30	20	25	1520	1	83	380
Flour, White (Softasilk)	4 oz	2	*	*	10	6	8	*	6	0-5	0	23	100
Flour, White (White Deer All-Purpose)	4 oz	15	*	*	45	25	30	2	25	0-5	1	87	400
Flour, White (Wondra)	4 oz	15	*	*	45	25	30	2	25	0-5	1	87	400
Flour, White, Thickening (Pillsbury's Best Sauce 'n Gravy)	2 tbsp	2	0	0	6	2	2	0	2	0-5	0	11	50
Flour, Whole Wheat (Gold Medal)	4 oz	25	*	*	35	8	30	2	25	0-5	2	78	390
Flour, Whole Wheat (Pillsbury's Best)	1 c	25	0	0	30	8	25	2	20	10	2	80	400
Frostings													
Banana (Betty Crocker Chiquita)	1/12 pkg prep	*	2	*	*	0	*	*	0	80	6	30	170

Product	Serving				% U.S. RDA							
Butter Brickle (Betty Crocker)	½ pkg prep	*	2	*	*	0	*	*	0	115	6	30	170
Butter Pecan (Betty Crocker)	½ pkg prep	*	2	*	*	0	*	*	0	100	6	30	170
Butter Pecan, rts* (Betty Crocker)	½ can prep	*	*	*	**	0	**	**	0	90	7	25	160
Cake and Cookie Decorator, All Colors (Pillsbury)	1 tbsp prep	0	0	0	0	0	0	0	0	5	2	12	70
Caramel (Pillsbury Rich 'n Easy)	for ½ cake prep	0	0	0	0	0	0	0	0	35	5	24	140
Caramel Pecan, rts (Pillsbury)	for ½ cake prep	0	0	0	0	0	0	0	0	70	8	21	160
Cherry, rts (Betty Crocker)	½ can prep	*	*	*	*	0	*	*	0	100	6	26	160
Cherry, Creamy (Betty Crocker)	½ pkg prep	*	2	*	**	0	**	**	0	100	6	30	170
Chocolate, rts (Betty Crocker)	½ can prep	*	*	*	*	2	*	*	2	100	8	23	170
Chocolate Almond Fudge (Betty Crocker)	½ pkg prep	*	2	*	*	2	*	*	2	75	7	27	180
Chocolate Chip, rts (Betty Crocker)	½ can prep	*	*	*	**	0	**	**	0	90	7	26	170
Chocolate Chocolate Chip, rts (Betty Crocker)	½ can prep	*	*	*	*	2	*	*	2	95	7	24	160
Chocolate Fudge (Betty Crocker)	½ pkg prep	*	2	*	*	2	*	*	2	75	6	30	170

*Ready to spread

Frostings	Amt.	Protein	A	C	B₁	B₂	Niacin	Calcium	Iron	Sodium (mg)	Fat (g)	Carbohydrate (g)	Calories
		% U.S. RDA											
Chocolate Fudge (Pillsbury Rich 'n Easy)	for ½ cake prep	0	0	0	0	0	0	0	0	70	4	27	150
Chocolate Fudge, rts (Pillsbury)	for ½ cake prep	0	0	0	0	0	0	0	0	80	6	24	150
Chocolate Mint, rts (Pillsbury)	for ½ cake prep	0	0	0	0	0	0	0	0	80	6	24	150
Chocolate Nut, rts (Betty Crocker)	½ can prep	*	*	*	*	0	*	*	4	100	8	22	160
Coconut Almond (Betty Crocker)	½ pkg prep	*	2	*	*	0	*	*	0	90	8	18	140
Coconut Almond (Pillsbury)	for ½ cake prep	2	2	0	0	2	0	2	0	85	10	16	160
Coconut Almond, rts (Pillsbury)	for ½ cake prep	0	0	0	0	0	0	0	0	60	9	17	150
Coconut Pecan (Betty Crocker)	½ pkg prep	*	2	*	*	0	*	*	0	100	8	18	140
Coconut Pecan (Pillsbury)	for ½ cake prep	0	0	0	0	0	0	2	0	105	7	20	150
Coconut Pecan, rts (Betty Crocker)	½ can prep	*	*	*	*	0	*	*	0	80	8	24	170
Coconut Pecan, rts (Pillsbury)	for ½ cake prep	0	0	0	0	0	0	0	0	60	10	17	160
Cream Cheese, rts (Betty Crocker)	½ can prep	*	*	*	*	0	*	*	0	100	6	26	160
Cream Cheese, rts (Pillsbury)	for ½ cake prep	0	0	0	0	0	0	0	0	115	6	26	160

		% U.S. RDA												
Cream Cheese and Nuts (Betty Crocker)	1/12 pkg prep	*	0	*	*	0	*	*	*	0	110	6	24	150
Dark Chocolate Fudge (Betty Crocker)	1/12 pkg prep	2	*	2	*	*	*	*	*	4	90	6	30	170
Dark Dutch Fudge, rts (Betty Crocker)	1/12 can prep	*	*	*	*	0	*	*	*	2	100	7	23	160
Double Dutch (Pillsbury Rich 'n Easy)	for 1/12 cake prep	0	0	0	0	0	0	0	0	0	80	4	26	150
Double Dutch, rts (Pillsbury)	for 1/12 cake prep	0	0	0	0	0	0	0	0	0	45	7	22	150
Lemon, Creamy (Betty Crocker)	1/12 pkg prep	2	*	2	*	0	*	*	*	0	100	6	30	170
Lemon (Pillsbury Rich 'n Easy)	for 1/12 cake prep	0	0	0	0	0	0	0	0	0	15	5	25	140
Lemon, rts (Betty Crocker)	1/12 can prep	*	*	*	*	0	*	*	*	0	100	6	26	160
Lemon, rts (Pillsbury)	for 1/12 cake prep	0	0	0	0	0	0	0	0	0	80	6	26	160
Milk Chocolate (Betty Crocker)	1/12 pkg prep	2	*	2	*	0	*	*	*	0	80	5	30	170
Milk Chocolate (Pillsbury Rich 'n Easy)	for 1/12 cake prep	0	0	0	0	0	0	0	0	0	55	5	26	150
Milk Chocolate, rts (Betty Crocker)	1/12 can prep	*	*	*	*	0	*	*	*	0	100	7	24	160
Milk Chocolate, rts (Pillsbury)	for 1/12 cake prep	0	0	0	0	0	0	0	0	0	60	6	23	150
Orange, rts (Betty Crocker)	1/12 can prep	*	*	*	*	0	*	*	*	0	90	6	26	160

Frostings	Amt.	Protein	A	C	B₁	B₂	Niacin	Calcium	Iron	Sodium (mg)	Fat (g)	Carbohydrate (g)	Calories
								% U.S. RDA					
Sour Cream Chocolate Fudge (Betty Crocker)	½ pkg prep	*	2	*	*	0	*	*	4	75	6	30	170
Sour Cream Chocolate, rts (Betty Crocker)	½ can prep	*	*	*	*	0	*	*	4	100	8	22	170
Sour Cream Vanilla, rts (Pillsbury)	for ½ cake prep	0	0	0	0	0	0	0	0	80	6	27	160
Sour Cream White (Betty Crocker)	½ pkg prep	*	2	*	*	0	*	*	0	100	5	31	170
Sour Cream White, rts (Betty Crocker)	½ can prep	*	*	*	*	0	*	*	0	100	6	26	160
Strawberry (Pillsbury Rich 'n Easy)	for ½ cake prep	0	0	0	0	0	0	0	0	55	5	25	140
Strawberry, rts (Pillsbury)	for ½ cake prep	0	0	0	0	0	0	0	0	75	6	26	160
Vanilla (Pillsbury Rich 'n Easy)	for ½ cake prep	0	0	0	0	0	0	0	0	30	5	25	150
Vanilla, rts (Betty Crocker)	½ can prep	*	*	*	*	0	*	*	0	100	6	27	160
Vanilla, rts (Pillsbury)	for ½ cake prep	0	0	0	0	0	0	0	0	75	6	26	160
White, Fluffy (Betty Crocker)	½ pkg prep	*	0	*	*	0	*	*	0	40	0	16	60
White, Creamy (Betty Crocker)	½ pkg prep	*	2	*	*	0	*	*	0	100	6	31	180
White, Fluffy (Pillsbury)	for ½ cake prep	0	0	0	0	0	0	0	0	65	0	15	60

158

Frozen Dinners

		% U.S. RDA											
Bean and Beef Burrito (Swanson 4-Compartment)	15¼ oz	40	30	10	30	25	25	15	25	1635	32	88	720
Beans and Franks (Swanson 3-Compartment)	12½ oz	25	4	10	10	10	10	10	20	1100	20	75	550
Beef (Swanson 4-Compartment)	11½ oz	50	25	10	10	15	25	2	25	1085	9	34	320
Beef, Chopped Sirloin (Swanson 4-Compartment)	11½ oz	40	120	15	4	15	30	10	30	915	18	32	370
Beef, Chopped Sirloin (Swanson Le Menu)	12¼ oz	50	*	15	6	20	30	15	25	1115	24	30	420
Beef Enchiladas (Swanson 4-Compartment)	15 oz	30	25	8	15	10	15	15	20	1415	23	57	510
Beef Sirloin Tips (Swanson Le Menu)	11½ oz	50	8	40	10	25	25	10	25	1100	18	24	390
Beef, Sliced (Swanson Hungry-Man)	16 oz	70	8	6	8	30	45	2	30	1250	11	60	490
Beef Steak, Chopped (Swanson Hungry-Man)	17¼ oz	60	30	30	6	25	45	6	35	2030	37	42	620
Chicken, Boneless (Swanson Hungry-Man)	17½ oz	100	20	8	30	30	50	8	40	1525	30	77	790
Chicken, Fried, Barbecue Flavored (Swanson 4-Compartment)	9½ oz	50	15	20	15	20	25	4	20	845	24	51	520

Frozen Dinners	Amt.	Pro-tein	A	C	B₁	B₂	Nia-cin	Cal-cium	Iron	Sodium (mg)	Fat (g)	Carbohy-drate (g)	Calories
							% U.S. RDA						
Chicken, Fried, Breast Portion (Swanson 4-Compartment)	10¾ oz	50	*	15	20	15	35	4	15	1425	32	62	650
Chicken, Fried, Breast Portions (Swanson Hungry-Man)	14 oz	70	*	25	25	25	45	10	20	2060	47	77	870
Chicken, Fried, Dark Meat (Swanson 4-Compartment)	10¼ oz	45	*	15	20	25	15	2	20	1345	31	55	600
Chicken, Fried, Dark Portions (Swanson Hungry-Man)	14 oz	60	10	25	15	30	50	6	35	1640	48	79	890
Chicken a la King (Swanson Le Menu)	10¼ oz	45	15	10	4	10	25	6	10	1170	13	29	320
Chicken Parmigiana (Swanson Hungry-Man)	20 oz	70	60	50	15	35	40	30	15	2205	52	55	820
Chicken, Breast of, Parmigiana (Swanson Le Menu)	11½ oz	40	15	35	10	15	35	15	15	950	21	26	410
Chicken, Sweet and Sour (Swanson Le Menu)	11¼ oz	45	50	15	8	15	30	8	10	960	22	45	460
Eggs, Scrambled, and Sausage w Hash Brown Potatoes (Swanson)	6¼ oz	20	*	4	15	20	8	6	15	790	34	17	420
Fish 'n Chips (Swanson)	5½ oz	15	*	4	10	8	10	2	10	585	16	31	310

160

		% U.S. RDA										
Fish 'n Chips (Swanson 4-Compartment)	10½ oz	30	8	8	20	10	20	4	15	970	30	59	590
Fish 'n Chips (Swanson Hungry-Man)	14¾ oz	45	10	10	40	30	25	6	25	1280	46	78	850
Lasagna (Swanson 4-Compartment)	13 oz	15	10	30	15	2	15	15	15	780	19	54	420
Lasagna w Meat (Swanson Hungry-Man)	18¾ oz	45	25	50	35	30	25	30	40	1395	24	90	680
Macaroni and Beef (Swanson 3-Compartment)	12 oz	20	8	15	4	10	15	10	15	925	15	46	370
Macaroni and Cheese (Swanson 3-Compartment)	12¼ oz	15	60	10	10	10	6	20	10	970	15	47	380
Meat Loaf (Swanson 4-Compartment)	11 oz	35	6	35	10	10	25	8	20	1010	26	49	510
Mexican (Swanson Hungry-Man)	22 oz	50	45	10	20	35	40	35	45	2000	42	103	910
Mexican Style Combination (Swanson 4-Compartment)	16 oz	30	30	15	15	6	15	10	15	1865	29	66	590
Noodles and Chicken (Swanson 3-Compartment)	10½ oz	15	6	10	10	6	15	2	10	805	9	37	270
Omelet w Cheese Sauce and Ham (Swanson)	7 oz	30	10	2	10	30	6	20	15	1180	32	11	400
Omelet, Spanish Style (Swanson)	8 oz	10	10	40	6	20	6	10	15	895	18	16	250

161

Frozen Dinners	Amt.	Pro-tein	A	C	B₁	B₂	Nia-cin	Cal-cium	Iron	Sodium (mg)	Fat (g)	Carbohy-drate (g)	Calories
					% U.S. RDA								
Pepper Steak (Swanson Le Menu)	11½ oz	40	20	20	4	15	20	4	25	1045	13	34	360
Polynesian Style (Swanson)	12 oz	30	6	*	10	10	20	8	15	1355	19	65	510
Pork, Loin of (Swanson 4-Compartment)	11¼ oz	40	50	20	35	8	25	2	10	635	13	26	310
Salisbury Steak (Swanson 4-Compartment)	11 oz	40	*	10	10	15	30	8	25	1055	21	46	460
Salisbury Steak (Swanson Hungry-Man)	16½ oz	70	130	10	10	30	45	20	35	1565	41	45	710
Spaghetti and Meatballs (Swanson 3-Compartment)	12½ oz	25	20	20	15	10	15	10	15	1065	14	57	410
Swiss Steak (Swanson 4-Compartment)	10 oz	45	*	10	15	15	15	10	25	830	14	38	360
Turkey (Swanson 4-Compartment)	11½ oz	40	6	10	15	10	35	4	15	1295	10	42	340
Turkey (Swanson Hungry-Man)	18½ oz	80	10	20	25	30	70	8	30	2110	17	80	630
Turkey, Breast of, Sliced, w Mushrooms (Swanson Le Menu)	11¼ oz	50	40	20	6	15	50	4	10	1165	24	36	470
Veal Parmigiana (Swanson 4-Compartment)	12¾ oz	40	25	20	15	20	25	15	15	1280	25	42	480

Food	Measure					Protein	Vit. A	Vit. C	Thiamine	Riboflavin	Niacin	Calcium	Iron
						% U.S. RDA							
Veal Parmigiana (Swanson Hungry-Man)	20 oz	560	64	23	2075	40	20	50	40	20	50	45	60
Western Style (Swanson)	12¼ oz	430	44	18	1040	25	6	20	10	6	10	30	70
Western Style (Swanson Hungry-Man)	17½ oz	650	61	29	1900	35	8	35	20	10	20	35	50
Yankee Pot Roast (Swanson Le Menu)	11 oz	360	29	15	830	25	4	25	15	8	15	130	50
Fruit, Fresh													
Apples, Raw w Skin	1 med (3 per lb)	80	20	1	1	2	*	*	2	2	10	2	2
Apricots, Raw w Skin	3 (12 per lb)	60	14	0–1	1	2	2	4	2	2	20	60	4
Avocado, Raw, California	½	190	7	19	4	4	2	8	8	8	25	6	8
Avocado, Raw, California, ½" Cubes	1 c	260	9	26	6	4	2	10	20	10	35	8	10
Avocado, Raw, Florida	½	200	14	17	6	4	2	10	20	10	35	8	8
Avocado, Raw, Florida, ½" Cubes	1 c	190	14	17	6	4	2	10	20	10	35	8	8
Bananas, Raw	1 med (8¾")	100	27	0–1	1	4	*	4	4	4	20	4	4
Bananas, Raw, Sliced	1 c	130	34	0–1	2	6	2	4	6	4	25	6	6
Banana Flakes	1 c	340	89	0–1	4	15	4	15	15	10	10	15	15
Blackberries, Raw	1 c	80	19	2	1	8	4	4	4	2	50	2	6
Blueberries, Raw	1 c	90	22	0–1	1	8	2	4	6	2	35	2	8
Cantaloupe, Raw	½ (5" diam)	80	21	0–1	33	6	4	8	4	8	50	180	4
Casaba Melon, Raw	2" × 7¾" wedge	40	9	0–1	17	4	2	4	2	4	30	*	2

163

Fruit, Fresh	Amt.	Pro-tein	A	C	B$_1$	B$_2$	Nia-cin	Cal-cium	Iron	Sodium (mg)	Fat (g)	Carbohy-drate (g)	Calories
		% U.S. RDA											
Cherries, Raw, Sour, Pitted	1 c	2	30	25	6	6	4	4	4	3	0-1	23	90
Cherries, Raw, Sweet, Whole	10	2	2	10	2	2	2	2	2	1	0-1	12	45
Cherries, Raw, Sweet, Pitted	1 c	2	4	25	4	6	4	4	4	3	0-1	26	100
Cranberries, Raw	1 c	*	*	15	2	2	*	2	2	2	1	11	45
Dates, Pitted, Chopped	1 c	6	2	*	10	10	20	10	30	2	1	130	490
Grapes, Raw, American Type (Slip Skin)	1 c	2	2	6	4	2	2	2	2	3	1	16	70
Grapes, Raw, European Type (Adherent Skin)	1 c	2	4	10	6	2	2	2	4	5	1	28	110
Grapefruit, Pink Seedless, Raw	½ med (3¾" diam)	*	10	70	4	2	*	2	2	1	0-1	13	50
Grapefruit, White Seedless, Raw	½ med	*	*	70	4	2	*	2	2	1	0-1	12	45
Grapefruit, Pink, Raw, Sections	1 c w 2 tbsp juice	2	20	140	6	2	2	4	4	2	0-1	24	90
Grapefruit, White, Raw, Sections	1 c w 2 tbsp juice	2	*	140	6	2	2	4	4	2	0-1	24	90
Honeydew Melon	7" × 2" wedge	2	2	60	4	2	4	2	4	18	0-1	12	50
Kumquats, Raw w Skin	1 med	*	2	10	*	2	*	2	*	1	0-1	3	12
Lemons, Raw	1 med (2⅛" diam)	2	*	70	2	*	*	2	2	1	0-1	6	20

Food	Serving							% U.S. RDA						Calories
Loganberries, Raw	1 c	2	6	60	2	4	4	4	10	1	1	22	90
Mango, Raw	1	2	190	120	6	6	10	2	4	NA	NA	NA	130
Nectarines, Raw w Skin	1 (2½" diam)	2	45	30	2	4	6	*	4	8	0–1	24	90
Oranges, Raw	1 (2⅝" diam)	2	6	110	8	2	2	6	2	1	0–1	NA	60
Oranges, Sections w/o Membranes	1 c	2	8	150	10	4	4	8	4	2	0–1	22	90
Papaya, Raw, ½" Cubes	1 c	2	50	130	4	4	2	2	2	4	0–1	14	55
Peaches, Raw	1 (2½" diam)	*	25	10	2	2	4	*	2	1	0–1	10	40
Peaches, Raw, Sliced	1 c	2	45	20	2	4	8	2	4	2	0–1	17	70
Pears, Raw w Skin	1 (3½" × 2½")	2	*	10	2	4	*	2	2	3	1	25	100
Pears, Raw, Sliced w Skin	1 c	2	*	10	2	4	*	2	2	3	1	26	100
Pineapple, Raw, Diced	1 c	*	2	45	10	2	2	4	4	2	0–1	22	80
Plums, Raw w Skin	1 (2⅛" diam)	*	4	6	2	2	2	*	2	1	0–1	8	30
Pomegranate, Raw	1 (3⅜" diam)	2	*	10	4	2	2	*	2	5	0–1	25	100
Prunes, "Softenized," Uncooked	10 med	2	20	4	4	6	4	4	15	5	0–1	44	160
Prunes, Cooked, Unsweetened	1 c w liq	4	30	4	4	9	8	6	20	9	1	67	250
Raisins, Seedless	1 c pressed down	6	*	4	10	8	4	10	30	45	0–1	128	480
Raspberries, Black, Raw	1 c	4	*	40	2	8	6	4	6	1	2	21	100
Raspberries, Red, Raw	1 c	2	4	50	2	6	6	2	6	1	0–1	17	70
Rhubarb, Cooked, Sweetened	1 c	2	4	25	4	8	4	20	8	5	0–1	98	380

Fruit, Fresh	Amt.	Pro-tein	A	C	B₁	B₂	Nia-cin	Cal-cium	Iron	Sodium (mg)	Fat (g)	Carbohy-drate (g)	Calories
		% U.S. RDA											
Strawberries, Raw, Whole, Capped	1 c	2	2	150	2	6	4	4	8	1	1	13	60
Tangelo, Raw	1 med (2⁹/₁₆″ diam)	*	8	45	4	2	*	2	2	0	0–1	9	40
Tangerines, Raw	1 (2³/₈″ diam)	2	8	45	4	2	*	4	2	2	0–1	10	40
Watermelon, Raw, Diced	1 c	2	20	20	4	2	2	2	4	2	0–1	10	40
Watermelon	¹/₁₆ (10″×16″ melon)	4	50	50	8	8	4	2	10	4	1	28	110
Fruit, Dried													
Apples, Dried, Cooked, Un-sweetened	1 c	2	*	*	2	4	2	2	8	3	1	52	200
Apples, Dried, Sliced, Un-cooked (Del Monte)	2 oz	0	*	*	*	6	2	*	4	0–50	0	37	140
Apricots, Dried, Uncooked	10 med halves	2	80	*	*	4	6	2	10	9	0–1	24	90
Apricots, Dried, Uncooked (Del Monte)	2 oz	2	90	*	*	4	8	2	15	0–10	0	35	140
Currants, Zante (Del Monte)	½ c	2	*	4	6	6	6	6	10	0–10	0	53	200
Dates, Chopped (Dromedary)	¼ c	*	*	*	*	4	2	2	4	NA	0	31	130
Dates, Pitted (Dromedary)	5	*	*	*	*	4	2	2	4	NA	0	23	100
Mixed (Carnation All Fruit Mix)	1 pouch	*	2	*	*	*	*	*	2	10	0	18	80
Mixed (Del Monte)	2 oz	*	25	*	*	4	2	2	8	10	0	34	130

Food	Serving												
		% U.S. RDA											
Peaches, Dried, Uncooked	1 c	8	120	50	2	20	45	8	60	26	1	110	420
Peaches, Dried, Cooked, Unsweetened	1 c w liq	4	60	8	*	8	20	4	25	13	1	54	210
Peaches, Dried, Uncooked (Del Monte)	2 oz	2	25	*	*	6	10	*	10	0–10	0	35	140
Pears, Dried, Uncooked	1 c	8	2	20	2	20	6	6	15	13	3	121	480
Pears, Dried, Cooked, Un-sweetened	1 c w liq	6	2	8	*	10	4	4	8	8	2	81	320
Prunes, Moist (Del Monte Moist-Pak)	2 oz	2	15	2	2	4	4	2	10	0–10	0	30	120
Prunes, Dried, Uncooked w Pits (Del Monte)	2 oz	2	15	2	2	4	4	2	6	0–10	0	31	120
Prunes, Dried, Uncooked, Pitted (Del Monte)	2 oz	2	15	2	2	4	4	2	6	0–10	0	35	140
Raisins, Golden (Del Monte)	3 oz	4	4	*	*	6	4	4	8	0–10	0	68	260
Raisins, Natural (Del Monte)	3 oz	4	*	*	8	6	6	4	10	15	0	68	250
Fruit, Canned and Frozen													
Apples, Frozen, Escalloped (Stouffer's)	4 oz	*	*	*	*	15	*	*	10	50	3	28	140
Applesauce, Canned (Del Monte)	½ c	0	0	2	*	*	*	0	2	0–5	0	24	90
Applesauce, Canned (Del Monte Lite)	½ c	0	0	15	15	*	*	0	*	0–10	0	13	50

Fruit, Canned and Frozen	Amt.	% U.S. RDA							Iron	Sodium (mg)	Fat (g)	Carbohy-drate (g)	Calories
		Pro-tein	A	C	B₁	B₂	Nia-cin	Cal-cium					
Applesauce, Canned (Mott's)	8 oz	*	*	10	2	4	*	*	2	3.4	0	55	230
Applesauce, Canned, Natural Style (Mott's)	8 oz	*	*	10	2	4	*	*	2	3.2	0	22	100
Apricots, Canned, Halves (Del Monte)	½ c	0	10	6	*	*	2	*	2	0-10	0	26	100
Apricots, Canned, Halves (Del Monte Lite)	½ c	0	10	6	*	*	2	*	*	0-10	0	16	60
Apricots, Canned, Whole (Del Monte)	½ c	0	10	4	*	*	2	*	2	0-10	0	27	100
Cherries, Canned, Dark, Sweet w Pits (Del Monte)	½ c	0	4	6	*	2	*	*	2	0-10	0	23	90
Cherries, Canned, Dark, Sweet, Pitted (Del Monte)	½ c	0	4	6	*	2	2	*	2	0-10	0	24	90
Cherries, Canned, Light, Sweet w Pits (Del Monte)	½ c	0	2	4	*	2	2	*	2	0-10	0	26	100
Figs, Canned, Whole (Del Monte)	½ c	0	*	2	*	2	2	2	*	0-10	0	28	100
Fruit Cocktail, Canned (Del Monte)	½ c	0	4	4	*	*	2	0	2	0-10	0	23	80

Food	Serving	% U.S. RDA											Calories
Fruit Cocktail, Canned (Del Monte Lite)	½ c	0	4	4	*	*	*	0	*	0–10	0	15	50
Fruit Compote, Canned (Rokeach)	4 oz	*	15	3	*	5	4	2	5	4	1	31	120
Fruits for Salad, Canned (Del Monte)	½ c	0	2	4	2	2	2	0	*	0–10	0	22	90
Fruit Salad, Canned (Del Monte Tropical)	½ c	0	2	30	2	2	2	*	2	0–10	0	26	90
Mandarin Oranges, Canned (Del Monte)	5½ oz	*	8	50	4	2	*	*	2	0–10	0	25	100
Mixed Fruit, Canned, Chunky (Del Monte)	½ c	0	4	4	*	2	2	0	2	0–10	0	23	80
Mixed Fruit, Canned, Chunky (Del Monte Lite)	½ c	0	4	4	*	2	2	0	*	0–10	0	14	50
Mixed Fruit, Canned, Individual Serving (Del Monte Fruit Cup)	5 oz	*	4	100	*	2	2	*	2	0–10	0	27	100
Mixed Fruit, Canned (Mother's)	4 oz	*	15	3	*	5	4	2	5	4	1	31	120
Mixed Fruit, Frozen, in Lite Syrup (Birds Eye Quick Thaw)	5 oz	*	8	45	*	4	2	*	2	5	0	27	100
Peaches, Canned, Cling (Del Monte)	½ c	0	6	4	*	*	4	0	*	0–10	0	22	80
Peaches, Canned, Cling, Halves or Slices (Del Monte Lite)	½ c	0	6	4	*	*	4	0	*	0–10	0	13	50

Fruit, Canned and Frozen	Amt.	Protein	A	C	B₁	B₂	Niacin	Calcium	Iron	Sodium (mg)	Fat (g)	Carbohydrate (g)	Calories
		%U.S. RDA											
Peaches, Canned, Cling, Individual Serving (Del Monte Fruit Cup)	5 oz	*	6	100	*	2	4	*	2	0–10	0	28	110
Peaches, Canned, Freestone, Halves or Slices (Del Monte)	½ c	0	2	2	*	*	4	0	*	0–10	0	23	90
Peaches, Canned, Freestone (Del Monte Lite)	½ c	0	2	2	*	*	4	0	*	0–10	0	13	60
Peaches, Canned, Spiced w Pits (Del Monte)	3½ oz	0	6	25	*	*	2	0	*	0–10	0	20	80
Pears, Canned, Bartlett, Halves or Slices (Del Monte)	½ c	0	0	2	*	*	*	0	*	0–10	0	22	80
Pears, Canned, Bartlett, Halves or Slices (Del Monte Lite)	½ c	0	0	2	*	*	*	0	*	0–10	0	14	50
Pineapple, Canned in Juice, Crushed, Chunk, Tidbits, or Slices (Del Monte)	½ c	0	*	6	6	*	*	*	*	0–10	0	18	70
Pineapple, Canned in Juice, Spears (Del Monte)	2 spears	0	2	4	6	2	2	2	2	10	0	14	50
Pineapple, Canned in Syrup, Crushed, Chunks, or Slices (Del Monte)	½ c	0	*	6	6	*	2	*	*	0–10	0	23	90

Food	Measure	% U.S. RDA												
Prunes, Canned, Stewed (Rokeach)	½ c	*	8	2	*	4	4	2	8	0	0–5	0	25	90
Raspberries, Red, Frozen, in Lite Syrup (Birds Eye Quick Thaw)	5 oz	*	*	30	*	4	4	2	6	0	0	0	26	100
Strawberries, Frozen, Halves, in Lite Syrup (Birds Eye Quick Thaw)	5 oz	*	*	110	*	4	2	*	4	0	5	0	16	60
Strawberries, Frozen, Halves, in Syrup (Birds Eye Quick Thaw)	5 oz	*	*	110	*	4	2	2	6	0	5	0	30	120
Strawberries, Frozen, Whole, in Lite Syrup (Birds Eye)	4 oz	*	*	120	*	4	*	*	4	0	0	0	14	60
Fruit Fillings														
Mincemeat, Condensed (None Such)	¼ pkg	2	*	*	*	4	4	4	10	2	330	2	50	220
Mincemeat w Brandy and Rum (None Such)	⅓ c	*	*	*	*	2	2	4	6	2	265	2	48	220
Fruit Juices														
Apple (Mott's)	6 fl oz	*	*	*	*	6	6	*	2	0	6	0	19	80
Apple (Mott's Natural Style)	6 fl oz	*	*	*	*	6	6	*	2	0	6	0	19	80
Apple Grape, Frozen, Reconstituted (Welch's Orchard)	6 fl oz	*	*	*	*	*	*	*	*	0	0–10	0	23	90

Fruit Juices	Amt.	Protein	A	C	B_1	B_2	Niacin	Calcium	Iron	Sodium (mg)	Fat (g)	Carbohydrate (g)	Calories
Apricot Nectar, Canned (Del Monte)	6 fl oz	*	40	50	2	2	2	*	4	0–10	0	26	100
Blend, Frozen, Reconstituted (Welch's Orchard Frozen Harvest)	6 fl oz	*	*	*	*	*	*	*	*	0–10	0	23	90
Grape, Bottled (Welch's)	6 fl oz	*	*	45	2	2	2	*	*	0–10	0	30	120
Grape, Red, Bottled (Welch's)	6 fl oz	*	*	45	2	*	2	2	2	0–10	0	30	120
Grape, White, Bottled (Welch's)	6 fl oz	*	*	45	*	*	*	2	2	0–10	0	30	120
Grape, Frozen, Reconstituted (Minute Maid)	6 fl oz	*	*	10	2	2	2	*	*	2	0–1	25	100
Grape, Frozen, Reconstituted (Welch's)	6 fl oz	*	*	45	*	*	*	*	*	NA	0	25	100
Grape, Frozen, Reconstituted (Welch's Orchard)	6 fl oz	*	*	*	*	*	*	*	*	0–10	0	30	120
Grape, Red, Sparkling (Welch's)	6 fl oz	*	*	*	2	*	*	2	2	NA	0	30	120
Grape, White, Sparkling (Welch's)	6 fl oz	*	*	*	*	*	*	2	2	NA	0	30	120
Grapefruit, Fresh	8 fl oz	2	4	160	6	2	2	2	2	2	0–1	23	100
Grapefruit (Ocean Spray)	6 fl oz	*	*	60	*	*	*	*	*	0–10	0	15	60

Food	Serving	% U.S. RDA										Calories
Grapefruit, Canned, Unsweetened (Del Monte)	6 fl oz	*	*	90	4	2	2	*	2	0–10	0	17	70
Grapefruit, Frozen, Reconstituted (Minute Maid)	6 fl oz	*	*	120	4	2	2	2	*	Trace	0–1	18	75
Grapefruit, Frozen, Reconstituted (Ocean Spray)	6 fl oz	*	*	70	*	*	*	2	*	0–10	0	16	70
Lemon, Fresh	8 fl oz	2	2	190	4	2	2	2	2	2	0–1	20	60
Lemon (ReaLemon)	2 tbsp	*	*	15	*	*	*	*	*	10	0	2	6
Lemon, Frozen, Reconstituted (Minute Maid)	6 fl oz	*	*	130	2	*	*	2	2	2	0–1	13	40
Lime, Fresh	8 fl oz	2	*	130	4	2	*	2	2	2	0–1	22	60
Lime (ReaLime)	2 tbsp	*	*	8	*	*	*	*	*	10	0	1	4
Orange, Fresh	8 fl oz	2	10	210	15	4	4	2	2	2	0–1	26	110
Orange, Canned, Unsweetened (Del Monte)	6 fl oz	*	4	120	6	2	2	2	4	0–10	0	19	80
Orange, Dairy Case (Minute Maid)	6 fl oz	2	6	90	10	2	*	2	*	1	0–1	20	85
Orange, Frozen, Reconstituted (Minute Maid)	6 fl oz	2	8	150	10	2	*	2	*	1	0–1	21	90
Orange, Imitation, Frozen, Reconstituted (Birds Eye Awake)	6 fl oz	*	*	100	*	45	*	2	*	15	0	21	80
Orange, Imitation, Frozen, Reconstituted (Birds Eye Orange Plus)	6 fl oz	*	*	100	10	2	*	2	*	10	0	24	100

Fruit Juices	Amt.	Pro-tein	A	C	B₁	B₂	Nia-cin	Cal-cium	Iron	Sodium (mg)	Fat (g)	Carbohy-drate (g)	Calories
Orange, Imitation (Bright and Early)	6 fl oz	*	20	180	15	*	*	*	*	0	2	22	100
Pineapple, Canned, Unsweetened (Del Monte)	6 fl oz	0	*	100	6	2	2	2	4	0–10	0	25	100
Prune, Canned, Unsweetened (Del Monte)	6 fl oz	*	*	10	2	*	6	*	8	0–10	0	33	120
Prune, Canned (Super Mott's)	6 fl oz	2	*	70	2	6	8	2	10	NA	0	30	120
Tangerine, Frozen, Reconstituted (Minute Maid)	6 fl oz	*	10	60	6	2	*	2	2	2	0–1	21	85
Fruit Drinks													
Apple (Hi-C)	6 fl oz	*	*	100	*	*	*	*	2	12	0	22	90
Apple, Mix (Kool-Aid)	8 fl oz	*	*	10	*	*	*	2	*	0	0	24	100
Apple, Mix (Wyler's Crystals)	8 fl oz	*	*	15	*	*	*	*	*	25	0	22	90
Black Cherry, Mix, Un-sweetened (Wyler's)	8 fl oz	*	*	15	*	*	*	*	*	NA	0	1	2
Cherry (Hi-C)	6 fl oz	*	*	100	*	*	*	*	*	4	0	23	90
Cherry, Mix (Kool-Aid)	8 fl oz	*	*	10	*	*	*	*	*	5	0	23	90
Cherry, Mix, Sugar Free (Kool-Aid)	8 fl oz	*	*	10	*	*	*	4	*	5	0	0	4
Citrus Cooler (Hi-C)	6 fl oz	*	*	100	*	*	*	*	*	4	0	23	90

% U.S. RDA

										% U.S. RDA			
Cranberry Juice Cocktail (Ocean Spray)	6 fl oz	*	*	100	*	*	*	*	*	*	*	0-10	0	26	110
Cranberry Juice Cocktail, Low Calorie (Ocean Spray)	6 fl oz	*	*	100	*	*	*	*	*	*	*	0-10	0	9	35
Cranberry Juice Cocktail, Frozen, Reconstituted (Ocean Spray)	6 fl oz	*	*	100	*	*	*	*	*	*	*	0-10	0	28	110
Cranberry Juice Cocktail, Frozen, Reconstituted (Welch's)	6 fl oz	*	*	45	*	*	*	*	*	*	*	NA	0	26	100
Cranberry Apple (Ocean Spray Cranapple)	6 fl oz	*	*	100	*	*	*	*	*	*	*	0-10	0	32	130
Cranberry Apple, Low Calorie (Ocean Spray)	6 fl oz	*	*	100	*	*	*	*	*	*	*	0-10	0	7	30
Cranberry Apple, Frozen, Reconstituted (Ocean Spray Cranapple)	6 fl oz	*	*	100	*	*	*	*	*	*	*	0-10	0	29	120
Cranberry Apple, Frozen, Reconstituted (Welch's)	6 fl oz	*	*	45	*	*	*	*	*	*	*	NA	0	30	120
Cranberry Apricot (Ocean Spray Cranicot)	6 fl oz	*	*	0	*	*	*	*	*	*	*	0-10	0	26	110
Cranberry Grape (Ocean Spray Cran-Grape)	6 fl oz	*	*	100	*	*	*	*	*	*	*	0-10	0	26	110
Cranberry Grape, Frozen, Reconstituted (Welch's)	6 fl oz	*	*	45	*	*	*	*	*	*	*	NA	0	27	110

Fruit Drinks	Amt.	Protein	A	C	B_1	B_2	Niacin	Calcium	Iron	Sodium (mg)	Fat (g)	Carbohydrate (g)	Calories
					% U.S. RDA								
Cranberry Orange, Frozen, Reconstituted (Ocean Spray Cranorange)	6 fl oz	*	*	100	*	*	*	*	*	0–10	0	25	100
Grape (Hi-C)	6 fl oz	*	*	100	*	*	*	*	*	0–1	0	23	100
Grape (Welchade)	6 fl oz	*	*	45	*	*	*	*	*	NA	0	23	90
Grape (Welch's Concord Juice Cocktail)	6 fl oz	*	*	45	*	*	*	*	*	0–10	0	27	110
Grape (Welch's Grape Juice Drink)	6 fl oz	*	*	45	*	*	*	*	*	NA	0	27	110
Grape, Frozen, Reconstituted (Welch's)	6 fl oz	*	*	45	*	*	*	*	*	NA	0	23	90
Grape, Mix (Kool-Aid)	8 fl oz	*	*	10	*	*	*	*	*	0	0	23	90
Grape, Mix (Tang)	6 fl oz	*	10	100	*	*	*	4	*	5	0	23	90
Grape, Mix, Sugar Free (Kool-Aid)	8 fl oz	*	*	10	*	*	*	4	*	0	0	0	4
Grape and Apple (Welch's Concord 'n Apple Juice Cocktail)	6 fl oz	*	*	45	*	*	*	*	*	0–10	0	27	110
Grapefruit, Mix (Tang)	6 fl oz	*	10	100	*	*	*	4	*	0	0	22	90
Lemonade, Frozen, Reconstituted (Minute Maid)	6 fl oz	*	*	15	*	*	*	*	*	1	0	20	75
Lemonade, Mix, Regular or Pink (Country Time)	8 fl oz	*	*	15	*	*	*	*	*	30	0	22	90

Food	Serving					% U.S. RDA						
Lemonade, Mix, Regular or Pink (Kool-Aid)	8 fl oz	*	*	10	*	*	4	*	0	0	22	90
Lemonade, Mix (Wyler's Crystals)	8 fl oz	*	*	15	*	*	*	*	NA	0	22	90
Lemonade, Mix, Sugar Free (Country Time)	8 fl oz	*	*	15	*	*	*	*	0	0	0	4
Lemonade, Mix, Sugar Free (Crystal Light)	8 fl oz	*	*	10	*	*	*	*	0	0	0	4
Lemonade, Mix, Sugar Free (Kool-Aid)	8 fl oz	*	*	10	*	*	4	*	0	0	0	4
Lemonade, Mix, Sugar Free (Wyler's)	8 fl oz	*	*	15	*	*	*	*	35	0	2	6
Lemon-Lime, Mix (Country Time)	8 fl oz	*	*	15	*	*	*	*	30	0	22	90
Lemon-Lime, Mix, Sugar Free (Crystal Light)	8 fl oz	*	*	10	*	*	*	*	0	0	0	4
Limeade, Frozen, Reconstituted (Minute Maid)	6 fl oz	*	*	8	*	*	*	*	0-1	0	20	75
Orange (Bama)	6 fl oz	*	*	50	*	*	*	*	NA	0	22	90
Orange (Hi-C)	6 fl oz	*	*	100	*	*	*	*	58	0	24	100
Orange, Mix (Borden Instant Breakfast Drink)	4 fl oz	*	20	100	*	*	4	*	40	0	16	60
Orange, Mix (Kool-Aid)	8 fl oz	*	*	10	*	*	*	*	0	0	22	90
Orange, Mix (Tang)	6 fl oz	*	10	100	*	*	4	*	0	0	22	90

Fruit Drinks	Amt.	% U.S. RDA Protein	A	C	B₁	B₂	Niacin	Calcium	Iron	Sodium (mg)	Fat (g)	Carbohydrate (g)	Calories
Orange, Mix, Sugar Free (Crystal Light)	8 fl oz	*	*	10	*	*	*	*	*	0	0	0	4
Orange, Mix, Unsweetened, (Wyler's)	8 fl oz	*	*	15	*	*	*	*	*	NA	0	1	2
Pineapple Grapefruit, Canned (Del Monte)	6 fl oz	*	*	100	2	*	2	*	2	50	0	24	90
Pineapple Orange, Canned (Del Monte)	6 fl oz	*	15	100	2	*	2	*	2	20	0	24	90
Pineapple Pink Grapefruit, Canned (Del Monte)	6 fl oz	*	*	100	2	*	2	*	2	50	0	24	90
Punch (Bama)	6 fl oz	*	*	50	*	*	*	*	*	NA	0	22	90
Punch, (Hi-C) Florida	6 fl oz	*	*	100	*	*	*	*	*	3	0	26	100
Punch, Mix (Kool-Aid Rainbow)	8 fl oz	*	*	10	*	*	*	*	*	5	0	25	100
Punch, Mix (Kool-Aid Sunshine)	8 fl oz	*	*	10	*	*	*	2	*	5	0	24	100
Punch, Mix (Kool-Aid Tropical)	8 fl oz	*	*	10	*	*	*	*	*	0	0	25	100
Punch, Mix (Wyler's Crystals Tropical)	8 fl oz	*	*	15	*	*	*	*	*	NA	0	22	90
Punch, Mix, Sugar Free (Crystal Light)	8 fl oz	*	*	10	*	*	*	*	*	0	0	0	4

Food	Serving	% U.S. RDA										Calories
Punch, Mix, Sugar Free (Kool-Aid)	8 fl oz	*	10	*	*	*	*	*		5	0	4
Punch, Mix, Sugar Free (Wyler's Tropical)	8 fl oz	*	15	*	*	*	*	*	30	0	1	4
Raspberry, Mix (Kool-Aid)	8 fl oz	*	10	*	*	*	*	*	0	0	22	90
Strawberry (Hi-C)	6 fl oz	*	100	*	*	*	*	*	0-1	0	23	100
Strawberry, Mix (Kool-Aid)	8 fl oz	*	10	*	*	*	*	*	0	0	22	90
Wild Berry (Hi-C)	6 fl oz	*	100	*	2	*	*	*	5	0	23	90
Wild Cherry, Mix (Wyler's Crystals)	8 fl oz	*	15	*	*	*	*	*	NA	0	22	90
Wild Cherry, Mix, Sugar Free (Wyler's)	8 oz	*	15	*	*	*	*	*	20	0	1	4
Wild Grape, Mix (Wyler's Crystals)	8 fl oz	*	15	*	*	*	*	*	NA	0	22	90
Wild Grape, Mix, Sugar Free (Wyler's)	8 fl oz	*	15	*	*	*	*	*	20	0	1	4
Gelatin												
All Flavors (Jell-O)	½ c	*	*	*	*	*	*	*	40-80	0	19	80
Low Calorie, All Flavors (D-Zerta)	½ c	*	*	*	*	*	*	*	5	0	0	8
Drinking Gelatin, Orange Flavor (Knox)	1 env	*	*	*	*	*	*	*	25	0	10	70
Drinking Gelatin, Unflavored (Knox)	1 env	*	*	*	*	*	*	*	10	0	0	25

Ice Cream, Ice Milk, and Frozen Confections	Amt.	% U.S. RDA								Sodium (mg)	Fat (g)	Carbohydrate (g)	Calories
		Protein	A	C	B₁	B₂	Niacin	Calcium	Iron				
Ice Cream, Regular (10% Fat), Hardened	1 c	15	10	2	4	15	*	20	*	84	14	28	260
Ice Cream, Regular (10% Fat), Soft-Serve	1 c	15	15	4	4	20	*	25	2	109	19	36	330
Ice Cream, Regular, Buttered Pecan (Lady Borden)	½ c	4	8	*	*	8	*	8	*	NA	12	16	180
Ice Cream, Regular, Chocolate (Lady Borden)	½ c	4	8	*	*	6	*	8	*	NA	10	16	160
Ice Cream, Regular, Chocolate (Meadow Gold)	½ c	4	4	*	*	8	*	8	*	NA	6	18	140
Ice Cream, Regular, Chocolate (Meadow Olde Fashioned Recipe)	½ c	6	6	*	2	8	*	10	*	NA	7	16	140
Ice Cream, Regular, Dutch Chocolate (Borden)	½ c	4	4	*	*	8	*	8	*	NA	6	16	130
Ice Cream, Regular, Dutch Chocolate Almond (Borden All Natural)	½ c	4	6	*	2	8	*	10	*	NA	9	18	160
Ice Cream, Regular, French Vanilla (Borden All Natural)	½ c	6	6	*	2	10	*	10	*	NA	8	16	150
Ice Cream, Regular, French Vanilla (Lady Borden)	½ c	6	6	*	2	10	*	10	*	NA	9	20	170

Food	Serving				% U.S. RDA				Sodium (mg)			Calories
Ice Cream, Regular, Strawberry (Borden)	½ c	4	4	*	*	6	*	6	*	NA	5	17	120
Ice Cream, Regular, Strawberry (Meadow Gold)	½ c	4	4	*	2	8	*	8	*	NA	6	19	140
Ice Cream, Regular, Vanilla (Borden All Natural)	½ c	6	6	*	2	10	*	10	*	NA	7	17	140
Ice Cream, Regular, Vanilla (Borden)	½ c	4	6	*	2	8	*	8	*	NA	7	15	130
Ice Cream, Regular, Vanilla Flavored (Meadow Gold)	½ c	4	6	*	2	10	*	10	*	NA	7	16	140
Ice Cream, Slices, Vanilla (Good Humor)	1	4	4	*	*	8	*	6	*	45	6	13	110
Ice Cream, Slices, Vanilla (Good Humor Cal-Control)	1	4	*	*	*	4	*	6	*	45	1	11	60
Ice Cream Bar, Chip Crunch (Good Humor)	1	4	4	*	*	6	*	6	*	35	14	16	200
Ice Cream, Bar, Chocolate Eclair (Good Humor)	1	2	2	*	*	4	*	4	*	70	9	24	180
Ice Cream Bar, Chocolate Fudge Cake (Good Humor)	1	4	4	*	*	6	*	6	*	95	16	25	260
Ice Cream Bar, Chocolate Malt (Good Humor)	1	4	4	*	*	6	*	6	*	50	13	16	190

Ice Cream, Ice Milk, and Frozen Confections	Amt.	Protein	A	C	B₁	B₂	Niacin	Calcium	Iron	Sodium (mg)	Fat (g)	Carbohydrate (g)	Calories
		% U.S. RDA											
Ice Cream Bar, Toasted Almond (Good Humor)	1	2	2	*	*	4	*	4	*	30	8	28	190
Ice Cream Bar, Toasted Caramel (Good Humor)	1	4	4	*	*	6	*	6	*	55	9	21	170
Ice Cream Bar, Vanilla (Good Humor)	1	4	4	*	*	6	*	6	*	40	11	16	170
Ice Cream Cookie Sandwich (Good Humor) 2.7 oz	1	6	6	*	2	8	*	6	4	195	11	42	290
Ice Cream Cookie Sandwich (Good Humor) 4 oz	1	8	8	*	4	10	2	8	6	270	16	59	400
Ice Cream Sandwich, Vanilla (Good Humor)	1	4	2	*	*	6	*	6	*	120	5	28	170
Ice Cream, Specialty (Bon Bon Ice Cream Nuggets, Chocolate)	5 nuggets	2	*	*	*	4	*	4	*	53	12.1	15.3	172
Ice Cream, Specialty (Bon Bon Ice Cream Nuggets, Vanilla)	5 nuggets	2	*	*	*	4	*	4	*	38	12	13.8	167
Ice Milk, Hardened	1 c	15	6	2	4	15	*	20	*	89	7	30	200
Ice Milk, Soft-Serve	1 c	20	8	4	6	25	*	25	2	119	9	40	270

		% U.S. RDA											
Ice Milk, Chocolate (Borden All Natural)	½ c	6	2	*	2	10	*	10	*	NA	3	17	110
Ice Milk, Strawberry (Borden All Natural)	½ c	6	2	*	2	8	*	10	*	NA	3	18	110
Ice Milk, Vanilla (Borden All Natural)	½ c	6	2	*	2	10	*	10	*	NA	3	16	100
Ice Water, Flavored	1 c	2	*	4	*	*	*	*	*	0-10	0-1	63	250
Good Humor Fat Frog	1	4	4	*	*	8	*	8	*	45	7	17	140
Good Humor Heart	1	6	4	*	*	8	*	8	*	60	12	21	200
Good Humor Shark	1	*	*	*	*	*	*	*	*	0	0	17	70
Good Humor Whammy	1	2	2	*	*	4	*	2	*	25	6	9	90
Jell-O Pudding Pops, All Flavors	1 bar	6	*	*	*	6	*	8	*	65-100	3	16	90
Pudding Stix (Good Humor)	1	8	*	*	*	2	*	10	*	65	2	15	90
Sherbet, Lemon (Borden)	½ c	*	*	*	*	4	*	4	*	NA	1	25	110
Sherbet, Orange (Borden)	½ c	*	*	*	*	4	*	4	*	NA	1	25	110
Jellies and Jams													
Butter, Apple (Bama)	2 tsp	*	*	*	*	*	*	*	*	5	0	6	25
Butter, Apple (Smucker's)	2 tsp	*	*	*	*	*	*	*	*	0-10	0	6	25
Butter, Peach (Smucker's)	2 tsp	*	*	*	*	*	*	*	*	0-10	0	8	30
Jam, Red Plum (Bama)	2 tsp	*	*	*	*	*	*	*	*	5	0	8	30

Jellies and Jams	Amt.	Pro-tein	A	C	B₁	B₂	Nia-cin	Cal-cium	Iron	Sodium (mg)	Fat (g)	Carbohy-drate (g)	Calories
		% U.S. RDA											
Jellies, Jams, and Preserves, All Flavors (Smucker's)	2 tsp	*	*	*	*	*	*	*	*	0-10	0	9	35
Jellies, Jams, and Preserves, All Flavors (Welch's)	2 tsp	*	*	*	*	*	*	*	*	NA	0	9	35
Jellies and Preserves, Single Service (Smucker's)	1 (½ oz)	*	*	*	*	*	*	*	*	0-10	0	9	40
Jellies, Imitation, All Flavors (Smucker's)	2 tsp	*	*	*	*	*	*	*	*	0-10	0	1	4
Jellies, Imitation, Single Service (Smucker's)	1 (⅜ oz)	*	*	*	*	*	*	*	*	0-10	0	1	4
Jellies and Jams, Low Calorie Imitation, All Flavors (Smucker's Slenderella)	2 tsp	*	*	*	*	*	*	*	*	0-10	0	4	16
Jelly, Grape (Bama)	2 tsp	*	*	*	*	*	*	*	*	5	0	8	30
Jelly, Mint Flavored Apple (Bama)	2 tsp	*	*	*	*	*	*	*	*	NA	0	8	30
Preserves, Apricot (Bama)	2 tsp	*	*	*	*	*	*	*	*	NA	0	8	30
Spreads, Low Sugar, All Flavors (Smucker's)	2 tsp	*	*	*	*	*	*	*	*	0-10	0	4	16
Spreads, All Flavors (Welch's Lite)	2 tsp	*	*	*	*	*	*	*	*	NA	0	5	20

Legumes

		% U.S. RDA											
Beans, Baked, Red Kidney (B & M)	8 oz	25	*	*	8	8	6	4	35	776	7	50	330
Beans, Baked, Small Pea (B & M)	8 oz	25	*	*	2	6	6	10	40	848	8	49	330
Beans, Baked, Yellow-Eyed (B & M)	8 oz	25	*	*	6	10	6	4	35	968	7	50	330
Beans, Baked Style (Campbell's Home Style)	8 oz	15	4	6	4	2	4	10	20	1150	4	48	270
Beans, Baked Style (Campbell's Old Fashioned)	8 oz	15	*	10	2	2	4	10	20	1065	3	49	270
Beans, Baked Style w Franks (Heinz Beans 'n' Franks)	7¾ oz	NA	NA	NA	NA	NA	NA	10	15	905	15	34	330
Beans, Baked Style w Pork (Campbell's)	8 oz	15	4	4	6	2	4	10	15	945	4	44	250
Beans, Baked Style w Pork (Heinz)	8 oz	NA	NA	NA	NA	NA	4	15	20	745	4	46	250
Beans, Baked Style w Pork (Hunt's)	4 oz	10	2	4	10	4	4	4	10	446	1	26	140
Beans, Baked Style, Vegetarian (Heinz)	8 oz	NA	NA	NA	NA	NA	4	10	20	980	2	43	230
Beans, Barbecue (Campbell's)	7⅞ oz	15	6	4	6	4	4	8	15	1110	4	43	250
Beans, Burrito Filling Mix (Del Monte)	½ c	10	0	15	6	6	*	4	10	900	1	20	110

185

Legumes	Amt.	Protein	A	C	B$_1$	B$_2$	Niacin	Calcium	Iron	Sodium (mg)	Fat (g)	Carbohydrate (g)	Calories
		% U.S. RDA											
Beans, Chili (Hunt-Wesson)	4 oz	10	10	2	15	4	4	4	10	455	1	18	100
Beans, Garbanzo (Old El Paso)	½ c	6	0	0	*	*	*	3	8	247	1.3	12	77
Beans, Great Northern, Dry, Cooked, Drained	1 c	30	*	*	15	8	6	8	25	13	1	39	210
Beans, Lima, Dry, Cooked, Drained	1 c	35	*	*	15	6	6	6	35	4	1	49	260
Beans, Navy, Pea, Dry, Cooked, Drained	1 c	35	*	*	20	8	6	10	30	13	1	41	220
Beans, Red Kidney, Dry, Cooked, Drained	1 c	30	*	*	15	6	6	6	25	6	1	40	220
Beans, Red Kidney (Hunt's)	4 oz	10	*	*	6	4	4	4	18	400	0	21	120
Beans, Refried (Del Monte)	½ c	10	0	10	4	4	2	4	10	530	.2	20	130
Beans, Refried (Old El Paso)	¼ c	6	0	0	3	*	*	3	7	296	.6	10	60
Beans, Refried, w Green Chilies (Old El Paso)	¼ c	5	0	0	*	2	2	*	7	203	.4	10	25
Beans, Refried, w Sausage (Old El Paso)	¼ c	6	0	0	*	2	4	*	8	177	8	8	117
Beans, Refried, Spicy (Del Monte)	½ c	10	0	10	4	4	2	4	10	480	2	20	130
Cowpeas (Black-eyed), Dry, Cooked, Drained	1 c	30	*	25	25	6	4	4	20	20	1	35	190

							% U.S. RDA						
Lentils, Dry, Cooked	1 c	210	38	0–1	NA	25	4	6	8	10	*	35
Peas, Split, Dry, Cooked	1 c	230	42	1	26	20	2	8	10	20	2	35
Meat												
Bacon, Canadian Style (Eckrich Calorie Watcher)	1 oz	35	1	1	460	2	*	6	2	10	10	8
Bacon, Canadian Style (Oscar Mayer)	1 sl	40	0	2	393	*	*	7	2	13	12	12
Bacon, Cooked (Oscar Mayer)	1 sl	35	.1	3.1	114	*	*	*	*	2	3	3
Bacon Bits (Oscar Mayer)	¼ oz	20	.2	1	189	*	*	3	*	2	*	5
Bacon, Imitation (Bac*Os)	1 tbsp	40	2	2	165	2	*	*	*	45	*	4
Bacon, Imitation (French's Crumbles)	1 tsp	6	0–.5	0–.5	55	0–.5	*	*	*	*	*	*
Bacon, Imitation (Morningstar Farms Breakfast Strips)	3 strips	110	4	9	445	4	NA	8	4	40	NA	NA
Banquet Loaf (Eckrich Beef Smorgas Pac)	1 sl	50	1	4	250	2	*	2	*	*	6	6
Bar-B Loaf (Eckrich Calorie Watcher)	1 sl	35	1	2	370	2	*	4	4	10	10	10
Bar-B-Q Loaf (Oscar Mayer)	1 sl	45	1.7	2.8	369	*	*	3	3	6	8	9
Beef Breakfast Strips (Oscar Mayer Lean 'n Tasty)	1 strip	40	2	3	202	*	*	3	*	*	5	6

Meat	Amt.	% U.S. RDA								Sodium (mg)	Fat (g)	Carbohydrate (g)	Calories
		Protein	A	C	B₁	B₂	Niacin	Calcium	Iron				
Beef, Chuck, Braised, Simmered, or Pot Roasted, Lean and Fat	3 oz	50	*	*	2	10	20	*	15	40	17	0	250
Beef, Chuck, Braised, Simmered, or Pot Roasted, Lean Only	3 oz	60	*	*	4	10	20	2	20	45	6	0	160
Beef, Chuck, Cooked, Diced, Lean and Fat	1 c	80	*	*	4	15	30	2	25	66	27	0	410
Beef, Chuck, Cooked, Diced, Lean Only	1 c	90	*	*	6	20	30	2	30	75	10	0	270
Beef, Dried or Chipped	1 oz	20	*	*	2	6	6	*	8	1219	2	0	60
Beef, Ground, Broiled Well-done, Lean	3 oz	50	*	*	6	10	25	**	15	57	10	0	190
Beef, Ground, Broiled Well-done, Regular	3 oz	50	*	*	4	10	25	*	15	50	18	0	270
Beef Plate, Simmered, Lean and Fat	3 oz	40	2	*	2	8	15	*	15	33	32	0	370
Beef Plate, Simmered, Lean Only	3 oz	60	*	*	2	10	20	2	20	45	7	0	170
Beef Roast, Rib, Cooked, Lean and Fat	3 oz	40	2	*	2	8	15	*	10	41	34	0	370
Beef Roast, Rib, Cooked, Lean Only	3 oz	60	*	*	4	10	20	*	15	59	12	0	210

Food	Serving	% U.S. RDA											Calories
Beef Roast, Rump, Cooked, Lean and Fat	3 oz	45	*	*	4	8	20	*	15	49	23	0	300
Beef Roast, Rump, Cooked, Lean Only	3 oz	60	*	*	4	10	20	*	15	61	8	0	180
Beef Roast, Rump, Cooked, Diced, Lean and Fat	1 c	70	2	*	6	15	30	2	25	81	38	0	490
Beef Roast, Rump, Cooked, Diced, Lean Only	1 c	90	*	*	6	20	35	2	30	100	13	0	290
Beef Roast, Rump, Cooked, Ground, Lean Only	1 c	70	*	*	6	15	30	2	25	78	10	0	230
Beef Roast, Spread, Canned (Underwood)	½ can (2.4 oz)	25	*	*	*	6	10	*	8	515	10	NA	140
Beef, Slender Sliced (Eckrich Calorie Watcher)	1 oz	10	*	10	*	2	6	*	4	560	2	1	40
Beef Steak, Club, Porterhouse, or T-Bone, Broiled, Lean and Fat	3 oz	35	2	*	4	8	20	*	10	41	36	0	400
Beef Steak, Club, Porterhouse, or T-Bone, Broiled, Lean Only	3 oz	60	*	*	4	10	25	*	15	63	9	0	190
Beef Steak, Flank, Cooked	3 oz	60	*	*	4	10	20	2	20	45	6	0	170
Beef Steak, Round, Braised, Broiled, or Sauteed, Lean and Fat	3 oz	60	*	*	4	10	25	*	15	60	13	0	220

189

Meat	Amt.	Pro-tein	A	C	B$_1$	B$_2$	Nia-cin	Cal-cium	Iron	Sodium (mg)	Fat (g)	Carbohy-drate (g)	Calories
		% U.S. RDA											
Beef Steak, Round, Braised, Broiled, or Sauteed, Lean Only	3 oz	60	*	*	4	10	25	2	15	65	5	0	160
Beef Steak, Sirloin, Broiled, Lean and Fat	3 oz	45	*	*	4	8	20	*	15	48	27	0	330
Beef Steak, Sirloin, Broiled, Lean Only	3 oz	60	*	*	6	10	25	2	20	67	7	0	180
Bologna (Eckrich)	1 sl	6	*	10	4	2	2	*	2	290	8	2	90
Bologna (Eckrich German Brand)	1 sl	8	*	10	4	2	2	*	2	350	7	1	80
Bologna (Eckrich Smorgas Pac) 12-oz pkg	1 sl	6	*	10	2	*	2	*	*	230	6	1	70
Bologna (Eckrich Smorgas Pac) 16-oz pkg	1 sl	8	*	10	4	2	2	*	2	310	8	2	90
Bologna, Beef (Eckrich Beef Smorgas Pac)	1 sl	6	*	8	*	*	2	*	2	230	6	1	70
Bologna, Chub (Eckrich German Brand)	1 oz	8	*	8	4	4	4	**	2	360	7	1	80
Bologna, Lunch, Chub (Eckrich)	1 oz	6	*	10	4	2	2	*	2	290	9	2	100
Bologna, Pickled Ring (Eckrich)	1 oz	6	*	6	2	2	4	**	2	290	8	2	90
Bologna, Ring (Eckrich)	1 oz	6	*	10	2	2	2	*	2	280	8	2	90

							% U.S. RDA						
Bologna, Sliced (Eckrich) 16-oz pkg	1 sl	6	*	10	4	2	2	*	2	290	8	2	90
Bologna (Oscar Mayer)	1 sl	5	NA	6	3	2	2	*	*	241	6.9	.4	75
Bologna, Beef (Eckrich)	1 sl	6	*	10	*	*	2	*	2	270	8	2	90
Bologna, Beef (Oscar Mayer)	1 sl	5	NA	6	*	*	2	*	*	239	6.7	.6	75
Bologna, Garlic (Eckrich)	1 sl	6	*	10	4	2	2	*	2	290	8	2	90
Bologna, Sandwich (Eckrich)	1 sl	6	*	10	4	2	2	*	2	310	8	2	90
Bologna, Sliced (Eckrich) 12-oz pkg	1 sl	6	*	10	4	2	2	*	2	290	8	2	90
Bologna, Thick Sliced (Eckrich)	1 sl	10	*	15	6	4	4	*	2	490	14	3	160
Bologna, Thick Sliced, Beef (Eckrich)	1 sl	10	*	15	2	4	4	*	4	400	12	2	140
Bologna, Thin Sliced (Eckrich)	2 sl	8	*	10	4	2	2	*	2	320	10	2	110
Bologna, Thin Sliced, Beef (Eckrich)	2 sl	8	*	10	*	2	2	*	2	320	9	2	110
Bologna w Cheese (Eckrich)	1 sl	6	*	10	6	2	2	*	2	290	8	2	90
Bologna and Cheese (Oscar Mayer)	1 sl	6	NA	6	3	*	2	*	*	247	7	.6	75
Braunschweiger (Oscar Mayer)	1 oz	8	86	4	4	25	11	*	15	330	9	.8	95

Meat	Amt.	% U.S. RDA								Sodium (mg)	Fat (g)	Carbohydrate (g)	Calories
		Protein	A	C	B₁	B₂	Niacin	Calcium	Iron				
Braunschweiger, Chub (Eckrich)	1 oz	8	*	4	4	25	10	*	15	400	6	1	70
Corn Dogs (Oscar Mayer)	1	15	NA	5	18	9	16	3	10	1252	20	27	330
Corned Beef, Fresh, Cooked	3 oz	20	*	*	*	6	6	*	10	802	26	0	320
Corned Beef Loaf, Jellied (Oscar Mayer)	1 sl	10	NA	3	*	*	2	*	3	286	2	0	45
Corned Beef, Slender Sliced (Eckrich Calorie Watcher)	1 oz	10	*	10	*	2	6	*	4	340	2	1	40
Corned Beef Spread, Canned (Underwood)	½ can (2¼ oz)	20	*	*	*	4	8	*	8	605	10	NA	120
Franks (Eckrich)	1	8	*	6	2	2	4	*	2	360	11	2	120
Franks, Beef (Eckrich)	1	10	*	10	*	2	4	*	2	380	10	2	110
Franks, Beef (Oscar Mayer)	1 link	11	NA	18	*	2	5	*	3	466	13	.9	145
Franks Beef, Jumbo (Eckrich)	1	10	*	10	2	4	6	*	4	620	17	3	190
Franks, Cheese (Eckrich)	1	15	*	20	8	4	6	2	4	650	17	3	190
Gourmet Loaf (Eckrich Beef Smorgas Pac)	1 sl	6	*	8	*	2	2	*	2	300	1	2	25
Gourmet Loaf (Eckrich Calorie Watcher)	1 sl	10	*	10	*	2	4	*	2	390	1	2	35

Food	Serving											
					% U.S. RDA							
Ham, Canned (Oscar Mayer Jubilee)	1 oz	11	NA	13	15	3	7	*	*	341	1	.1	30
Ham, Chopped (Eckrich Calorie Watcher)	1 sl	10	*	4	10	2	4	*	2	330	2	1	45
Ham, Chopped (Eckrich Smorgas Pac)	1 sl	8	*	*	10	2	4	*	2	250	2	1	35
Ham, Chopped (Oscar Mayer)	1 sl	10	NA	9	13	3	5	*	*	373	4	.8	65
Ham, Cooked, Sliced (Eckrich)	1 sl	10	*	10	15	2	10	*	2	470	1	1	30
Ham, Cooked, Sliced (Eckrich Calorie Watcher)	1 sl	10	*	10	15	2	8	*	2	470	1	1	30
Ham, Cooked, Smoked (Oscar Mayer)	1 sl	8	NA	8	13	2	5	*	*	282	1	0	25
Ham, Cured, Roasted, Lean and Fat	3 oz	40	*	*	25	8	15	*	10	NA	19	0	250
Ham, Cured, Roasted, Lean Only	3 oz	50	*	*	35	10	20	*	15	790	8	0	160
Ham, Cured, Roasted, Diced, Lean and Fat	1 c	70	*	*	45	15	25	2	20	NA	30	0	410
Ham, Cured, Roasted, Diced, Lean Only	1 c	80	*	*	60	20	30	2	25	1540	12	0	260
Ham, Cured, Roasted, Ground, Lean Only	1 c	60	*	*	45	15	25	2	20	1210	10	0	210
Ham, Deviled, Canned (Underwood)	½ can (2¼ oz)	20	*	*	4	4	6	*	6	640	20	NA	220

| Meat | Amt. | % U.S. RDA | | | | | | | | Sodium (mg) | Fat (g) | Carbohydrate (g) | Calories |
		Protein	A	C	B_1	B_2	Niacin	Calcium	Iron				
Ham, Fresh, Roasted, Lean and Fat	3 oz	45	*	*	30	10	20	*	15	NA	26	0	320
Ham, Fresh, Roasted, Lean Only	3 oz	60	*	*	35	15	25	2	20	NA	8	0	180
Ham, Fresh, Roasted, Diced, Lean and Fat	1 c	70	*	*	45	20	30	2	25	79	43	0	520
Ham, Fresh, Roasted, Diced, Lean Only	1 c	90	*	*	60	25	40	2	30	102	14	0	300
Ham, Fresh, Roasted, Ground, Lean Only	1 c	70	*	*	45	20	30	2	25	80	11	0	240
Ham, Imported Danish (Eckrich)	1 oz	10	*	15	10	2	6	*	2	390	1	1	25
Ham Loaf (Eckrich)	1 sl	10	*	10	10	2	4	*	2	330	6	1	70
Ham Salad (The Spreadables)	¼ can	10	*	*	10	4	6	*	6	335	8	4	110
Ham Slice (Oscar Mayer Jubilee)	1 oz	12	NA	14	16	3	6	*	*	373	1	0	30
Ham, Smoked, Boneless (Oscar Mayer Jubilee)	1 oz	11	NA	13	15	4	7	*	*	386	3	.2	50
Ham, Smoked, Slender Sliced (Eckrich Calorie Watcher)	1 oz	10	*	10	10	2	6	*	2	360	3	1	45

Food	Portion	% U.S. RDA											
Ham, Smoked, Sweet (Eckrich Calorie Watcher)	1 sl	*	8	15	10	2	4	*	*	270	1	1	25
Ham Steaks (Oscar Mayer Jubilee)	1 sl	NA	25	31	31	7	14	*	3	741	3	0	70
Ham and Cheese Loaf (Eckrich)	1 sl	*	8	10	8	2	4	*	2	350	5	1	60
Ham and Cheese Loaf (Oscar Mayer)	1 sl	NA	10	10	11	3	4	*	*	365	6	.6	75
Hamburger, Imitation (Morningstar Farms Grillers)	1 patty	NA	NA	NA	40	10	30	4	15	345	13	5	190
Head Cheese (Oscar Mayer)	1 sl	NA	6	10	*	2	*	*	2	352	4	0	55
Heart, Beef, Braised, Lean	3 oz	*	60	2	15	60	35	*	30	87	5	0-1	160
Heart, Beef, Braised, Diced, Lean	1 c	*	100	2	25	100	60	*	50	151	9	1	270
Honey Loaf (Oscar Mayer)	1 sl	NA	10	8	12	4	4	*	*	373	1	1	35
Honey Style Loaf (Eckrich Calorie Watcher)	1 sl	*	10	10	8	4	4	*	2	350	2	3	40
Honey Style Loaf (Eckrich Smorgas Pac) 12-oz pkg	1 sl	*	6	10	6	2	2	*	2	280	1	2	30
Honey Style Loaf (Eckrich Smorgas Pac) 16-oz pkg	1 sl	*	10	10	8	2	4	*	2	370	1	3	35
Kidney, Beef, Braised	3 oz	20	60	*	30	240	45	2	60	215	10	0-1	210

Meat	Amt.	Protein	A	C	B₁	B₂	Niacin	Calcium	Iron	Sodium (mg)	Fat (g)	Carbohydrate (g)	Calories
		% U.S. RDA											
Kielbasa (Eckrich Polska)	1 oz	8	*	8	4	2	4	*	2	260	9	1	95
Kielbasa, Links, Skinless (Eckrich Polska)	2 links (2 oz)	16	*	16	4	4	4	*	4	500	16	2	180
Kielbasa, Skinless, Links (Eckrich Polska)	1 link (2 oz)	15	*	20	8	6	6	2	4	490	15	2	180
Lamb Chop, Loin, Cooked, Lean and Fat	3½ oz	50	*	*	8	15	25	*	8	53	29	0	360
Lamb Chop, Loin, Cooked, Lean Only	2.3 oz	40	*	*	6	10	20	*	8	45	5	0	120
Lamb Chop, Rib, Cooked, Lean and Fat	3.2 oz	40	*	*	8	10	20	*	6	45	33	0	370
Lamb Chop, Rib, Cooked, Lean Only	2 oz	35	*	*	6	8	15	*	6	38	6	0	120
Lamb, Leg, Roasted, Lean and Fat	3 oz	50	*	*	8	15	25	*	8	53	16	0	240
Lamb, Leg, Roasted, Lean Only	3 oz	60	*	*	10	15	25	2	10	60	6	0	160
Lamb, Leg, Roasted, Diced, Lean and Fat	1 c	80	*	*	15	20	40	2	15	87	27	0	390
Lamb, Leg, Roasted, Diced, Lean Only	1 c	90	*	*	15	25	45	2	15	98	10	0	260
Lamb, Shoulder, Roasted, Lean and Fat	3 oz	40	*	*	8	10	20	*	6	45	23	0	290

Food	Serving			% U.S. RDA								
Lamb, Shoulder, Roasted, Lean Only	3 oz	50	*	*	8	15	25	*	8	56	9	0	170
Lamb, Shoulder, Roasted, Diced, Lean and Fat	1 c	70	*	*	10	20	35	*	10	74	38	0	470
Lamb, Shoulder, Roasted, Diced, Lean Only	1 c	80	*	*	15	25	40	*	15	92	14	0	290
Liver, Beef, Fried	3 oz	50	910	40	15	210	70	*	40	156	9	5	200
Liver, Calf, Fried	3 oz	60	560	50	15	210	70	2	70	100	11	4	220
Liver, Hog, Fried	3 oz	60	250	30	20	220	100	2	140	94	10	2	210
Liver Cheese (Oscar Mayer)	1 sl	12	156	*	5	49	21	*	25	456	10	.6	115
Liverwurst Spread, Canned (Underwood)	½ can (2.4 oz)	20	80	*	8	50	15	*	25	570	19	3	220
Luncheon Meat (Oscar Mayer)	1 sl	8	NA	6	5	2	4	*	*	358	9	.4	95
Luxury Loaf (Oscar Mayer)	1 sl	11	NA	9	12	4	4	*	*	328	1	1.5	40
Macaroni-Cheese Loaf (Eckrich)	1 sl	6	*	2	4	4	2	2	2	370	6	3	70
Old Fashion Loaf (Eckrich)	1 sl	8	*	10	4	2	2	2	2	330	6	3	70
Old Fashion Loaf (Eckrich Smorgas Pac) 12-oz pkg	1 sl	6	*	8	2	2	2	2	*	250	4	2	50
Old Fashion Loaf (Eckrich Smorgas Pac) 16-oz pkg	1 sl	8	*	10	4	2	2	2	2	340	6	2	70

Meat	Amt.	Pro-tein	A	C	B$_1$	B$_2$	Nia-cin	Cal-cium	Iron	Sodium (mg)	Fat (g)	Carbohy-drate (g)	Calories
						% U.S. RDA							
Old Fashioned Loaf (Oscar Mayer)	1 sl	9	NA	6	7	5	3	3	*	101	4	2	65
Olive Loaf (Eckrich)	1 sl	6	*	10	2	4	2	2	2	370	7	2	80
Olive Loaf (Oscar Mayer)	1 sl	7	NA	4	5	4	2	3	*	400	4	3	65
Pastrami, Slender Sliced (Eckrich Calorie Watcher)	1 oz	10	*	10	*	2	6	*	4	360	2	1	40
Paté, Liver (Underwood Sell's)	½ can	20	80	*	8	50	15	*	25	570	19	3	220
Peppered Loaf (Eckrich Calorie Watcher)	1 sl	10	*	10	8	4	4	*	2	390	2	1	40
Peppered Loaf (Oscar Mayer)	1 sl	10	NA	10	7	4	4	*	*	399	2	1.3	40
Pepperoni, Sliced (Eckrich)	2 oz	20	*	*	8	8	10	2	6	NA	24	2	270
Pickle Loaf (Eckrich)	1 sl	6	*	10	4	2	2	2	2	320	7	2	80
Pickle Loaf (Eckrich Smorgas Pac)	1 sl	6	*	10	4	2	2	2	2	320	8	2	90
Pickle Loaf, Beef (Eckrich Beef Smorgas Pac)	1 sl	6	*	8	*	2	2	2	*	260	5	1	50
Pickle and Pimiento Loaf (Oscar Mayer)	1 sl	8	NA	4	6	4	3	3	*	382	4	3	65
Picnic Loaf (Oscar Mayer)	1 sl	9	NA	7	7	3	3	3	*	320	4	1.5	65

		% U.S. RDA											
Pork Breakfast Strips (Oscar Mayer Lean 'n Tasty)	1 strip	7	NA	7	5	2	3	0-1	1	220	3	.2	45
Pork Chop, Loin, Broiled, Lean and Fat	2.7 oz (3 chops per lb)	45	*	*	50	15	25	*	15	47	25	0	310
Pork Chop, Loin, Broiled, Lean Only	2 oz (3 chops per lb)	40	*	*	40	10	20	*	10	42	9	0	150
Pork, Cured, Boston Butt or Picnic, Roasted, Lean and Fat	3 oz	45	*	*	30	10	20	*	15	NA	22	0	280
Pork, Cured, Boston Butt or Picnic, Roasted, Lean Only	3 oz	50	*	*	35	10	20	*	15	790	12	0	210
Pork, Cured, Boston Butt or Picnic, Roasted, Diced, Lean Only	1 c	90	*	*	60	20	35	2	30	1300	20	0	340
Pork, Cured, Boston Butt or Picnic, Roasted, Ground, Lean Only	1 c	70	*	*	45	15	30	2	20	1023	15	0	270
Pork, Loin, Baked or Roasted, Lean and Fat	3 oz	45	*	*	50	15	25	*	15	51	24	0	310
Pork, Loin, Baked or Roasted, Lean Only	3 oz	60	*	*	60	15	30	2	20	61	12	0	220
Pork, Loin, Baked or Roasted, Diced, Lean and Fat	1 c	80	*	*	90	20	40	2	25	84	40	0	510

Meat	Amt.	% U.S. RDA								Sodium (mg)	Fat (g)	Carbohydrate (g)	Calories
		Protein	A	C	B₁	B₂	Niacin	Calcium	Iron				

Meat	Amt.	Protein	A	C	B1	B2	Niacin	Calcium	Iron	Sodium (mg)	Fat (g)	Carbohydrate (g)	Calories
Pork, Loin, Baked or Roasted, Diced, Lean Only	1 c	90	*	*	100	25	45	2	30	101	20	0	360
Pork, Shoulder, Roasted, Lean and Fat	3 oz	40	*	*	30	10	20	*	15	47	24	0	300
Pork, Shoulder, Roasted, Lean Only	3 oz	50	*	*	35	15	20	*	15	56	12	0	210
Pork, Shoulder, Roasted, Diced, Lean and Fat	1 c	70	*	*	45	20	30	2	25	77	40	0	490
Pork, Shoulder, Roasted, Diced, Lean Only	1 c	80	*	*	60	20	35	2	25	93	20	0	340
Pork, Shoulder, Roasted, Ground, Lean Only	1 c	70	*	*	45	20	30	2	20	73	16	0	270
Pork, Smoked, Slender Sliced (Eckrich Calorie Watcher)	1 oz	10	*	10	10	4	4	*	2	350	3	1	45
Salami, Beer, Sliced (Eckrich)	1 sl	8	*	*	4	2	4	*	2	350	6	1	70
Salami, Cooked (Chub) (Eckrich)	1 oz	8	*	*	2	2	2	*	2	360	6	1	70
Salami, Cotto (Eckrich)	1 sl	8	*	*	4	2	4	*	2	340	5	1	70
Salami, Cotto (Oscar Mayer)	1 sl	7	NA	6	4	5	4	*	3	245	4	4	50

Food	Serving				% U.S. RDA							
Salami, Cotto, Beef (Eckrich)	2 sl	10	*	10	*	4	4	2	4	480	8	2	100
Salami, Cotto, Beef (Oscar Mayer)	1 sl	8	NA	6	2	3	4	*	2	279	4	.6	50
Salami for Beer (Oscar Mayer)	1 sl	7	NA	11	8	2	3	*	*	282	4	.4	55
Salami for Beer, Beef (Oscar Mayer)	1 sl	6	NA	6	*	*	3	*	*	234	7	.2	75
Salami, Hard (Oscar Mayer)	1 sl	4	NA	3	3	*	2	*	*	167	3	.2	35
Salami, Hard, Sliced (Eckrich)	1 oz	10	*	*	4	4	6	*	2	600	12	1	130
Sandwich Spread (Oscar Mayer)	1 oz	5	NA	*	3	2	2	*	*	275	5	3.2	65
Sausage (Oscar Mayer New England Brand)	1 sl	8	NA	8	9	3	3	*	*	295	2	.6	35
Sausage, Cheese, Smoked (Eckrich)	2 oz	15	*	20	6	6	6	4	4	500	15	2	180
Sausage, Ham Roll (Oscar Mayer)	1 sl	9	NA	8	13	2	5	*	*	270	2	.5	35
Sausage, Honey Roll, Beef (Oscar Mayer)	1 sl	9	NA	6	*	2	5	*	2	304	2	.7	40
Sausage, Luncheon Roll (Oscar Mayer)	1 sl	8	NA	8	11	2	4	*	*	244	2	.2	35
Sausage, Minced Roll (Eckrich)	1 sl	8	*	10	4	2	2	*	2	340	7	1	80

| | | % U.S. RDA | | | | | | | | | | | |
Meat	Amt.	Protein	A	C	B₁	B₂	Niacin	Calcium	Iron	Sodium (mg)	Fat (g)	Carbohydrate (g)	Calories
Sausage, New England Brand (Eckrich Calorie Watcher)	1 sl	10	*	10	10	4	4	*	2	440	2	1	35
Sausage, Patty, Fresh (Eckrich)	1 patty	15	*	*	10	4	10	*	4	NA	26	1	240
Sausage, Pork (Eckrich)	2 oz	10	*	*	10	4	8	*	2	NA	26	1	260
Sausage, Pork (Oscar Mayer Little Friers)	1 link	7	NA	*	6	2	4	*	*	223	8	.2	80
Sausage, Pork, Links (Eckrich)	2 links	15	*	*	10	4	10	*	4	NA	20	1	220
Sausage, Pork, Patties (Oscar Mayer Southern Brand)	1 patty	12	NA	*	9	3	9	*	3	282	11	0	125
Sausage, Pork, Roll, Hot, Fresh (Eckrich)	2 oz	15	*	*	10	4	10	*	4	NA	26	1	240
Sausage, Pressed Luncheon (Oscar Mayer)	1 sl	8	NA	8	6	3	3	*	*	281	2	.7	35
Sausage, Smoked (Eckrich)	2 oz	15	*	15	6	4	8	*	4	530	17	1	190
Sausage, Smoked, Beef (Eckrich)	2 oz	15	*	20	2	4	6	*	6	520	17	1	190
Sausage, Smoked, Links, Hot (Eckrich)	1 link	20	*	26	10	5	5	*	5	640	21	3	240
Sausage, Smoked, Links, Skinless (Eckrich)	1 link	15	*	20	8	6	6	2	4	490	15	2	180

		% U.S. RDA											
Sausage, Smoked, w Cheese (Eckrich)	1 link	20	*	25	10	8	8	4	6	670	20	2	240
Sausage, Smoked, Skinless (Eckrich)	1 oz	8	*	10	4	2	2	*	2	250	7	1	90
Sausage, Imitation (Morningstar Farms Breakfast Links)	3 links	NA	NA	NA	40	15	25	2	15	675	14	5	200
Sausage, Imitation (Morningstar Farms Breakfast Patties)	2 patties	NA	NA	NA	40	15	30	4	15	870	14	7	220
Smokies, Beef (Oscar Mayer)	1 link	13	NA	8	*	3	6	*	4	455	12	.9	130
Smokies, Cheese (Oscar Mayer)	1 link	13	NA	12	7	4	6	2	2	450	13	.4	140
Smokie Links (Oscar Mayer)	1 link	12	NA	13	8	3	5	*	2	396	12	.6	135
Smok-y-Links, Beef (Eckrich)	2 links	15	*	15	*	4	6	2	4	400	12	2	140
Smok-y-Links, Ham (Eckrich)	2 links	10	*	15	8	4	4	2	2	560	13	2	150
Smok-y-Links, Maple Flavored (Eckrich)	2 links	10	*	15	6	4	6	2	4	400	13	2	150
Smok-y-Links, Skinless (Eckrich)	2 links	10	*	10	6	4	6	2	4	410	13	2	150
Spareribs, Braised, Lean and Fat	3 oz	40	*	*	25	10	15	*	10	31	34	0	370

| Meat | Amt. | % U.S. RDA | | | | | | | | Sodium (mg) | Fat (g) | Carbohy-drate (g) | Calories |
		Pro-tein	A	C	B₁	B₂	Nia-cin	Cal-cium	Iron				
Summer Sausage (Eckrich Smoky Tang)	1 oz	8	*	*	2	2	4	*	2	350	7	1	80
Summer Sausage (Oscar Mayer)	1 sl	7	NA	10	3	3	5	*	2	340	7	.2	75
Summer Sausage, Beef (Oscar Mayer)	1 sl	7	NA	8	2	4	4	*	2	317	6	.7	70
Summer Sausage, Sliced (Eckrich)	1 sl	10	*	2	4	2	4	*	2	380	7	1	90
Sweetbreads, Beef, Braised	3 oz	50	*	*	4	8	15	*	8	99	20	0	270
Tongue, Beef, Braised, Medium Fat	1 oz	15	*	*	*	4	4	*	4	17	5	0-1	70
Veal, Boneless Cuts, Braised, Pot Roasted, or Stewed, Medium Fat	3 oz	60	*	*	6	15	25	*	15	41	11	0	200
Veal, Boneless Cuts, Braised, Pot Roasted, or Stewed, Medium Fat, Chopped	1 c	90	*	*	8	25	45	2	25	68	18	0	330
Veal, Cutlet, Braised or Broiled, Medium Fat	3 oz	50	*	*	4	10	25	*	15	56	10	0	180
Veal, Loin, Braised or Broiled, Medium Fat	3 oz	50	*	*	4	10	25	*	15	55	12	0	200
Veal, Loin, Braised or Broiled, Diced, Medium Fat	1 c	80	*	*	6	20	40	2	25	91	19	0	330

		% U.S. RDA											
Veal, Rib, Roasted	3 oz	50	*	*	8	15	35	*	15	57	15	0	230
Veal, Rib, Roasted, Diced	1 c	80	*	*	10	25	60	2	25	93	24	0	380
Veal, Rib, Roasted, Ground	1 c	70	*	*	10	20	45	2	20	73	19	0	300
Wieners (Oscar Mayer)	1 link	11	NA	19	6	2	5	*	2	459	13	.8	145
Wieners w Cheese (Oscar Mayer)	1 link	12	NA	15	5	3	4	2	2	510	13	.7	145
Milk													
Buttermilk, Made from Skim Milk	1 c	20	*	4	6	25	*	30	2	319	0-1	13	90
Buttermilk, Cultured (Borden)	1 c	20	*	4	6	25	*	30	*	NA	1	11	90
Chocolate Milk (Meadow Gold)	1 c	20	4	4	6	25	*	30	*	NA	8	26	210
Chocolate Milk, Dutch (Borden)	1 c	20	4	4	6	25	*	30	*	NA	8	26	210
Chocolate Milk, Lowfat (Dutch Brand)	1 c	20	10	4	6	25	*	30	*	NA	3	26	160
Chocolate Milk, Lowfat (Meadow Gold)	1 c	20	10	4	6	25	*	30	*	NA	2	25	160
Condensed Milk, Sweetened (Carnation)	4 fl oz	25	10	6	8	35	*	40	*	196	13	83	490
Condensed Milk, Sweetened (Eagle Brand)	1/3 c	15	4	4	4	25	*	30	*	120	9	52	320

Milk	Amt.	Protein	A	C	B$_1$	B$_2$	Niacin	Calcium	Iron	Sodium (mg)	Fat (g)	Carbohydrate (g)	Calories
		% U.S. RDA											
Condensed Sweetened Filled Dairy Blend (Magnolia)	⅓ c	15	10	*	2	25	*	30	*	120	9	54	320
Evaporated Milk (Carnation)	4 fl oz	20	4	*	2	20	*	30	*	133	10	12	170
Evaporated Milk (Pet)	½ c	20	4	*	2	20	*	30	*	NA	10	12	170
Evaporated Milk, Lowfat (Carnation)	½ c	20	10	*	2	20	*	30	*	138	3	12	110
Evaporated Milk, Skim (Carnation)	½ c	20	10	*	2	20	*	35	*	140	0	14	100
Evaporated Milk, Skim (Pet)	½ c	20	10	*	2	20	*	35	*	NA	0	14	100
Milk, Dry, Nonfat, Reconstituted (Carnation)	1 c	20	10	2	6	25	*	30	*	124	0	12	80
Milk, Whole, 3.5% Fat	1 c	20	6	4	4	25	*	30	*	122	9	12	160
Milk, Partly Skimmed (2% Fat), Nonfat Milk Solids Added	1 c	25	4	4	6	30	*	35	2	150	5	15	150
Milk, Nonfat (Skim)	1 c	20	*	4	6	25	*	30	*	127	0–1	13	90
Milk, Homogenized (Borden)	1 c	20	4	4	6	25	*	30	*	NA	8	11	150
Milk, Homogenized (Meadow Gold)	1 c	20	4	4	6	25	*	30	*	NA	8	11	150
Milk, Homogenized, Skim (Borden)	1 c	20	10	4	8	30	*	30	*	NA	0	12	90

Food	Serving	% U.S. RDA										
Milk, Homogenized, Skim (Meadow Gold)	1 c	20	10	4	8	30	*	30	*	NA	1	12	90
Milk, Lowfat (2%) (Meadow Gold Viva)	1 c	20	10	4	6	25	*	30	*	NA	5	11	120
Milk, Nonfat, Protein Fortified (Borden Skimline)	1 c	25	10	6	20	30	10	35	15	NA	1	13	100
Milk, 2% Milkfat, Protein Fortified (Borden Hi-Protein Brand)	1 c	25	10	6	8	30	*	35	*	NA	5	13	140
Milk Beverages													
Alba '77 Fit'n Frosty, Chocolate or Chocolate Marshmallow	1 env	NA	NA	NA	NA	NA	NA	20	*	170	1	11	70
Alba '77 Fit'n Frosty, Strawberry or Vanilla	1 env	NA	NA	NA	NA	NA	NA	20	*	170	0	11	70
Carnation Slender, Canned, All Flavors	1 can	25	25	25	25	25	25	25	25	430-530	4	34	220
Chocolate (Borden Frosted)	8 fl oz	10	2	*	2	25	*	25	8	205	11	36	260
Chocolate, Mix (Carnation Instant Breakfast)	1 env, dry	10	35	45	20	4	25	10	25	135	1	23	130
Chocolate, Mix (Carnation Slender)	1 env, dry	10	20	25	20	5	25	5	25	110	1	21	110
Chocolate, Mix (Ovaltine)	¾ oz	2	45	45	45	45	45	8	15	NA	0-1	16	80
Chocolate, Mix (Pillsbury Instant Breakfast)	1 pouch, dry	10	30	30	15	15	25	8	25	185	0	26	130

Milk Beverages	Amt.	Pro-tein	A	C	B₁	B₂	Nia-cin	Cal-cium	Iron	Sodium (mg)	Fat (g)	Carbohy-drate (g)	Calories
		% U.S. RDA											
Chocolate Malt, Mix (Carnation Instant Breakfast)	1 env, dry	10	35	45	20	4	25	10	25	160	1	22	130
Chocolate Malt, Mix (Pillsbury Instant Breakfast)	1 pouch, dry	10	30	30	25	15	25	8	25	190	0	26	130
Chocolate Malt, Mix (Carnation Instant)	3 heap tsp	2	*	*	2	2	2	*	2	47.25	1	18	85
Coffee, Mix (Carnation Instant Breakfast)	1 env, dry	15	35	45	20	4	25	10	25	130	0	24	130
Dutch Chocolate, Mix (Carnation Slender)	1 env, dry	10	20	25	20	5	25	5	25	110	1	21	110
Eggnog, Mix (Carnation Instant Breakfast)	1 env, dry	15	35	45	20	4	25	10	25	185	0	23	130
French Vanilla, Mix (Carnation Slender)	1 env, dry	10	20	25	20	5	25	5	25	110	.5	22	110
Malt, Mix (Ovaltine)	4–5 heap tsp, dry	2	45	45	45	45	45	8	15	NA	0–1	17	80
Malt, Mix (Carnation Instant Natural)	3 heap tsp	6	*	*	8	10	4	6	*	97.7	1.7	15.6	90
Strawberry (Borden Frosted)	8 fl oz	20	*	*	4	15	*	25	*	190	10	36	270
Strawberry, Mix (Carnation Instant Breakfast)	1 env, dry	15	35	45	20	4	25	10	25	195	0	24	130
Strawberry, Mix (Pillsbury Instant Breakfast)	1 pouch, dry	10	30	30	25	15	25	8	25	180	0	27	130

		% U.S. RDA											
Vanilla, Mix (Carnation Instant Breakfast)	1 env, dry	15	35	45	20	4	25	10	25	135	0	24	130
Vanilla, Mix (Pillsbury Instant Breakfast)	1 pouch, dry	10	30	30	25	15	25	8	25	195	0	27	130
Muffins													
Blueberry (Pepperidge Farm)	1	2	0	2	0	2	0	2	2	250	7	27	180
Blueberry (Thomas' Toast-r-Cakes)	1	4	*	*	6	4	4	2	2	197	4	17	110
Bran (Thomas' Toast-r-Cakes)	1	4	*	*	6	4	6	2	6	245	4	17	110
Bran w Raisins (Pepperidge Farm)	1	4	0	0	4	6	8	2	8	295	7	28	180
Carrot Walnut (Pepperidge Farm)	1	8	0	0	20	15	15	4	10	220	4	27	170
Cinnamon Swirl (Pepperidge Farm)	1	4	0	0	2	4	6	2	2	170	6	30	190
Corn (Pepperidge Farm)	1	4	0	0	4	6	4	2	2	260	7	27	180
Corn (Thomas' Toast-r-Cakes)	1	4	*	*	6	4	4	2	2	208	4	19	120
English (Pepperidge Farm)	1	8	0	0	15	10	10	2	6	220	1	26	135
English (Thomas')	1	6	*	*	10	8	6	8	10	208	1	26	130
English (Wonder)	1	6	0	0	15	8	10	8	8	280	1	26	130
English, Bacon and Cheese (Pepperidge Farm)	1	8	0	0	20	10	10	2	10	370	2	25	140

Muffins	Amt.	Pro-tein	A	C	B₁	B₂	Nia-cin	Cal-cium	Iron	Sodium (mg)	Fat (g)	Carbohy-drate (g)	Calories
				% U.S. RDA									
English, Cinnamon Apple (Pepperidge Farm)	1	6	0	0	10	10	10	4	8	200	2	27	140
English, Cinnamon Chip (Pepperidge Farm)	1	8	0	0	20	8	8	2	10	250	3	28	160
English, Cinnamon Raisin (Pepperidge Farm)	1	8	0	0	15	10	10	4	6	190	2	28	150
English, Honey Wheat (Thomas')	1	6	*	*	15	2	10	2	6	228	1	27	128
English, Raisin (Thomas')	1	6	*	*	8	8	10	2	8	187	1	30	153
English, Sourdough (Pepperidge Farm)	1	6	0	0	15	10	10	4	6	260	1	27	140
English, Wheat, Stone Ground (Pepperidge Farm)	1	8	0	0	15	6	8	2	8	210	1	26	130
Mix, Apple Cinnamon (Betty Crocker)[1]	½ pkg	4	*	*	4	4	2	2	2	135	4	18	120
Mix, Corn (Betty Crocker)	½ pkg	4	*	*	8	6	4	4	4	315	5	25	160
Mix, Corn (Dromedary)	1 muffin	2	2	*	8	4	2	2	2	NA	5	20	130
Mix, Tart Cherry (Betty Crocker)	½ pkg	4	*	*	4	4	2	2	2	120	4	18	120
Mix, Wild Blueberry (Betty Crocker)	½ pkg	4	*	*	4	4	2	4	2	150	4	18	120

Food	Serving						% U.S. RDA						
Orange-Cranberry (Pepperidge Farm)	1	190	30	7	200	2	2	0	4	2	2	0	2
Raisin Rounds (Wonder)	1	150	28	3	230	8	8	8	10	15	0	0	6
Sour Dough (Wonder)	1	130	27	1	255	8	8	10	8	15	0	0	6
Nuts and Seeds													
Almonds, in Shell	10	60	2	6	Trace	2	2	2	6	2	*	*	4
Almonds, Shelled, Whole	1 c	850	28	77	6	35	35	25	80	25	*	*	60
Almonds, Shelled, Sliced	1 c	570	19	52	4	25	20	15	50	15	*	*	40
Brazil Nuts, Shelled	1 c (about 32)	920	16	94	1	25	25	10	10	90	*	*	45
Cashews, Oil Roasted	1 c	790	41	64	21	30	6	15	20	40	*	2	60
Chestnuts, Fresh, Shelled	1 c	310	68	3	10	15	4	4	20	25	*	*	10
Filberts, Shelled, Whole Kernels	1 c	860	23	84	3	25	30	6	*	40	*	*	40
Mixture (Carnation Deluxe Trail Mix)	1 pouch	130	9	8	10	4	2	6	4	4	*	*	6
Mixture (Carnation Raisins & Nuts)	1 pouch	130	11	7	10	2	2	10	2	*	*	*	6
Mixture (Carnation Tropical Fruit & Nuts)	1 pouch	100	16	3	10	2	*	4	2	2	*	*	4
Peanuts, Roasted in Shell, Jumbo	10	110	6	13	2	2	2	15	2	4	*	*	10
Peanuts, Salted, Whole or Halves	1 c	840	27	72	601	15	10	120	10	30	*	*	80

211

Nuts and Seeds	Amt.	% U.S. RDA								Sodium (mg)	Fat (g)	Carbohy-drate (g)	Calories
		Pro-tein	A	C	B₁	B₂	Nia-cin	Cal-cium	Iron				
Pecans, Halves	1 c	20	2	4	60	8	4	8	15	Trace	77	16	740
Pumpkin Seeds, Dry, Hulled	1 c	90	2	*	25	15	15	8	90	NA	65	21	770
Squash Seeds, Dry, Hulled	1 c	90	2	*	25	15	15	8	90	NA	65	21	770
Sunflower Seeds, Dry, Hulled	1 c	80	2	*	190	20	40	15	60	44	68	29	810
Walnuts, Black, Chopped or Broken Kernels	1 c	60	8	*	20	8	4	*	40	4	75	19	790
Walnuts, English, Halves	1 c (about 50)	35	*	4	20	8	4	10	15	2	64	16	650
Walnuts, English, Pieces or Chips	1 c	40	*	4	25	10	6	10	20	2	77	19	780
Pancakes, Waffles, and Similar Breakfast Foods													
French Toast w Sausages, Frozen (Swanson)	6½ oz pkg	30	*	*	40	25	20	10	25	820	26	37	450
Pancake Mix (Golden Blend)	3 4" cakes	10	4	0	15	15	8	15	10	500	7	26	200
Pancake Mix (Golden Blend Complete)	3 4" cakes	8	0	0	25	10	15	15	20	915	5	43	240
Pancake Mix (Hungry Jack Complete, Bulk)	3 4" cakes	6	0	0	20	10	10	10	15	730	2	39	190
Pancake Mix (Hungry Jack Complete, Packets)	3 4" cakes	6	0	0	15	10	10	15	10	675	3	35	180

Product	Serving	% U.S. RDA											
Pancake Mix (Hungry Jack Extra Lights)	3 4" cakes	10	4	0	15	10	6	15	8	485	7	30	210
Pancake Mix (Panshakes)	3 4" cakes	10	2	0	30	35	15	15	10	880	6	43	250
Pancake Mix, Blueberry (Hungry Jack)	3 4" cakes	10	4	2	15	15	8	10	10	815	15	40	320
Pancake Mix, Buttermilk (Betty Crocker)	3 4" cakes	15	4	*	15	15	10	15	8	810	10	39	280
Pancake Mix, Buttermilk (Betty Crocker Complete)	3 4" cakes	8	*	*	15	10	8	10	6	580	3	41	210
Pancake Mix, Buttermilk (Hungry Jack)	3 4" cakes	10	4	0	15	20	10	6	6	570	11	29	240
Pancake Mix, Buttermilk (Hungry Jack Complete, Bulk)	3 4" cakes	6	0	0	20	10	10	15	15	730	2	39	190
Pancake Mix, Potato (French's)	3 3" cakes	4	2	4	*	4	4	10	2	490	5	17	130
Pancakes and Blueberry Sauce, Frozen (Swanson)	7-oz pkg	10	*	10	20	15	10	6	10	800	9	70	400
Pancakes and Sausages, Frozen (Swanson)	6-oz pkg	25	*	*	30	20	20	8	15	950	22	50	460
Waffles, Frozen (Eggo Homestyle)	1	4	10	0	10	10	10	2	10	NA	5	16	120
Waffles, Frozen, Apple Cinnamon (Eggo)	1	4	10	0	10	10	10	2	10	NA	7	20	150

Pancakes, Waffles, and Similar Breakfast Foods	Amt.	Pro-tein	A	C	B₁	B₂	Nia-cin	Cal-cium	Iron	Sodium (mg)	Fat (g)	Carbohy-drate (g)	Calories
							% U.S. RDA						
Waffles, Frozen, Blueberry Flavored (Eggo)	1	4	10	0	10	10	10	2	10	NA	5	16	120
Waffles, Frozen, Butter-milk (Eggo)	1	4	10	0	10	10	10	2	10	NA	5	15	110
Waffles, Frozen, Straw-berry Flavored (Eggo)	1	4	10	0	10	10	10	2	10	NA	5	18	120
Pasta and Pasta Dishes													
Egg Noodle and Cheese, Mix (Kraft Dinner)	⅔ c prep	10	8	*	8	10	8	4	6	555	14	25	250
Egg Noodle w Chicken, Mix (Kraft Dinner)	¾ c prep	10	4	*	8	6	8	4	8	960	10	30	240
Fettuccine Alfredo, Frozen (Buitoni)	10 oz	15	4	6	20	15	15	50	15	1119	26	36	440
Fettuccine Alfredo, Frozen (Stouffer's)	5 oz	10	15	*	6	10	4	15	2	1195	18	19	270
Fettuccine Alfredo, Mix (Betty Crocker Inter-national Noodles)	¼ pkg	10	6	*	15	10	6	10	4	490	11	23	220
Fettuccine Carbonara, Fro-zen (Buitoni)	10 oz	12	6	4	20	25	15	40	20	1062	28	36	440
Fettuccine Primavera, Fro-zen (Buitoni)	10 oz	9	10	25	25	15	15	10	15	1099	7	86	440
Franco-American UFOs	7½ oz	8	10	15	15	10	15	2	10	780	3	35	180

Food	Serving												
		\% U.S. RDA											
Franco-American UFOs w Meteors	7½ oz	15	10	10	10	10	15	2	10	790	8	31	230
Lasagna, Frozen (Green Giant)	9½ oz	25	15	15	20	25	20	15	15	1145	6	42	290
Lasagna, Frozen (Stouffer's)	10½ oz	40	20	*	15	15	15	35	15	1200	14	36	385
Lasagna, Mix (Hamburger Helper)	⅕ pkg	40	4	*	20	15	25	2	15	925	14	29	320
Lasagna, Chicken, Frozen (Green Giant)	12 oz	60	40	2	30	80	30	80	15	1215	32	47	640
Lasagna, Deep Dish, Frozen (Buitoni)	11 oz	19	35	15	15	30	45	25	10	1535	10	55	390
Lasagna, Deep Dish w Meat Sauce, Frozen (Buitoni)	10½ oz	24	30	2	10	30	20	10	20	410	14	45	400
Lasagna Florentine, Frozen (Buitoni)	9½ oz	20	30	*	15	15	10	50	10	1100	29	36	480
Lasagna w Meat, Frozen (Swanson Hungry-Man)	12¾ oz	40	20	90	25	25	20	20	35	1250	16	63	480
Lasagna w Meat, Frozen (Swanson Main Course)	13¼ oz	35	15	25	20	25	15	25	15	1160	23	45	480
Lasagna w Meat Sauce, Frozen (Buitoni)	14 oz	28	30	*	20	35	25	35	15	1850	18	64	540
Lasagna w Meat Sauce, Frozen (Green Giant)	10½ oz	40	20	15	8	35	20	45	20	1515	16	45	430

Pasta and Pasta Dishes	Amt.	% U.S. RDA								Sodium (mg)	Fat (g)	Carbohydrate (g)	Calories
		Protein	A	C	B_1	B_2	Niacin	Calcium	Iron				
Lasagna w Meat Sauce, Frozen (Green Giant Single Serve)	12 oz	50	20	20	10	40	25	50	20	1660	20	44	490
Lasagna, Spinach, Frozen (Green Giant)	12 oz	30	100	40	20	45	10	45	25	1455	14	41	540
Lasagna, Zucchini, Frozen (Stouffer's Lean Cuisine)	11 oz	30	50	10	8	15	10	30	8	1040	7	28	260
Linguini w Clam Sauce, Frozen (Stouffer's)	10½ oz	25	*	*	20	10	10	2	15	1010	8	36	285
Macaroni, Dry (American Beauty)	2 oz	10	0	0	35	15	20	0	10	0-5	0-1	43	200
Macaroni, High Protein, Dry (Buitoni)	2 oz	12	*	*	35	15	15	*	10	NA	1	37	210
Macaroni and Beef, Canned (Franco-American BeefyOs)	7½ oz	15	10	8	10	10	15	2	10	1250	8	30	220
Macaroni and Beef, Canned (Heinz Mac 'n Beef)	7¼ oz	8 g	NA	NA	NA	NA	NA	2	10	850	8	23	200
Macaroni and Beef w Tomatoes, Frozen (Stouffer's)	5¾ oz	15	10	*	8	10	10	4	10	810	8	20	190
Macaroni and Cheese, Canned (Franco-American)	7⅜ oz	8	10	*	15	10	10	8	8	960	5	24	170

| | | % U.S. RDA | | | | | | | | | | | |
Food	Portion									Sodium (mg)			Calories
Macaroni and Cheese, Canned (Heinz)	7½ oz	NA	NA	NA	NA	NA	NA	10	10	1105	8	26	190
Macaroni, Elbow, and Cheese, Canned (Franco-American)	7⅜ oz	8	15	*	15	10	10	8	8	960	6	23	170
Macaroni and Cheese, Frozen (Green Giant)	9 oz	20	6	15	15	15	6	20	8	1115	10	36	290
Macaroni and Cheese, Frozen (Stouffer's)	6 oz	20	4	*	10	10	4	25	6	780	12	24	260
Macaroni and Cheese, Frozen (Swanson Main Course)	12 oz	25	30	8	10	20	4	25	15	1815	22	43	440
Macaroni and Cheese, Mix (Creamette)	2 oz	15	*	*	35	15	15	10	10	NA	2	47	220
Macaroni and Cheese (Cheddar), Mix (Golden Grain)	¼ pkg dry	10	*	*	30	15	10	8	8	NA	2	38	200
Macaroni and Cheese, Mix (Kraft Dinner)	¾ c prep	15	10	*	15	15	8	8	10	655	14	34	300
Macaroni and Cheese, Mix (Kraft Dinner), Family Size	¾ c prep	10	10	*	20	10	10	10	8	605	14	36	300
Macaroni and Cheese, Mix (Kraft Deluxe Dinner)	¾ c prep	15	8	*	15	15	8	10	10	650	8	36	260
Macaroni and Cheese, Spiral, Mix (Kraft Dinner)	¾ c prep	15	15	*	20	15	8	10	10	770	16	32	300

Pasta and Pasta Dishes	Amt.	Pro-tein	A	C	B₁	B₂	Nia-cin	Cal-cium	Iron	Sodium (mg)	Fat (g)	Carbohy-drate (g)	Calories
			% U.S. RDA										
Macaroni and Cheese, Mix (Lipton), Prep w Butter or Margarine	½ c prep	8	4	*	20	10	8	6	4	580	10	25	210
Macaroni in Pizza Sauce, Canned (Franco-American PizzOs)	7½ oz	6	15	10	10	10	10	2	8	1060	2	35	170
Macaroni, Spinach Ribbons, Dry (Creamette)	2 oz	10	*	*	35	15	15	2	15	NA	1	40	200
Manicotti, Jumbo, Frozen (Buitoni)	6 oz	17	8	2	15	20	10	35	6	625	9	31	270
Manicotti w Sauce, Frozen (Buitoni)	13 oz	24	45	6	15	15	2	30	40	1680	12	55	420
Noodles, Egg, Dry (American Beauty)	2 oz	10	0	0	35	15	20	0	10	10	3	41	220
Noodles, Egg, Dry (Buitoni)	2 oz	8	*	*	40	15	20	2	10	NA	3	40	220
Noodles, Egg, Dry (Creamette)	2 oz	10	*	*	35	15	15	2	10	NA	3	40	220
Noodles, Egg, Dry, All Varieties (Pennsylvania Dutch Brand)	2 oz	10	*	*	30	10	15	*	10	15	3	40	220
Noodles, Parisienne, Mix (Betty Crocker International Noodles)	¼ pkg	8	4	*	10	8	6	2	4	570	4	28	170

Food	Measure	% U.S. RDA									Sodium (mg)			Calories
Noodles Romanoff, Frozen (Stouffer's)	4 oz	8	15	*	8	8	4	8	8	4	675	9	16	170
Noodles Romanoff, Mix (Betty Crocker International Noodles)	¼ pkg	10	6	*	8	8	8	8	4	4	705	12	23	230
Noodles, Spinach, Dry (Buitoni)	2 oz	12	*	*	15	15	35	15	*	10	NA	1	37	210
Noodles and Beef in Sauce, Canned (Heinz)	7½ oz	NA	NA	NA	NA	NA	NA	NA	2	10	825	8	17	170
Noodles and Cheese, Mix (Noodle Roni Parmesano)	⅓ pkg dry	8	*	*	20	8	10	*	2	6	NA	2	23	130
Noodles and Chicken, Canned (Heinz)	7½ oz	NA	NA	NA	NA	NA	NA	NA	2	4	930	7	19	160
Noodles and Sauce, Alfredo (Lipton Deluxe), Prep w Butter or Margarine and Whole Milk	½ c prep	10	8	*	20	8	8	8	10	6	535	11	22	220
Noodles and Sauce, Beef Flavor (Lipton), Made w Butter or Margarine	½ c prep	8	4	*	15	4	4	10	*	4	550	7	26	190
Noodles and Sauce, Butter Flavor (Lipton), Made w Butter or Margarine	½ c prep	8	4	*	15	4	4	10	*	4	550	9	24	190
Noodles and Sauce, Butter and Herb (Lipton), Made w Butter or Margarine	½ c prep	8	4	*	15	6	10	10	*	4	515	9	23	180

Pasta and Pasta Dishes	Amt.	% U.S. RDA								Sodium (mg)	Fat (g)	Carbohydrate (g)	Calories
		Protein	A	C	B₁	B₂	Niacin	Calcium	Iron				
Noodles and Sauce, Cheese Flavor (Lipton), Made w Butter or Margarine	½ c prep	8	4	*	15	8	8	4	4	485	9	24	200
Noodles and Sauce, Chicken Bombay (Lipton Deluxe), Made w Butter or Margarine and Whole Milk	½ c prep	10	20	*	20	8	8	4	6	525	9	22	190
Noodles and Sauce, Chicken Flavor (Lipton), Made w Butter or Margarine	½ c prep	6	4	*	15	6	8	*	4	460	9	25	190
Noodles and Sauce, Parmesano (Lipton Deluxe), Made w Butter or Margarine and Whole Milk	½ c prep	10	6	*	20	10	8	6	4	445	11	22	210
Noodles and Sauce, Sour Cream and Chives (Lipton), Made w Butter or Margarine	½ c prep	8	4	*	15	6	10	*	4	460	9	23	190
Noodles and Sauce, Stroganoff (Lipton Deluxe), Made w Butter or Margarine and Whole Milk	½ c prep	10	4	*	20	8	8	4	8	495	10	22	200
Noodles and Tuna, Canned (Heinz)	7½ oz	NA	NA	NA	NA	NA	NA	2	6	950	5	20	170
Pasta Romana, Dry (Buitoni)	2 oz	7	*	*	35	15	15	*	10	NA	1	41	210

		% U.S. RDA											
Ravioli, Beef, Canned (Franco-American)	7½ oz	15	30	4	10	10	10	2	10	1095	5	36	230
Ravioli, Cheese, Frozen (Buitoni)	3¾ oz	10	6	*	8	10	10	10	8	245	5	44	260
Ravioli, Cheese, Parmesan, Frozen (Buitoni)	12 oz	26	25	25	20	20	6	15	15	1240	12	57	440
Ravioli, Cheese, Round, Frozen (Buitoni)	5½ oz	18	10	*	30	20	10	30	10	405	8	42	310
Ravioli, Meat, Frozen (Buitoni)	3¾ oz	12.5	*	*	20	6	15	8	8	365	4	43	265
Ravioli, Meat, Parmesan, Frozen (Buitoni)	12 oz	15	8	*	25	35	25	30	15	1785	18	75	520
Ravioli, Meat, Round, Frozen (Buitoni)	5½ oz	16	2	*	35	30	30	4	20	655	5	58	340
RavioliOs, Canned (Franco-American)	7½ oz	15	30	2	10	8	10	2	10	1030	5	34	210
Shells, Baked, w Sauce, Frozen (Buitoni)	10½ oz	14	8	20	40	40	10	10	30	1520	5	55	320
Shells, Dry (American Beauty)	2 oz	10	0	0	35	15	20	0	10	0–5	0–1	43	200
Shells, Stuffed, w Sauce, Frozen (Buitoni)	10 oz	21	25	6	15	30	6	45	8	1330	12	39	350
Shells, Stuffed w Beef and Spinach, w Tomato Sauce, Frozen (Stouffer's)	9 oz	30	45	35	15	15	15	15	15	1315	11	28	290

Pasta and Pasta Dishes	Amt.	Pro-tein	A	C	B₁	B₂	Nia-cin	Cal-cium	Iron	Sodium (mg)	Fat (g)	Carbohy-drate (g)	Calories
					% U.S. RDA								
Shells, Stuffed w Broccoli, Frozen (Buitoni)	5 oz	6	2	2	15	10	10	15	15	617	3	24	150
Shells, Stuffed w Cheese, w Meat Sauce, Frozen (Stouffer's)	9 oz	30	25	25	10	20	10	40	10	1310	14	30	320
Shells, Stuffed w Chicken, w Cheese Sauce, Frozen (Stouffer's)	9 oz	40	30	*	10	30	20	50	10	1060	22	24	400
Shells, Stuffed w Spinach and Cheese, Frozen (Buitoni)	5½ oz	8	10	*	10	15	8	20	10	579	4	24	160
Spaghetti, Dry (American Beauty)	2 oz	10	0	0	35	15	20	0	10	0-5	0-1	43	200
Spaghetti, Dry (Creamette)	2 oz	10	*	*	30	10	15	*	10	0-5	1	42	210
Spaghetti, Mix (Hamburger Helper)	⅓ pkg	40	10	*	20	15	25	2	20	1045	14	31	330
Spaghetti, Mix (Kraft American Style Dinner)	1 c prep	10	30	2	20	10	15	6	10	575	7	44	270
Spaghetti, Mix (Kraft Tangy Italian Style Dinner)	1 c prep	15	15	2	20	8	15	6	8	780	7	42	270
Spaghetti w Beef and Mushroom Sauce, Frozen (Stouffer's Lean Cuisine)	11½ oz	25	15	10	10	10	20	6	10	1450	7	38	280

							% U.S. RDA						
Spaghetti, in Meat Sauce, Canned (Franco-American)	7½ oz	15	15	8	10	10	15	2	10	110	8	26	210
Spaghetti w Meat Sauce, Frozen (Stouffer's)	14 oz	30	50	*	25	20	30	10	25	1970	12	62	445
Spaghetti w Meat Sauce, Mix (Kraft Dinner)	¾ c prep	15	10	2	15	8	10	6	8	765	10	31	250
Spaghetti w Meatballs in Tomato Sauce, Canned (Franco-American)	7⅜ oz	15	10	6	10	10	15	2	10	950	8	27	220
Spaghetti w Meatballs in Tomato Sauce, Canned (Franco-American SpaghettiOs)	7⅜ oz	15	6	4	10	10	15	2	10	1035	8	25	210
Spaghetti w Sliced Beef Franks in Tomato Sauce, Canned (Franco-American SpaghettiOs)	7⅜ oz	15	8	4	10	10	15	2	10	1070	9	26	220
Spaghetti, in Tomato Sauce w Cheese, Canned (Franco-American)	7⅜ oz	6	10	*	15	10	10	2	6	940	2	36	180
Spaghetti, in Tomato Sauce w Cheese, Canned (Heinz)	7¾ oz	NA	NA	NA	NA	NA	NA	2	4	1105	2	30	160
Spaghetti, in Tomato and Cheese Sauce, Canned (Franco-American SpaghettiOs)	7½ oz	6	10	*	10	8	10	2	6	895	2	33	170

Pasta and Pasta Dishes	Amt.	Protein	A	C	B$_1$	B$_2$	Niacin	Calcium	Iron	Sodium (mg)	Fat (g)	Carbohydrate (g)	Calories
		% U.S. RDA											
Spaghetti, in Tomato Sauce w Breaded Veal, Frozen (Swanson)	8¼ oz	30	10	15	15	10	25	2	15	915	11	29	270
Spaghetti, in Tomato Sauce w Meat, Canned (Heinz)	7½ oz	NA	NA	NA	NA	NA	NA	2	10	965	6	21	170
Stroganoff, Mix (Betty Crocker International Noodles)	¼ pkg	10	6	*	15	10	8	6	6	605	12	26	240
Tortellini, Guido, Frozen (Buitoni)	10 oz	20	8	*	25	25	20	40	15	1133	9	55	380
Ziti, Baked, Frozen (Buitoni)	10½ oz	14	10	20	10	25	4	15	45	1020	5	64	360
Pastries													
Apple Criss Cross (Pepperidge Farm)	2 oz	2	0	0	0	0	2	0	0	140	9	24	180
Donette, Chocolate Coated (Hostess)	1	0	0	0	2	2	0	0	2	50	3	6	60
Donette, Powdered (Hostess)	1	0	0	0	2	0	0	0	0	40	2	5	40
Donut, Chocolate (Dolly Madison)	1	2	*	*	4	4	4	2	6	240	8	18	150
Donut, Chocolate Coated (Hostess)	1	2	0	0	2	2	2	0	2	150	8	14	130

		% U.S. RDA											
Donut, Cinnamon (Hostess)	1	2	0	0	2	2	2	2	2	140	6	15	110
Donut, Krunch (Hostess)	1	2	0	0	2	2	2	2	2	130	4	16	110
Donut, Old Fashioned (Hostess)	1	2	0	0	6	4	2	2	2	220	10	22	180
Donut, Old Fashioned, Glazed (Hostess)	1	4	0	0	6	4	2	2	4	200	12	30	230
Donut, Plain (Hostess)	1	2	0	0	4	2	2	2	2	135	7	12	110
Donut, Powdered Sugar (Dolly Madison)	1	2	*	*	6	4	4	4	4	240	6	19	140
Donut, Powdered Sugar (Hostess)	1	2	0	0	2	2	2	0	2	140	5	15	110
Dumpling, Apple, Frozen (Pepperidge Farm)	3 oz	2	0	2	2	2	2	0	2	240	14	33	260
Eclair, Mix, Chocolate Flavored (Betty Crocker Classics)	⅙ pkg	8	2	*	2	8	*	15	4	455	12	54	340
Fruit Squares, Apple, Frozen (Pepperidge Farm)	1	2	0	2	0	0	0	0	2	180	12	27	230
Fruit Squares, Blueberry, Frozen (Pepperidge Farm)	1	2	0	8	0	2	2	0	4	190	11	29	220
Fruit Squares, Cherry, Frozen (Pepperidge Farm)	1	2	0	6	0	2	2	0	4	190	12	29	230
Strudel, Apple, Frozen (Pepperidge Farm)	3 oz	2	0	2	0	2	2	0	4	220	11	35	240

Pastries	Amt.	Protein	A	C	B₁	B₂	Niacin	Calcium	Iron	Sodium (mg)	Fat (g)	Carbohydrate (g)	Calories
								% U.S. RDA					
Turnover, Apple, Frozen (Pepperidge Farm)	1	4	0	2	2	2	2	0	4	220	17	35	310
Turnover, Apple (Pillsbury)	1	2	0	0	6	4	4	0	2	305	8	23	170
Turnover, Blueberry, Frozen (Pepperidge Farm)	1	4	0	10	2	2	2	0	4	240	19	32	320
Turnover, Blueberry (Pillsbury)	1	2	0	0	6	4	4	0	2	305	8	22	170
Turnover, Cherry, Frozen (Pepperidge Farm)	1	4	0	8	2	2	2	0	4	290	19	32	310
Turnover, Cherry (Pillsbury)	1	2	0	6	6	4	4	0	2	310	8	24	170
Turnover, Peach, Frozen (Pepperidge Farm)	1	4	6	50	2	2	2	0	2	260	19	34	320
Turnover, Raspberry, Frozen (Pepperidge Farm)	1	4	0	15	2	2	2	0	4	270	18	37	320
Pastry Shells													
Patty Shells, Frozen (Pepperidge Farm)	1	4	0	0	2	2	2	0	2	180	15	17	210
Pie Crust (Pillsbury All Ready), Refrigerated	⅛ of double crust	2	0	0	0	0	0	0	0	275	15	23	240
Pie Crust, Mix (Betty Crocker)	1/16 pkt	2	*	*	4	2	2	*	*	140	8	10	120
Pie Crust, Mix and Sticks (Pillsbury)	⅙ of 2-crust pie	6	0	0	20	8	10	0	6	425	17	25	270

Food	Serving	% U.S. RDA											
Pie Crust, Sticks (Betty Crocker)	⅛ stick	2	*	*	4	2	2	*	4	140	8	10	120
Puff Pastry Sheets, Frozen (Pepperidge Farm)	¼ sheet	6	0	0	2	2	2	0	4	290	17	45	255
Toaster Pastries													
Pop-Tarts, Blueberry (Kellogg's)	1	4	10	0	10	10	10	0	10	220	5	36	210
Pop-Tarts, Blueberry (Kellogg's Frosted)	1	4	10	0	10	10	10	0	10	220	5	38	200
Pop-Tarts, Brown Sugar Cinnamon (Kellogg's)	1	4	10	0	10	10	10	0	10	215	8	33	210
Pop-Tarts, Brown Sugar Cinnamon (Kellogg's Frosted)	1	4	10	0	10	10	10	0	10	205	7	34	210
Pop-Tarts, Cherry (Kellogg's)	1	4	10	0	10	10	10	0	10	230	5	36	210
Pop-Tarts, Cherry (Kellogg's Frosted)	1	4	10	0	10	10	10	0	10	230	5	37	210
Pop-Tarts, Chocolate Fudge (Kellogg's Frosted)	1	4	10	0	10	10	10	0	10	230	4	36	200
Pop-Tarts, Chocolate Vanilla (Kellogg's Frosted)	1	4	10	0	10	10	10	0	10	220	6	37	220
Pop-Tarts, Concord Grape (Kellogg's Frosted)	1	4	10	0	10	10	10	0	10	215	6	36	210
Pop-Tarts, Dutch Apple (Kellogg's Frosted)	1	4	10	0	10	10	10	0	10	215	6	36	210

Toaster Pastries	Amt.	Protein	A	C	B₁	B₂	Niacin	Calcium	Iron	Sodium (mg)	Fat (g)	Carbohydrate (g)	Calories
						% U.S. RDA							
Pop-Tarts, Raspberry (Kellogg's Frosted)	1	4	10	0	10	10	10	0	10	215	6	36	210
Pop-Tarts, Strawberry (Kellogg's)	1	4	10	0	10	10	10	0	10	225	4	37	200
Pop-Tarts, Strawberry (Kellogg's Frosted)	1	4	10	0	10	10	10	0	10	215	5	38	200
Toaster Strudel, Blueberry (Pillsbury)	1	2	0	0	8	6	6	0	4	205	8	28	190
Toaster Strudel, Cinnamon (Pillsbury)	1	2	0	0	8	6	6	0	4	200	8	26	190
Toaster Strudel, Raspberry (Pillsbury)	1	2	0	0	8	6	6	0	4	205	8	27	190
Toaster Strudel, Strawberry (Pillsbury)	1	2	0	0	8	6	6	0	4	205	8	27	190
Toastettes, All Varieties (Nabisco)	1	2	10	10	10	10	10	0	10	NA	5	35	190
Peanut Butter													
Bama Creamy	2 tbsp	10	*	*	*	2	15	*	2	160	16	7	200
Bama Crunchy	2 tbsp	10	*	*	*	2	15	2	2	135	16	6	200
Skippy Creamy	2 tbsp	15	*	*	*	*	20	*	2	150	17	4	190
Skippy Super Chunk	2 tbsp	15	*	*	*	*	20	*	2	150	17	4	190
Goober Grape (Smucker's)	2 tbsp	8	0	0	0	0	15	0	2	120	10	18	180

Pies

Pies	Portion	% U.S. RDA									
Apple, Frozen (Mrs. Smith's), 10"	1/8	NA	NA	NA	NA	NA	NA	590	17	56	390
Apple, Frozen (Mrs. Smith's Natural Juice), 9"	1/2	NA	NA	NA	NA	NA	NA	370	22	52	420
Apple Streusel, Frozen (Mrs. Smith's Natural Juice), 9"	1/2	NA	NA	NA	NA	NA	NA	365	16	67	420
Blueberry, Frozen (Mrs. Smith's), 10"	1/8	NA	NA	NA	NA	NA	NA	535	17	54	380
Boston Cream, Frozen (Mrs. Smith's), 10"	1/8	NA	NA	NA	NA	NA	NA	225	8	44	260
Boston Cream, Mix (Betty Crocker Classics)	1/8 pkg	2	6	8	2	15	2	405	6	48	260
Apple, Frozen (Mrs. Smith's)	1/8	4	2	4	2	*	4	590	17	56	390
Apple, Frozen (Mrs. Smith's Natural Juice)	1/2	4	*	2	*	*	8	370	22	52	420
Apple, Frozen (Mrs. Smith's Old Fashioned)	1/8	6	2	4	6	*	4	620	27	64	515
Apple Lattice, Frozen (Mrs. Smith's)	1/8	2	4	2	4	*	2	440	13	58	350
Apple Streusel, Frozen (Mrs. Smith's Natural Juice)	1/2	4	*	2	*	2	4	365	16	67	420

Pies	Amt.	Protein	A	C	B₁	B₂	Niacin	Calcium	Iron	Sodium (mg)	Fat (g)	Carbohydrate (g)	Calories
		% U.S. RDA											
Banana Cream, Frozen (Mrs. Smith's)	⅛	2	*	*	2	8	2	4	2	180	12	31	240
Blueberry, Frozen (Mrs. Smith's)	⅛	6	4	*	*	2	2	*	2	535	17	54	380
Boston Cream, Frozen (Mrs. Smith's)	⅛	2	2	*	*	10	2	2	2	225	8	44	260
Cherry, Frozen (Mrs. Smith's)	⅛	6	2	*	2	4	*	2	4	445	16	60	400
Cherry, Frozen (Mrs. Smith's Natural Juice)	⅐	6	2	*	4	4	2	*	6	380	18	59	410
Cherry Lattice, Frozen (Mrs. Smith's)	⅛	4	10	*	*	6	*	*	2	490	11	59	350
Chocolate Cream, Frozen (Mrs. Smith's)	⅛	2	2	*	2	2	4	2	2	235	13	35	270
Coconut Cream, Frozen (Mrs. Smith's)	⅛	2	*	*	2	4	*	2	2	220	14	33	270
Coconut Custard, Frozen (Mrs. Smith's)	⅛	12	2	*	2	20	4	10	6	550	15	40	330
Egg Custard, Frozen (Mrs. Smith's)	⅛	15	*	*	4	20	*	15	4	490	9	45	300
Lemon Cream, Frozen (Mrs. Smith's)	⅛	2	2	*	2	4	2	*	2	185	12	32	245
Lemon Meringue, Frozen (Mrs. Smith's)	⅛	2	4	*	4	2	2	*	2	315	10	52	310

| | | % U.S. RDA | | | | | | | | | | | |
Food	Serving												
Peach, Frozen (Mrs. Smith's)	1/8	6	2	*	4	*	2	*	4	435	16	53	365
Pecan, Frozen (Mrs. Smith's)	1/8	6	6	*	2	4	6	*	4	510	23	70	510
Pumpkin Custard, Frozen (Mrs. Smith's)	1/8	10	30	*	4	*	15	8	4	495	11	46	310
Pies, Snack													
Apple (Hostess)	1	4	0	2	10	8	8	2	8	540	20	45	390
Apple (Drake's)	1	4	*	*	6	4	2	*	4	230	10	30	220
Apple, Fried (Dolly Madison)	1	4	*	*	10	8	6	8	15	450	27	59	490
Berry (Hostess)	1	6	0	4	10	10	8	4	10	490	20	48	390
Blueberry (Hostess)	1	4	0	4	10	8	8	2	8	450	20	49	390
Cherry (Hostess)	1	6	0	2	10	8	8	2	8	530	20	55	390
Cherry, Fried (Dolly Madison)	1	4	*	*	10	6	6	6	15	450	27	53	470
Lemon (Hostess)	1	4	0	0	10	8	8	2	8	470	22	53	400
Peach (Hostess)	1	6	0	2	10	10	10	4	10	445	20	53	400
Strawberry (Hostess)	1	4	0	25	10	8	8	2	6	400	14	56	340
Pizza, Frozen													
Buitoni 6 Slice	4 oz	10	2	*	15	20	15	20	15	620	4	35	220
Canadian Bacon (Totino's Party Pizza)	1/2	20	20	4	20	30	15	20	10	875	13	40	340

Pizza, Frozen	Amt.	Protein	A	C	B₁	B₂	Niacin	Calcium	Iron	Sodium (mg)	Fat (g)	Carbohydrate (g)	Calories
					% U.S. RDA								
Canadian Style Bacon, (Totino's My Classic)	⅓	21 g	30	4	25	45	20	35	15	1405	18	49	440
Cheese (Buitoni)	2 oz	5	*	2	10	10	4	10	6	285	3	20	130
Cheese (Stouffer's French Bread Pizza)	5³⁄₁₆ oz	15	10	*	25	10	15	25	15	850	13	43	330
Cheese (Totino's Party Pizza)	½	25	8	4	15	20	10	25	8	635	16	41	350
Cheese, Deluxe (Totino's My Classic)	⅓	22 g	15	8	20	25	15	45	10	960	23	50	490
Combination, Deluxe (Totino's My Classic)	⅓	25 g	45	25	35	55	20	45	20	1435	34	50	610
Deluxe (Stouffer's French Bread Pizza)	6³⁄₁₆ oz	20	15	*	20	20	20	20	15	1150	18	46	400
Hamburger (Stouffer's French Bread Pizza)	6⅛ oz	25	15	*	20	20	15	20	15	1100	20	39	400
Pepperoni, Frozen (Fox Deluxe)	½	15	10	4	25	25	20	10	10	900	10	36	280
Pepperoni (Stouffer's French Bread Pizza)	5⅝ oz	15	15	*	20	15	15	20	15	1190	20	44	410
Pepperoni (Totino's Party Pizza)	½	20	20	4	20	30	15	20	10	1030	17	40	370
Pepperoni, Deluxe (Totino's My Classic)	⅓	23 g	45	25	25	55	20	45	20	1600	30	51	560

					% U.S. RDA								
Sausage (Stouffer's French Bread Pizza)	6 oz	25	15	*	25	20	15	20	15	1320	20	44	420
Sausage (Totino's Party Pizza)	½	20	20	4	25	30	15	20	10	1130	20	41	400
Sausage, Deluxe (Totino's My Classic)	⅓	22 g	40	25	35	50	20	40	20	1200	30	50	560
Sausage and Mushroom (Stouffer's French Bread Pizza)	6¼ oz	25	10	*	25	20	15	20	15	1220	18	40	395
Sausage and Pepperoni Combination (Totino's Party Pizza)	½	25	20	4	20	30	15	20	10	1120	19	41	400
Poultry and Game													
Chicken, Broiled, w/o skin	3 oz	45	2	*	2	10	40	*	8	56	4	0	120
Chicken, Fried, Breast, w Bone (2½-lb Fryer)	½	60	2	*	2	10	60	*	8	NA	5	2	160
Chicken, Fried, Drumstick, w Bone (2½-lb Fryer)	1	25	2	*	2	8	15	*	4	NA	4	0-1	90
Chicken, Fried, Thigh, w Bone (2½-lb Fryer)	1	35	2	*	2	15	20	*	6	NA	6	1	120
Chicken, Roasted, Dark Meat w/o Skin	3 oz	60	2	*	6	10	25	2	8	75	6	0	160
Chicken, Roasted, Dark Meat w/o Skin, Diced	1 c	90	4	*	10	15	35	2	15	123	9	0	260
Chicken, Roasted, Light Meat w/o Skin	3 oz	60	2	*	4	4	50	*	6	56	4	0	160

Poultry and Game	Amt.	Pro-tein	A	C	B₁	B₂	Nia-cin	Cal-cium	Iron	Sodium (mg)	Fat (g)	Carbohy-drate (g)	Calories
		% U.S. RDA											
Chicken, Roasted, Light Meat w/o Skin, Diced	1 c	100	4	*	8	8	80	2	10	92	7	0	260
Chicken, Stewed, Dark Meat w/o Skin	3 oz	60	4	*	4	10	35	2	8	55	8	0	180
Chicken, Stewed, Dark Meat w/o Skin, Diced	1 c	90	8	*	6	15	60	2	15	90	14	0	290
Chicken, Stewed, Light Meat w/o Skin	3 oz	60	2	*	2	4	45	*	6	41	4	0	150
Chicken, Stewed, Light Meat w/o Skin, Diced	1 c	100	4	*	2	8	80	2	10	67	7	0	250
Chicken, Breast (Eckrich Calorie Watcher), Re-frigerated	2 sl	15	*	6	2	2	10	*	2	420	1	1	40
Chicken, Chunk, Canned (Swanson)	2½ oz	30	*	*	*	4	15	*	4	270	6	0	110
Chicken, Chunk Style, Canned (Swanson Mixin')	2½ oz	25	*	*	*	4	15	2	4	225	8	0	130
Chicken, Frozen, Fried, As-sorted Pieces (Swanson)	3¼ oz	30	*	*	8	10	20	2	8	655	16	13	260
Chicken, Frozen, Fried, As-sorted Pieces (Swanson Take-Out)	3¼ oz	40	*	*	8	8	20	*	10	730	17	10	270
Chicken, Frozen, Fried, Breast Portions (Swanson)	4½ oz	50	*	*	10	10	35	2	15	865	19	20	350

Food	Serving	% U.S. RDA											
Chicken, Frozen, Fried, Thighs and Drumsticks (Swanson)	3¼ oz	35	*	*	6	10	15	2	8	550	19	11	280
Chicken, Slender Sliced (Eckrich Calorie Watcher), Refrigerated	1 oz	10	*	10	*	*	6	*	*	390	3	2	45
Chicken, White, Chunk, Canned (Swanson)	2½ oz	30	*	*	*	4	20	*	2	235	4	0	100
Chicken Salad, Canned (The Spreadables)	¼ can	15	*	*	*	2	10	*	*	230	9	4	120
Chicken Spread, Canned (Swanson)	1 oz	8	*	*	2	2	4	6	2	140	4	2	60
Chicken Spread, Canned (Underwood Chunky)	½ can (2.4 oz)	25	2	4	4	6	15	*	4	575	11	3	150
Goose, Domesticated, Roasted	3 oz	60	8	6	6	8	40	2	8	105	9	0	200
Liver, Chicken, Simmered	1 (about 2" × 2" × ⅝")	15	60	2	2	40	15	*	10	15	1	1	40
Liver, Chicken, Simmered, Chopped	1 c	80	340	15	15	220	80	2	70	85	6	5	230
Rabbit, Domesticated, Stewed	3 oz	60	*	*	2	4	50	2	8	39	9	0	180
Turkey, Roasted, Dark Meat w/o Skin	3 oz	60	4	*	2	10	20	2	10	84	7	0	170
Turkey, Roasted, Dark Meat w/o Skin, Diced	1 c	90	6	4	4	20	30	2	20	138	12	0	280

Poultry and Game	Amt.	Protein	A	C	B₁	B₂	Niacin	Calcium	Iron	Sodium (mg)	Fat (g)	Carbohydrate (g)	Calories
						% U.S. RDA							
Turkey, Roasted, Light Meat w/o Skin	3 oz	60	2	*	2	8	45	*	6	70	4	0	150
Turkey, Roasted, Light Meat w/o Skin, Diced	1 c	100	2	*	4	10	80	2	10	115	6	0	250
Turkey, Boneless, Canned	1 c	100	6	*	2	15	50	2	15	NA	26	0	410
Turkey, Breast (Louis Rich), Fresh	1 oz cooked	19	NA	NA	*	2	9	*	*	25	2	0	45
Turkey, Breast, Barbecued (Louis Rich)	1 oz	14	NA	NA	*	*	12	*	*	156	1	0	40
Turkey, Breast, Hickory Smoked (Louis Rich)	1 oz	13	NA	NA	*	2	13	*	*	208	1	.6	35
Turkey, Breast, Oven Roasted (Louis Rich)	1 sl	12	NA	NA	*	2	11	*	*	214	1	.1	30
Turkey, Breast, Slices (Louis Rich), Fresh	1 oz cooked	19	NA	NA	*	2	10	*	*	24	1	0	40
Turkey, Breast, Smoked (Louis Rich)	1 sl	8	NA	NA	*	*	8	*	*	181	0–1	.1	20
Turkey, Breast Tenderloins (Louis Rich), Fresh	1 oz cooked	20	NA	NA	*	2	10	*	*	29	1	0	40
Turkey, Drumsticks (Louis Rich), Fresh	1 oz cooked	18	NA	NA	*	4	4	*	3	24	3	0	60
Turkey, Drumsticks, Smoked (Louis Rich)	1 oz	13	NA	NA	*	4	6	*	2	399	2	.1	40

Food	Serving					% U.S. RDA							
Turkey, Ground (Louis Rich), Fresh	1 oz cooked	16	NA	NA	*	4	8	*	2	32	4	0	65
Turkey, Smoked, Slender Sliced (Eckrich Calorie Watcher)	1 oz	10	*	10	*	2	6	*	2	400	2	2	40
Turkey, Smoked (Louis Rich)	1 sl	11	NA	NA	*	*	9	NA	NA	272	1	.2	30
Turkey, Wings (Louis Rich), Fresh	1 oz cooked	16	NA	NA	*	2	5	*	*	21	3	0	55
Turkey, Wings, Smoked (Louis Rich Drumettes)	1 oz	15	NA	NA	*	2	9	*	*	285	2	.4	45
Turkey Bologna (Louis Rich)	1 sl	8	NA	NA	*	2	5	3	2	214	4	.6	60
Turkey Breakfast Sausage (Louis Rich)	1 oz cooked	13	NA	NA	*	4	7	*	2	191	4	0	65
Turkey Cotto Salami (Louis Rich)	1 sl	9	NA	NA	*	5	6	*	2	251	4	.2	50
Turkey Franks (Louis Rich)	1 link	12	NA	NA	*	4	8	5	4	454	9	1	100
Turkey Ham (Cured Turkey Thigh Meat) (Louis Rich)	1 sl	11	NA	NA	*	4	8	*	*	262	1.1	.4	35
Turkey Ham, Chopped (Louis Rich)	1 sl	11	NA	NA	*	4	7	*	*	250	2.2	.2	40
Turkey Luncheon Loaf (Louis Rich)	1 sl	10	NA	NA	*	*	7	*	*	287	2	.4	40

Poultry and Game	Amt.	Pro-tein	A	C	B₁	B₂	Nia-cin	Cal-cium	Iron	Sodium (mg)	Fat (g)	Carbohy-drate (g)	Calories
			% U.S. RDA										
Turkey Pastrami (Louis Rich)	1 sl	11	NA	NA	*	4	7	*	2	272	1	.4	35
Turkey Salad, Canned (The Spreadables)	¼ can	15	*	*	*	*	10	*	*	245	8	3	110
Turkey Smoked Sausage (Louis Rich)	1 oz	10	NA	NA	*	3	5	*	2	219	4	.3	55
Turkey Summer Sausage (Louis Rich)	1 sl	10	NA	NA	2	6	7	*	2	304	3	.3	50
Puddings													
Banana, Canned (Del Monte Pudding Cup)	5 oz	6	*	*	2	10	*	10	*	285	5	30	180
Banana, Canned (Hunt's Snack Pack)	5 oz	4	*	*	*	6	*	4	*	215	11	26	210
Banana Cream, Mix (Jell-O Instant), w Whole Milk	½ c prep	8	2	*	2	10	*	15	*	440	4	30	170
Banana Cream Pie Filling, Mix (Jell-O)	⅙ of prep mix	6	2	*	2	8	*	10	*	165	3	17	100
Butter Pecan, Mix (Jell-O Instant), w Whole Milk	½ c prep	10	2	*	4	10	*	15	*	440	5	29	170
Butterscotch, Canned (Del Monte Pudding Cup)	5 oz	6	*	*	2	10	*	10	*	285	5	31	180
Butterscotch, Canned (Hunt's Snack Pack)	5 oz	4	*	*	*	6	*	4	*	235	9	30	210

Food	Serving	% U.S. RDA										Calories
Butterscotch, Mix (D-Zerta), w Nonfat Milk	½ c prep	10	4	2	10	*	15	*	115	0	12	70
Butterscotch, Mix (Jell-O), w Whole Milk	½ c prep	8	2	*	10	*	15	*	245	4	30	170
Butterscotch, Mix (Jell-O Instant), w Whole Milk	½ c prep	8	2	*	10	*	15	*	475	4	30	170
Chocolate, Canned (Del Monte Pudding Cup)	5 oz	8	*	*	10	2	10	2	280	6	31	190
Chocolate, Canned (Hunt's Snack Pack)	5 oz	4	*	*	4	2	4	2	160	9	30	210
Chocolate, Mix (D-Zerta), w Nonfat Milk	½ c prep	10	4	2	10	*	15	*	115	0	11	60
Chocolate, Mix (Jell-O), w Whole Milk	½ c prep	10	2	*	10	*	15	*	170	4	28	160
Chocolate, Mix (Jell-O Instant), w Whole Milk	½ c prep	10	2	*	10	*	15	*	515	4	31	180
Chocolate Fudge, Canned (Del Monte Pudding Cup)	5 oz	8	*	*	10	4	10	4	260	6	31	190
Chocolate Fudge, Canned (Hunt's Snack Pack)	5 oz	4	*	*	4	2	2	2	165	10	28	200
Chocolate Fudge, Mix (Jell-O), w Whole Milk	½ c prep	10	2	2	10	*	15	*	170	4	28	160
Chocolate Fudge, Mix (Jell-O Instant), w Whole Milk	½ c prep	10	2	2	15	2	15	2	480	5	32	180

Puddings	Amt.	Protein	A	C	B₁	B₂	Niacin	Calcium	Iron	Sodium (mg)	Fat (g)	Carbohydrate (g)	Calories
								% U.S. RDA					
Chocolate Marshmallow, Canned (Hunt's Snack Pack)	5 oz	4	*	*	*	4	*	*	2	155	9	30	200
Coconut Cream, Mix (Jell-O Instant), w Whole Milk	½ c prep	10	2	*	4	10	*	15	*	355	7	28	180
Coconut Cream Pie Filling (Jell-O)	⅙ prep	6	2	*	2	8	*	10	*	140	4	16	110
Egg Custard, Golden, Mix (Jell-O Americana), w Whole Milk	½ c prep	10	4	*	6	15	*	20	2	220	5	23	160
French Vanilla, Mix (Jell-O), w Whole Milk	½ c prep	8	2	*	2	10	*	15	*	200	4	30	170
French Vanilla, Mix (Jell-O Instant), w Whole Milk	½ c prep	8	2	*	2	10	*	15	*	435	4	30	170
German Chocolate, Canned (Hunt's Snack Pack)	5 oz	4	*	*	*	4	*	*	2	155	9	35	220
Lemon, Canned (Hunt's Snack Pack)	5 oz	*	*	*	*	*	*	*	*	80	4	36	180
Lemon, Mix (Jell-O Instant), w Whole Milk	½ c prep	8	2	*	2	10	*	15	*	385	4	31	180
Lemon Pie Filling (Jell-O)	⅙ prep	4	2	*	*	4	*	*	*	90	2	38	170

Food	Serving												
		% U.S. RDA											
Milk Chocolate, Mix (Jell-O), w Whole Milk	½ c prep	10	2	*	2	10	2	*	15	*	170	4	28	170
Milk Chocolate, Mix (Jell-O Instant), w Whole Milk	½ c prep	10	2	*	4	10	4	*	15	*	505	5	31	180
Pineapple Cream, Mix (Jell-O Instant), w Whole Milk	½ c prep	8	2	*	2	10	2	*	15	*	390	4	30	170
Pistachio, Mix (Jell-O Instant), w Whole Milk	½ c prep	10	2	*	2	10	2	*	15	*	425	5	30	180
Rice, Canned (Hunt's Snack Pack)	5 oz	6	*	*	2	6	2	2	6	*	230	12	27	220
Rice, Mix (Jell-O Americana), w Whole Milk	½ c prep	10	2	*	6	10	2	2	15	2	155	4	30	170
Tapioca, Canned (Del Monte Pudding Cup)	5 oz	6	*	*	2	10	2	2	10	*	250	4	30	180
Tapioca, Canned (Hunt's Snack Pack)	5 oz	6	*	*	*	6	*	*	6	*	170	6	27	140
Tapioca, Chocolate, Mix (Jell-O Americana), w Whole Milk	½ c prep	10	2	*	4	15	4	*	15	2	170	5	28	170
Tapioca, Vanilla, Mix (Jell-O Americana), w Whole Milk	½ c prep	8	2	*	2	10	2	*	15	*	170	4	27	160
Vanilla, Canned (Del Monte Pudding Cup)	5 oz	6	*	*	2	10	2	2	10	*	285	5	32	180

| | | % U.S. RDA | | | | | | | | | | | |
Puddings	Amt.	Pro-tein	A	C	B₁	B₂	Nia-cin	Cal-cium	Iron	Sodium (mg)	Fat (g)	Carbohy-drate (g)	Calories
Vanilla, Canned (Hunt's Snack Pack)	5 oz	4	*	*	*	6	*	4	*	195	9	31	210
Vanilla, Mix (D-Zerta), w Nonfat Milk	½ c prep	10	4	2	2	10	*	15	*	105	0	12	70
Vanilla, Mix (Jell-O), w Whole Milk	½ c prep	8	2	*	2	10	*	15	*	200	4	27	160
Vanilla, Mix (Jell-O Instant), w Whole Milk	½ c prep	8	2	*	2	10	*	15	*	420	4	29	170
Rice and Rice Dishes													
Brown, Long Grain	1 c hot	8	*	*	10	2	15	2	6	550	2	50	230
Brown, Frozen in Beef Stock (Green Giant)	1 c	8	*	15	2	8	4	2	4	NA	8	55	300
White, Enriched, Cooked	1 c hot	6	*	*	15	2	10	2	10	767	0-1	50	220
White, Enriched, Instant, Cooked	1 c hot	6	*	*	15	2	8	*	8	450	Trace	40	180
White, Enriched, Parboiled, Long Grain, Cooked	1 c hot	6	*	*	10	*	6	*	6	627	0-1	50	190
White, Unenriched, Cooked	1 c hot	6	*	*	2	2	4	2	2	767	0-1	50	220
White (Minute Rice)	⅔ c	4	*	*	10	*	6	*	6	2	0	27	120
Long Grain and Wild (Minute), prep w Butter	½ c prep	4	4	4	10	4	8	2	6	570	4	25	150

Food	Amount	% U.S. RDA							Sodium	Fat	Carb.	Cal.
Long Grain White and Wild, Frozen (Green Giant Rice Originals)	½ c	4	0	15	0	10	0	8	565	1	23	110
Beef Flavor (Rice-a-Roni)	½ pkg dry	6	*	25	8	8	*	6	NA	1	27	130
Beef Flavor (Minute), Prep w Butter	½ c prep	4	2	20	*	8	*	6	720	4	25	150
Chicken Flavor (Rice-a-Roni)	⅓ pkg dry	4	*	20	6	6	*	8	NA	1	33	160
Chicken Flavor (Minute), Prep w Butter	½ c prep	4	2	15	*	8	*	6	685	4	25	150
Fried (Minute), Prep w Oil	½ c prep	4	*	15	*	8	*	6	635	5	25	160
Spanish, Canned (Heinz)	7¼ oz	NA	NA	NA	NA	NA	2	6	1045	5	26	150
Spanish, Mix (Rice-a-Roni)	½ pkg dry	4	*	15	6	10	*	6	NA	1	26	120
Rice, Frozen (Green Giant Rice Originals Medley)	½ c	4	2	25	2	8	0	6	280	3	20	120
Rice, Frozen, Chinese Fried Style (Birds Eye)	3.6 oz	4	15	4	*	4	*	4	425	0	23	100
Rice, Frozen, French Style (Birds Eye)	3.6 oz	4	*	4	*	2	*	6	635	0	25	120
Rice, Frozen, w Herb Butter Sauce (Green Giant Rice Originals)	½ c	4	6	8	2	6	0	6	420	6	21	150
Rice, Frozen, Italian Style (Birds Eye)	3.6 oz	6	6	15	*	4	*	6	385	1	28	130

Rice and Rice Dishes	Amt.	Protein	A	C	B₁	B₂	Niacin	Calcium	Iron	Sodium (mg)	Fat (g)	Carbohydrate (g)	Calories
		% U.S. RDA											
Rice, Frozen, Oriental Style (Birds Eye)	3.6 oz	4	10	10	4	*	4	*	4	460	1	27	130
Rice, Frozen, Spanish Style (Birds Eye)	3.6 oz	6	8	45	6	*	4	*	4	495	1	26	120
Rice and Broccoli, Frozen, in Flavored Cheese Sauce (Green Giant Rice Originals)	½ c	4	15	8	15	2	8	4	6	405	6	19	140
Rice and Peas, Frozen, w Mushrooms (Birds Eye)	2.3 oz	6	8	15	10	8	8	*	4	320	0	23	110
Rice Pilaf, Frozen (Green Giant Rice Originals)	½ c	4	0	2	15	2	10	0	8	520	2	23	120
Rice and Sauce, Beef Flavor (Lipton), Prep w Butter or Margarine	½ c prep	4	2	*	8	4	4	*	4	665	4	27	160
Rice and Sauce, Chicken Flavor (Lipton), Prep w Butter or Margarine	½ c prep	4	2	*	8	4	4	*	4	525	4	26	150
Rice and Sauce, Herb and Butter (Lipton), Prep w Butter or Margarine	½ c prep	4	2	*	8	4	4	*	4	500	5	25	160
Rice and Sauce, Spanish (Lipton), Prep w Butter or Margarine	½ c prep	4	6	2	8	4	4	*	4	520	3	26	140

					% U.S. RDA							
White Rice and Spinach, Frozen, in Cheese Sauce, Italian Blend (Green Giant Rice Originals)	½ c	6	30	8	10	4	6	6	6	460	7	21	160

Rolls and Buns

Bagels, Egg	1 (3″ diam)	10	*	*	10	6	6	*	6	NA	NA	NA	165
Bagels, Water	1 (3″ diam)	10	*	*	10	6	8	*	6	NA	NA	NA	165
Breadsticks, Soft (Pillsbury)	1 stick	4	0	0	8	4	6	0	4	240	2	18	100
Buns, Frankfurter (Pepperidge Farm)	1	8	0	0	10	10	10	4	6	320	3	23	140
Buns, Hamburger (Butter-Nut)	1	4	*	*	8	4	4	4	4	170	1	14	80
Buns, Hamburger (Eddy's)	1	4	*	*	8	4	4	4	4	170	1	14	80
Buns, Hamburger (Millbrook)	1	4	*	*	8	4	4	4	4	170	1	14	80
Buns, Hamburger (Pepperidge Farm)	1	6	0	0	15	8	8	4	6	260	3	21	130
Buns, Hamburger (Sweetheart)	1	4	*	*	8	4	4	4	4	170	1	14	80
Buns, Hamburger (Weber's)	1	4	*	*	8	4	4	4	4	170	1	14	80

Rolls and Buns	Amt.	Protein	A	C	B₁	B₂	Niacin	Calcium	Iron	Sodium (mg)	Fat (g)	Carbohydrate (g)	Calories
					% U.S. RDA								
Buns, Hamburger (Wonder)	1	6	0	0	10	6	6	6	6	230	3	22	120
Buns, Hot Dog (Butter-Nut)	1	4	*	*	8	4	4	4	4	170	1	14	80
Buns, Hot Dog (Eddy's)	1	4	*	*	8	4	4	4	4	170	1	14	80
Buns, Hot Dog (Millbrook)	1	4	*	*	8	4	4	4	4	170	1	14	80
Buns, Hot Dog (Sweetheart)	1	4	*	*	8	4	4	4	4	170	1	14	80
Buns, Hot Dog (Weber's)	1	4	*	*	8	4	4	4	4	170	1	14	80
Buns, Hot Dog (Wonder)	1	6	0	0	10	6	6	6	6	230	3	22	120
Buns, Sandwich, Cracked Wheat (Pepperidge Farm)	1	8	0	0	10	10	10	4	8	200	3	25	150
Buns, Sandwich, Mustard Bran (Pepperidge Farm)	1	10	0	2	8	10	10	4	8	220	3	21	130
Buns, Sandwich, Onion w Poppy Seeds (Pepperidge Farm)	1	8	0	0	15	8	8	4	10	240	3	26	150
Buns, Sandwich w Poppy Seeds (Pepperidge Farm)	1	8	0	0	15	8	8	6	6	435	3	22	130
Buns, Sandwich, w Sesame Seeds (Pepperidge Farm)	1	8	0	0	20	10	8	4	10	210	3	23	130

					% U.S. RDA								
Croissants, All Butter (Pepperidge Farm)	1	6	10	0	6	8	4	4	2	310	13	19	200
Croissants (Pepperidge Farm All Butter Tray)	1	6	10	0	6	8	4	4	2	310	13	19	200
Croissants (Pepperidge Farm Petite All-Butter)	1	4	6	0	6	8	6	4	6	160	7	14	130
Rolls (Wonder Gem Style)	2	6	0	0	15	8	10	6	8	310	5	27	170
Rolls (Wonder Half & Half)	2	6	0	0	15	8	10	6	8	145	5	25	160
Rolls (Wonder Home Bake)	2	6	0	0	15	8	10	6	8	230	5	26	170
Rolls, Brown and Serve (Butter-Nut)	1	4	*	*	8	4	4	4	4	185	3	11	90
Rolls, Brown and Serve (Eddy's)	1	4	*	*	8	4	4	4	4	185	3	11	90
Rolls, Brown and Serve (Millbrook)	1	4	*	*	8	4	4	4	4	185	3	11	90
Rolls, Brown and Serve (Sweetheart)	1	4	*	*	8	4	4	4	4	185	3	11	90
Rolls, Brown and Serve (Weber's)	1	4	*	*	8	4	4	4	4	185	3	11	90
Rolls, Butter Crescent (Pepperidge Farm)	1	4	0	0	10	6	6	2	4	160	6	13	110
Rolls w Buttermilk (Wonder)	2	6	0	0	15	8	10	6	8	280	5	26	170
Rolls, Club, Brown and Serve (Pepperidge Farm)	1	6	0	0	15	10	10	4	6	220	1	20	100

Rolls and Buns	Amt.	Pro-tein	A	C	B$_1$	B$_2$	Nia-cin	Cal-cium	Iron	Sodium (mg)	Fat (g)	Carbohy-drate (g)	Calories
		% U.S. RDA											
Rolls, Dinner (Home Pride)	2	8	0	0	15	10	10	8	8	340	4	28	170
Rolls, Dinner (Pepperidge Farm)	1	2	0	0	6	4	4	2	2	90	2	10	60
Rolls, Dinner (Wonder)	2	8	0	0	20	10	10	2	10	375	4	34	200
Rolls, Dinner, Butterflake (Pillsbury)	1	4	0	0	8	4	4	0	4	410	4	16	110
Rolls, Dinner, Country White, Bakery Style (Pillsbury)	1	4	0	0	8	6	6	0	6	350	1	20	100
Rolls, Dinner, Crescent (Pillsbury)	2	4	0	0	10	6	6	0	6	460	11	22	200
Rolls, Dinner, Parkerhouse (Pillsbury)	2	4	0	0	15	8	8	0	6	595	3	27	150
Rolls, Finger w Poppy Seeds (Pepperidge Farm)	1	2	0	0	6	4	4	2	2	95	2	8	60
Rolls, Finger w Sesame Seeds (Pepperidge Farm)	1	2	0	0	6	4	4	2	2	80	2	9	60
Rolls, French, Brown and Serve (2) (Pepperidge Farm)	½ roll	10	0	0	25	10	15	6	8	420	2	36	180
Rolls, French, Brown and Serve (3) (Pepperidge Farm)	½ roll	6	0	0	15	8	10	4	6	300	1	24	120

		% U.S. RDA										
Rolls, French, Brown and Serve (Wonder)	2	6	0	15	8	10	6	8	300	5	27	150
Rolls, French Style (Pepperidge Farm), 2" size	1 (1.3 oz)	6	0	15	8	10	4	4	250	1	19	110
Rolls, French Style, Brown and Serve (Pepperidge Farm Hearth)	1	2	0	6	4	6	2	2	100	1	10	50
Rolls, Kaiser (Wonder)	1	25	0	45	25	30	25	25	870	8	82	460
Rolls, Layered, Brown and Serve (Pepperidge Farm Golden Twist)	1	4	0	8	4	6	2	4	160	6	14	110
Rolls, Mix (Pillsbury Hot Roll Mix)	2	8	0	10	8	6	0	4	250	4	34	200
Rolls, Old Fashioned (Pepperidge Farm)	1	2	0	6	4	4	2	2	90	2	7	50
Rolls, Pan (Wonder)	2	8	0	20	10	10	10	10	375	4	34	200
Rolls, Parker House (Pepperidge Farm)	1	2	0	6	4	4	2	2	90	1	9	50
Rolls, Party (Pepperidge Farm)	1	2	0	4	2	2	0	2	50	1	5	30
Rolls, Party w Poppy Seeds (Pepperidge Farm)	1	2	0	4	2	2	0	2	55	4	22	45
Rolls, Soft Family (Pepperidge Farm)	1	6	0	8	8	6	4	4	200	2	18	100
Rolls, Sourdough French Style (Pepperidge Farm)	1 (1.3 oz)	6	0	15	8	8	2	6	240	1	19	100

Rolls and Buns	Amt.	Pro-tein	A	C	B$_1$	B$_2$	Nia-cin	Cal-cium	Iron	Sodium (mg)	Fat (g)	Carbohy-drate (g)	Calories
					% U.S. RDA								
Rolls, Wheat Loaf (Pillsbury) 1" sl Pipin' Hot		4	0	0	6	4	4	0	2	170	2	12	80
Rolls, White Loaf (Pillsbury) 1" sl Pipin' Hot		4	0	0	6	4	4	0	2	170	2	13	80
Wiener Wrap (Pillsbury)	1	2	0	0	4	2	2	0	2	430	2	10	60
Wiener Wrap, Cheese (Pillsbury)	1	2	0	0	6	4	4	0	2	395	2	10	60
Rolls, Sweet													
Almond Danish (Pepperidge Farm)	1	6	0	2	6	6	8	2	6	260	10	33	240
Apple Danish (Hostess)	1	6	0	0	10	10	10	6	10	410	20	43	360
Apple Danish (Pepperidge Farm)	1	4	0	2	4	4	4	2	6	240	7	28	180
Apple Danish (Pillsbury) Pipin' Hot	1	4	0	0	8	6	4	0	4	250	12	33	250
Blueberry Danish (Pepperidge Farm)	1	4	0	4	6	4	6	2	6	250	8	30	200
Butterhorn Danish (Hostess)	1	8	0	0	40	20	25	2	8	520	18	39	330
Caramel Danish w Nuts (Pillsbury)	2	6	0	0	10	6	8	0	6	490	16	39	310
Cheese Danish (Pepperidge Farm)	1	8	0	2	6	8	6	2	6	310	13	35	280

Food	Serving	% U.S. RDA											
Cherry (Dolly Madison)	1	4	*	*	6	6	6	2	6	165	4	33	180
Cherry Danish (Pepperidge Farm)	1	4	0	2	4	6	6	2	6	250	8	29	200
Cinnamon (Dolly Madison)	1	4	*	*	10	8	6	2	6	220	6	28	180
Cinnamon (Pillsbury Pipin' Hot)	1	4	0	0	10	8	6	0	4	360	11	27	220
Cinnamon w Icing (Hungry Jack Butter Tastin')	2	4	0	0	10	8	6	0	4	570	14	37	290
Cinnamon w Icing (Pillsbury)	2	4	0	0	10	8	6	0	6	520	9	34	230
Cinnamon Raisin Danish w Icing (Pillsbury)	2	4	0	0	10	6	6	0	4	450	14	39	290
Croissant, Almond (Pepperidge Farm)	1	8	6	0	8	8	4	6	4	260	11	21	210
Croissant, Chocolate (Pepperidge Farm)	1	6	10	0	6	4	4	6	4	330	16	25	260
Croissant, Cinnamon (Pepperidge Farm)	1	6	0	0	15	10	8	6	10	220	9	28	210
Croissant, Raisin (Pepperidge Farm)	1	4	8	0	10	8	6	4	6	270	10	24	200
Croissant, Walnut (Pepperidge Farm)	1	6	8	0	10	8	6	4	4	280	12	21	210
Honey Buns (Hostess)	1	8	0	0	8	8	8	2	8	650	27	49	450
Orange Danish w Icing (Pillsbury)	2	4	0	2	10	6	8	0	4	485	14	39	290

Rolls, Sweet	Amt.	% U.S. RDA								Sodium (mg)	Fat (g)	Carbohy-drate (g)	Calories
		Pro-tein	A	C	B₁	B₂	Nia-cin	Cal-cium	Iron				
Raspberry Danish (Hostess)	1	6	0	0	40	18	10	16	10	360	10	48	300
Salad Dressings													
Blue Cheese (Wish-Bone Chunky)	1 tbsp	*	*	*	*	*	*	*	*	150	8	0–1	70
Blue Cheese (Wish-Bone Lite Chunky)	1 tbsp	*	*	*	*	*	*	*	*	190	3	3	40
Buttermilk (Wish-Bone)	1 tbsp	*	*	*	*	*	*	*	*	150	5	2	50
Buttermilk and Onion (Hidden Valley Ranch)	1 tbsp	*	*	*	*	*	*	*	*	127	7	2	70
Caesar (Wish-Bone)	1 tbsp	*	*	*	*	*	*	*	*	250	8	0–1	70
Cheddar and Bacon (Wish-Bone)	1 tbsp	*	*	*	*	*	*	*	*	110	7	1	70
Cucumber, Creamy (Wish-Bone)	1 tbsp	*	*	*	*	*	*	*	*	125	8	1	80
Cucumber, Creamy (Wish-Bone Lite)	1 tbsp	*	*	*	*	*	*	*	*	165	4	1	40
French (Wish-Bone Deluxe)	1 tbsp	*	*	*	*	*	*	*	*	80	5	2	50
French (Wish-Bone Sweet 'n Spicy)	1 tbsp	*	*	*	*	*	*	*	*	150	6	3	70
French, Garlic (Wish-Bone)	1 tbsp	*	*	*	*	*	*	*	*	150	6	2	60
French, Herbal (Wish-Bone)	1 tbsp	*	*	*	*	*	*	*	*	130	6	2	60

Food	Serving	% U.S. RDA												
French Style (Wish-Bone Lite)	1 tbsp	*	*	*	*	*	*	*	*	*	70	2	2	30
French Style (Wish-Bone Lite Sweet 'n Spicy)	1 tbsp	*	*	*	*	*	*	*	*	*	150	2	4	30
Garden Herb (Hidden Valley Ranch)	1 tbsp	*	*	*	*	*	*	*	*	*	125	7	2	.70
Garlic, Creamy (Wish-Bone)	1 tbsp	*	*	*	*	*	*	*	*	*	170	8	0–1	80
Italian (Wish-Bone)	1 tbsp	*	*	*	*	*	*	*	*	*	240	7	1	70
Italian (Wish-Bone Lite)	1 tbsp	*	*	*	*	*	*	*	*	*	210	3	1	30
Italian (Wish-Bone Robusto)	1 tbsp	*	*	*	*	*	*	*	*	*	340	8	1	80
Italian, Mix (Good Seasons Low Calorie)	1 tbsp	*	*	*	*	*	*	*	*	*	160	0	2	8
Italian, Creamy (Wish-Bone)	1 tbsp	*	*	*	*	*	*	*	*	*	145	6	1	60
Italian, Creamy (Wish-Bone Lite)	1 tbsp	*	*	*	*	*	*	*	*	*	200	3	1	30
Italian, Herbal (Wish-Bone)	1 tbsp	*	*	*	*	*	*	*	*	*	240	7	1	70
Mayonnaise (Bama)	1 tbsp	*	*	*	*	*	*	*	*	*	70	11	0	100
Mayonnaise (Hellmann's/ Best Foods)	1 tbsp	*	*	*	*	*	*	*	*	*	80	11	0	100
Mayonnaise (Mrs. Filbert's)	1 tbsp	*	*	*	*	*	*	*	*	*	70	11	0	100
Mayonnaise, Imitation (Mrs. Filbert's)	1 tbsp	*	*	*	*	*	*	*	*	*	110	4	1	40
Onion 'n Chive (Wish-Bone Lite)	1 tbsp	*	*	*	*	*	*	*	*	*	160	3	3	40

Salad Dressings	Amt.	Pro-tein	A	C	B₁	B₂	Nia-cin	Cal-cium	Iron	Sodium (mg)	Fat (g)	Carbohy-drate (g)	Calories
		% U.S. RDA											
Ranch, Original (Hidden Valley Ranch)	1 tbsp	*	*	*	*	*	*	*	*	125	7	2	70
Russian (Wish-Bone)	1 tbsp	*	*	*	*	*	*	*	*	140	2	6	45
Russian (Wish-Bone Lite)	1 tbsp	*	*	*	*	*	*	*	*	140	0–1	5	25
Salad Dressing (Bama)	1 tbsp	*	*	*	*	*	*	*	*	120	4	3	50
Salad Dressing (Mrs. Filbert's)	1 tbsp	*	*	*	*	*	*	*	*	115	6	2	70
Sour Cream and Bacon (Wish-Bone)	1 tbsp	*	*	*	*	*	*	*	*	95	7	1	70
Thousand Island (Wish-Bone)	1 tbsp	*	*	*	*	*	*	*	*	130	6	2	60
Thousand Island (Wish-Bone Lite)	1 tbsp	*	*	*	*	*	*	*	*	160	2	3	25
Thousand Island (Wish-Bone Southern Recipe)	1 tbsp	*	*	*	*	*	*	*	*	90	6	3	70
Thousand Island w Bacon (Wish-Bone)	1 tbsp	*	*	*	*	*	*	*	*	95	6	2	60
Sauces and Gravies All entries are bottled or canned, unless otherwise noted.													
Barbecue Sauce (French's Cattlemen's Regular)	1 tbsp	*	*	*	*	*	*	*	*	255	0	5	25
Barbecue Sauce (French's Cattlemen's Smoky)	1 tbsp	*	*	*	*	*	*	*	*	295	0	5	25

Food	Serving	% U.S. RDA									
Barbecue Sauce (Heinz Regular)	1 tbsp	0	NA	NA	NA	NA	*	140	0	4	20
Barbecue Sauce (Heinz Onion)	1 tbsp	0	NA	NA	NA	NA	*	130	0	5	20
Barbecue Sauce (Heinz Hickory Smoke)	1 tbsp	0	NA	NA	NA	NA	*	135	0	5	20
Barbecue Sauce (Heinz Mushroom)	1 tbsp	0	NA	NA	NA	NA	*	130	0	5	20
Barbecue Sauce (Heinz Hot)	1 tbsp	0	NA	NA	NA	NA	*	120	0	5	20
Barbecue Sauce (Hunt's All Natural Hickory)	1 tbsp	*	4	6	*	*	*	195	0	6	25
Barbecue Sauce (Hunt's All Natural Hot & Zesty)	1 tbsp	*	4	4	*	*	*	195	0	6	25
Barbecue Sauce (Hunt's All Natural Original)	1 tbsp	*	4	4	*	*	*	195	0	5	20
Barbecue Sauce w Onion (Hunt's All Natural)	1 tbsp	*	4	4	*	*	*	195	0	5	20
Burrito Salsa (Del Monte)	¼ c	0	0	2	*	*	0	355	0	4	20
Cheese Sauce, Mix (French's)	¼ c prep	4	*	*	8	10	*	425	4	7	80
Chili Sauce (Del Monte)	¼ c	2	6	10	4	2	4	835	0	17	70
Chili Sauce (Heinz)	1 tbsp	*	NA	NA	NA	NA	NA	191	0-1	3.8	17
Enchilada Sauce, Green Chili (Old El Paso)	¼ c	*	0	0	*	*	6	400	0	4	17

Sauces and Gravies	Amt.	Pro-tein	A	C	B₁	B₂	Nia-cin	Cal-cium	Iron	Sodium (mg)	Fat (g)	Carbohy-drate (g)	Calories
					% U.S. RDA								
Enchilada Sauce, Hot (Del Monte)	½ c	2	15	10	2	4	6	2	4	1090	0	11	45
Enchilada Sauce, Hot (Old El Paso)	¼ c	*	0	*	*	5	*	*	20	247	1	4	27
Enchilada Sauce, Mild (Del Monte)	½ c	2	15	6	2	4	4	2	6	1150	0	11	45
Enchilada Sauce, Mild (Old El Paso)	¼ c	*	0	*	*	2	3	*	6	250	1	4	25
57 Sauce (Heinz)	1 tbsp	*	NA	NA	NA	NA	NA	NA	NA	265	0	3	15
Gravy, Au Jus (Franco-American)	2 fl oz	*	*	*	*	*	2	*	*	290	0	1	5
Gravy, Beef (Franco-American)	2 oz	*	*	*	*	*	2	*	*	315	1	3	25
Gravy, Brown w Onions (Franco-American)	2 oz	*	*	*	*	*	*	*	*	340	1	4	25
Gravy, Chicken (Franco-American)	2 oz	*	2	*	*	*	*	*	*	320	4	3	50
Gravy, Chicken Giblet (Franco-American)	2 oz	*	*	*	*	*	*	*	*	320	2	3	30
Gravy, Mushroom (Franco-American)	2 oz	*	*	*	*	*	*	*	*	320	1	3	25
Gravy, Turkey (Franco-American)	2 oz	*	*	*	*	*	2	*	*	300	2	3	30

Food	Portion	% U.S. RDA											
Gravy, Pork (Franco-American)	2 oz	*	*	*	*	*	*	*	*	350	3	3	40
Gravy, Mix, Au Jus (French's)	¼ c prep	*	*	*	*	*	*	*	*	265	0	2	8
Gravy, Mix, Brown (French's)	¼ c	*	*	*	*	*	*	*	*	280	1	3	20
Gravy, Mix, Brown (Pillsbury)	¼ c prep	0	0	0	0	0	0	0	0	305	0	3	15
Gravy, Mix, Brown (Spatini Family Style)	1 fl oz prep	*	*	*	*	*	*	*	*	205	0	2	8
Gravy, Mix, for Chicken (French's)	¼ c	*	*	*	*	*	*	*	*	300	1	4	25
Gravy, Mix, Chicken (Pillsbury)	¼ c prep	0	0	0	0	0	0	0	0	230	0	4	25
Gravy, Mix, Home Style (French's)	¼ c prep	*	*	*	*	*	*	*	*	335	1	4	25
Gravy, Mix, Home Style (Pillsbury)	¼ c prep	0	0	0	0	0	0	0	0	300	0	3	15
Gravy, Mix, Mushroom (French's)	¼ c prep	*	*	*	*	*	*	*	*	305	1	3	20
Gravy, Mix, Onion (French's)	¼ c prep	*	*	*	*	*	*	*	*	350	1	4	25
Gravy, Mix, for Pork (French's)	¼ c prep	*	*	*	*	*	*	*	*	280	1	3	20
Gravy, Mix, for Turkey (French's)	¼ c prep	*	*	*	*	*	*	*	*	380	1	4	25

Sauces and Gravies	Amt.	% U.S. RDA								Sodium (mg)	Fat (g)	Carbohydrate (g)	Calories
		Protein	A	C	B₁	B₂	Niacin	Calcium	Iron				
Green Chili Salsa, Mild (Del Monte)	¼ c	0	4	4	2	*	2	2	*	590	0	3	20
Hollandaise Sauce, Mix (French's)	3 tbsp prep	*	*	*	*	2	*	2	*	290	4	2	45
Pizza Sauce (Contadina Original Quick & Easy)	¼ c	*	8	10	2	*	4	*	2	395	2	5	40
Pizza Sauce w Cheese (Contadina)	¼ c	*	10	8	2	2	4	2	2	380	2	5	40
Pizza Sauce w Pepperoni (Contadina)	¼ c	*	10	8	2	2	4	*	2	360	2	5	45
Pizza Sauce w Tomato Chunks (Contadina)	¼ c	*	8	10	*	*	2	2	2	300	0	5	25
Salsa Picante, Hot (Del Monte)	¼ c	0	4	4	2	*	2	2	2	385	0	4	20
Salsa Picante, Hot and Chunky (Del Monte)	¼ c	0	6	6	2	0	0	2	2	405	0	3	15
Salsa Roja, Mild (Del Monte)	¼ c	0	4	2	0	0	0	0	2	510	0	4	20
Sauce for Potatoes, Au Gratin, Mix (French's)	⅙ pkg dry	*	*	*	*	*	*	*	*	670	3	5	55
Sauce for Potatoes, Scalloped, Mix (French's)	⅙ pkg dry	*	*	*	*	*	*	*	*	650	0	8	40

		% U.S. RDA												
Sauce for Potatoes, Sour Cream & Chives, Mix (French's)	½ pkg dry	*	*	*	*	*	*	*	*	*	800	4	6	65
Seafood Cocktail Sauce (Del Monte)	¼ c	2	10	8	2	2	4	*	*	2	765	0	17	70
Sloppy Joe Sauce (Hunt's Manwich, Original)	5 tbsp	2	20	25	2	*	4	4	*	6	405	0	10	40
Sloppy Joe Sauce (Hunt's Manwich, Mexican)	5 tbsp	2	25	20	4	2	2	4	*	6	470	0	9	40
Sour Cream Sauce, Mix (French's)	2½ tbsp prep	2	*	*	*	4	4	*	6	*	130	5	5	60
Spaghetti Sauce (Hunt's No Salt Added)	4 fl oz	2	30	35	6	4	6	6	2	10	30	2	13	80
Spaghetti Sauce (Prego)	4 fl oz	2	15	20	2	2	6	2	2	4	670	6	20	140
Spaghetti Sauce (Prego No Salt Added)	4 fl oz	2	30	25	4	4	8	4	6	6	25	6	10	100
Spaghetti Sauce, Meat Flavored (Prego)	4 fl oz	2	20	25	2	2	8	8	2	4	680	6	21	150
Spaghetti Sauce w Mushrooms (Prego)	4 fl oz	2	20	25	2	2	6	6	2	6	640	5	21	140
Spaghetti Sauce, Mix (Spatini)	1 fl oz prep	*	10	10	2	*	2	2	*	4	130	0	4	20
Spaghetti Sauce, Mix, Italian Style (French's)	5 fl oz prep	2	35	30	6	4	6	6	2	8	900	4	15	100
Spaghetti Sauce, Mix, w Mushrooms (French's)	5 fl oz prep	2	35	30	6	4	6	6	4	8	1045	4	13	100

Sauces and Gravies	Amt.	Protein	A	C	B₁	B₂	Niacin	Calcium	Iron	Sodium (mg)	Fat (g)	Carbohydrate (g)	Calories
		% U.S. RDA											
Spaghetti Sauce, Mix, Thick Homemade Style (French's)	⅞ c prep	4	50	50	10	6	10	2	10	1455	7	24	170
Stroganoff Sauce, Mix (French's)	⅓ c prep	6	2	*	8	6	*	10	*	490	5	11	110
Sweet 'n Sour Sauce (Contadina)	4 fl oz	*	4	*	2	*	*	2	2	500	3	30	150
Sweet 'n Sour Sauce, Mix (French's)	½ c prep	*	*	*	*	*	*	*	*	135	0	14	55
Taco Sauce, Hot (Del Monte)	¼ c	0	6	2	0	2	0	0	2	440	0	4	15
Taco Sauce, Hot (Old El Paso)	2 tbsp	*	0	*	*	*	*	*	*	131	0	2	11
Taco Sauce, Mild (Del Monte)	¼ c	0	4	0	0	0	0	0	2	480	0	4	15
Taco Sauce, Mild (Old El Paso)	2 tbsp	*	0	2	*	*	*	*	*	125	0	2	11
Taco Starter (Del Monte)	8 fl oz	4	100	15	8	20	10	6	15	2180	1	28	140
Teriyaki Sauce, Mix (French's)	2 tbsp prep	*	*	*	*	*	*	2	4	1180	0	7	35
Tomato Catsup (Del Monte)	¼ c	*	10	15	2	2	4	*	2	675	0	16	60
Tomato Catsup (Del Monte No Salt Added)	¼ c	*	10	15	2	2	4	*	2	25	0	16	60

Food	Serving				% U.S. RDA								
Tomato Catsup (Heinz)	1 tbsp	*	NA	NA	NA	NA	*	*	*	180	0-1	4	18
Tomato Catsup (Heinz Hot)	1 tbsp	*	NA	NA	NA	NA	*	*	*	180	0-1	4	18
Tomato Catsup (Heinz Lite)	1 tbsp	*	NA	NA	NA	NA	*	*	*	110	0-1	2	8
Tomato Catsup (Heinz Low Sodium Lite)	1 tbsp	*	NA	NA	NA	NA	*	*	*	90	0-1	2	8
Tomato Catsup (Hunt's)	1 tbsp	2	2	4	*	*	2	*	*	160	0	4	16
Tomato Catsup (Hunt's No Salt Added)	1 tbsp	2	2	4	*	*	4	*	*	0-5	0	5	20
Tomato Sauce Canned (Contadina)	½ c	2	25	15	4	2	6	*	4	NA	0	9	45
Tomato Sauce Canned (Del Monte)	1 c	4	50	80	10	6	10	2	10	1330	1	16	70
Tomato Sauce Canned (Del Monte No Salt Added)	1 c	4	50	80	10	6	10	2	10	50	1	16	70
Tomato Sauce (Hunt's)	½ c	2	20	25	4	2	6	*	15	665	0	7	30
Tomato Sauce (Hunt's No Salt Added)	½ c	2	25	30	4	2	6	*	15	25	0	8	35
Tomato Sauce, Italian Style Canned (Contadina)	½ c	*	20	8	2	2	4	*	2	NA	0	8	40
Tomato Sauce, Italian (Hunt's)	½ c	2	30	35	6	4	15	2	8	515	2	11	60
Tomato Sauce w Bits (Hunt's)	½ c	2	25	30	4	2	6	2	6	695	0	7	30
Tomato Sauce w Cheese (Hunt's)	½ c	4	20	25	4	4	6	6	6	795	1	8	45

Sauces and Gravies	Amt.	% U.S. RDA								Sodium (mg)	Fat (g)	Carbohydrate (g)	Calories
		Protein	A	C	B₁	B₂	Niacin	Calcium	Iron				
Tomato Sauce w Mushrooms (Hunt's)	½ c	2	20	25	4	2	4	*	6	710	0	6	25
Tomato Sauce w Onions (Del Monte)	1 c	4	35	60	10	6	10	2	10	1150	1	23	100
Tomato Sauce w Onions (Hunt's)	½ c	2	20	30	4	2	6	2	6	670	0	9	40
Tomato Sauce, Special (Hunt's)	½ c	2	20	25	4	2	6	*	6	315	0	8	35
Tomato Herb Sauce (Hunt's)	½ c	2	25	30	6	2	6	2	8	495	4	11	80
Welsh Rarebit Cheese Sauce (Snow's)	½ c	15	*	*	2	4	*	25	2	460	11	10	170
Worcestershire Sauce, Regular (French's)	1 tbsp	*	*	*	*	*	*	*	*	165	0	2	10
Worcestershire Sauce, Smoky (French's)	1 tbsp	*	*	*	*	*	*	*	*	165	0	2	10
Seasonings													
Barbecue Seasoning (French's)	1 tsp	*	*	*	*	*	*	*	*	70	0	1	6
Beef Stew Seasoning (French's)	⅙ pkg	*	*	*	*	2	*	2	2	765	0	5	25
Celery Salt (French's)	1 tsp	*	*	*	*	*	*	*	*	1505	0	0	2
Chili-O (French's)	⅙ pkg	*	*	*	*	2	*	*	*	630	0	5	25

Food	Serving	% U.S. RDA								Sodium (mg)			
Enchilada Seasoning (French's)	¼ pkg	*	*	*	*	2	2	2	*	1130	1	5	30
Garlic Salt (French's)	1 tsp	*	*	*	*	*	*	*	*	2050	0	1	4
Garlic Salt, Parslied (French's)	1 tsp	*	*	*	*	*	*	*	*	1125	0	1	6
Ground Beef Seasoning w Onions (French's)	¼ pkg	*	*	*	*	*	*	*	*	440	0	6	25
Hamburger Seasoning (French's)	¼ pkg	*	2	*	*	*	*	*	*	450	0	5	25
Hickory Smoke Salt (French's)	1 tsp	*	*	*	*	*	*	*	*	1145	0	0	2
Lemon and Pepper (French's)	1 tsp	*	*	*	*	*	*	*	*	805	0	1	6
Meat Marinade (French's)	⅛ pkg	*	*	*	*	*	*	*	*	540	0	2	10
Meat Tenderizer (French's)	1 tsp	*	*	*	*	*	*	*	*	1760	0	0	2
Meat Tenderizer, Seasoned (French's)	1 tsp	*	*	*	*	*	*	*	*	1550	0	0	2
Meatball Seasoning (French's)	¼ pkg	*	*	*	*	*	*	*	2	825	0	7	35
Meat Loaf Mix (Contadina)	1 tbsp rounded	2	*	2	2	2	2	2	NA	430	0–1	7	35
Meat Loaf Seasoning (French's)	⅛ pkg	*	*	*	*	*	*	*	*	615	0	5	20
Onion Salt (French's)	1 tsp	*	*	*	*	*	*	*	*	1590	0	1	6
Pepper, Seasoned (French's)	1 tsp	*	*	*	*	*	*	*	*	5	0	1	8
Pizza Seasoning (French's)	1 tsp	*	*	*	*	*	*	*	*	400	0	1	4

Seasonings	Amt.	Protein	A	C	B₁	B₂	Niacin	Calcium	Iron	Sodium (mg)	Fat (g)	Carbohydrate (g)	Calories
					% U.S. RDA								
Salad Onions, Instant (French's)	1 tbsp	*	*	*	*	*	*	*	*	2	0	3	15
Salad Seasoning (French's)	1 tsp	*	*	*	*	*	*	*	*	630	0	1	6
Salt, Imitation Butter Flavor (French's)	1 tsp	*	*	*	*	*	*	*	*	1125	1	0	8
Seafood Seasoning (French's)	1 tsp	*	*	*	*	*	*	*	*	1410	0	0	2
Seasoning Salt (French's)	1 tsp	*	*	*	*	*	*	*	*	1280	0	1	2
Sloppy Joe Seasoning (French's)	⅛ pkg	*	*	*	*	*	*	*	*	390	0	4	16
Stock Base, Beef Flavor (French's)	1 tsp	*	*	*	*	*	*	*	*	500	0	2	8
Stock Base, Chicken Flavor (French's)	1 tsp	*	*	*	*	*	*	*	*	475	0	1	8
Taco Seasoning (French's)	½ pkg	*	*	*	*	*	*	*	*	365	0	4	20
Taco Seasoning (Old El Paso)	1 pkg	2	0	*	*	0	*	3	12	3569	1	21	100
Vegetable Flakes, Dehydrated (French's)	1 tbsp	*	*	*	*	*	*	*	*	20	0	3	12
Snacks													
Bugles	1 oz	2	*	*	4	2	4	*	4	285	8	18	150
Bugles, Nacho Cheese	1 oz	2	*	*	4	2	4	*	4	285	10	16	160

					% U.S. RDA								
Cheddar Sticks (Flavor Tree)	1 oz	4	*	*	2	*	4	6	2	445	11	12	160
Cheese Balls, Baked (Guy's)	1 oz	2	*	*	*	2	*	2	2	320	11	14	160
Cheese 'n Crunch (Nabisco)	1 oz	2	*	*	2	*	2	2	*	NA	11	14	160
Cheese Snacks (Lite-line Puffed Cheese Curls)	1 oz	2	4	6	6	6	*	2	4	NA	5	19	130
Cheez Doodles, Crunchy	1 oz	2	4	6	6	6	6	2	4	NA	10	16	160
Cheez Doodles, Puffed	1 oz	2	6	8	10	8	8	2	4	NA	10	16	160
Cheez Waffies	1 oz	4	*	*	8	*	*	6	*	NA	8	14	140
Chipsters (Nabisco)	1 oz	2	*	2	*	4	*	*	2	NA	6	19	130
Corn Chips (Flavor Tree)	1 oz	2	*	2	*	*	4	4	2	260	8	17	150
Corn Diggers (Nabisco)	1 oz	2	*	*	*	*	*	*	*	NA	9	17	150
Corn & Sesame Chips (Nabisco)	1 oz	4	*	4	*	2	2	4	2	NA	10	15	160
Corn Sticks (Flavor Tree)	1 oz	2	*	2	*	*	2	2	2	220	10	15	160
Cracker Jack	1 oz	2	*	*	2	2	2	*	4	85	3	22	120
Crispy Chinese TV Snacks (Mother's)	1 oz	4	*	6	4	4	*	2	2	NA	7	17	140
Doo Dads (Nabisco)	1 oz	4	*	6	4	8	2	2	4	NA	7	17	140
Flings (Nabisco)	1 oz	2	*	*	4	4	*	4	*	NA	11	14	160
Fruit Rolls, Apricot (Flavor Tree)	1 roll	*	*	*	*	2	*	4	4	20	0	23	100

265

Snacks	Amt.	Pro-tein	A	C	B₁	B₂	Nia-cin	Cal-cium	Iron	Sodium (mg)	Fat (g)	Carbohy-drate (g)	Calories
		% U.S. RDA											
Fruit Rolls, Apple, Cherry, Grape, Fruit Punch, Orange, Raspberry, Strawberry (Flavor Tree)	1 roll	*	*	*	*	*	*	*	*	25–35	0	23	90
Fruit Rolls, Peach (Flavor Tree)	1 roll	*	*	4	*	*	*	*	2	30	0	23	90
Fruit Roll, Plum (Flavor Tree)	1 roll	*	*	*	*	*	2	*	4	15	0	23	90
Fruit Rolls, All Flavors (Sunkist)	1 roll	*	*	*	*	*	*	*	*	15	0	11	45
Fruit Roll-Ups, Apple, Cherry, Grape, Strawberry	1 roll	*	*	*	*	*	*	*	*	5	0–1	12	50
Fruit Roll-Ups, Apricot	1 roll	*	2	*	*	*	*	*	*	5	0–1	12	50
Granola Nuts (Flavor Tree)	1 oz	6	*	*	8	2	*	*	4	195	13	9	170
Granola Snack, Cinnamon (Nature Valley Light & Crunchy)	1 pouch	2	*	*	4	*	*	*	4	170	5	19	130
Granola Snack, Honey Nut (Nature Valley Light & Crunchy)	1 pouch	2	*	*	2	2	*	*	4	160	6	19	140
Granola Snack, Oats and Honey (Nature Valley Light & Crunchy)	1 pouch	2	*	*	4	*	*	*	4	170	5	19	130

							% U.S. RDA						
Granola Snack, Peanut Butter (Nature Valley Light & Crunchy)	1 pouch	6	*	*	4	2	4	2	6	240	10	23	200
Granola Snack, Raspberry Glaze (Nature Valley Light & Crunchy)	1 pouch	4	*	*	4	2	2	4	6	220	8	27	190
Granola Snack, Vanilla Glaze (Nature Valley Light & Crunchy)	1 pouch	4	*	*	2	2	2	2	6	220	8	28	190
Korkers (Nabisco)	1 oz	2	*	*	*	*	2	2	2	NA	10	16	160
Party Mix (Flavor Tree)	1 oz	6	*	*	2	*	6	6	2	400	11	11	160
Party Mix, No Salt Added (Flavor Tree)	1 oz	6	*	*	2	*	6	4	2	10	11	11	160
Popcorn, Popped, Plain, Large Kernel	1 c	2	*	*	2	*	*	*	2	NA	0-1	5	25
Popcorn, Popped, w Oil and Salt, Large Kernel	1 c	2	*	*	2	*	*	*	2	175	2	6	40
Popcorn, Popped, Plain (Orville Redenbacher Gourmet)	4 c	4	*	*	*	2	2	4	4	.2	1	18	90
Popcorn, Popped, w Oil and Salt (Orville Redenbacher Gourmet)	4 c	4	*	*	2	*	4	4	4	700	8	21	160
Popcorn, Microwave, Popped, Plain (Totino's)	4 c	6	0	6	2	2	2	2	6	405	15	28	260

Snacks	Amt.	% U.S. RDA								Sodium (mg)	Fat (g)	Carbohydrate (g)	Calories
		Protein	A	C	B₁	B₂	Niacin	Calcium	Iron				
Popcorn, Microwave, Popped, No Salt (Totino's)	4 c	4	2	2	2	2	0	0	6	6	8	26	190
Popcorn, Microwave, Popped, Butter Flavor (Orville Redenbacher Gourmet)	4 c	4	*	*	*	2	2	*	4	210	7	17	140
Popcorn, Microwave, Popped, Butter Flavor (Totino's)	4 c	6	2	4	2	2	2	0	6	405	14	29	260
Popcorn, Microwave, Popped, Natural Flavor (Orville Redenbacher Gourmet)	4 c	4	*	*	*	2	2	*	4	285	8	16	140
Popcorn, Butter Flavor (Wise)	½ oz	2	10	*	*	*	*	*	*	NA	4	8	70
Popcorn, Cheese Flavor (Wise Cheez)	½ oz	*	15	*	*	*	*	*	*	NA	6	7	90
Potato Chips (Wise)	1 oz	2	*	10	2	*	6	*	2	240	11	14	160
Potato Chips, Barbecue Flavored, Rippled (Morton's Ridgies)	1 oz	2	*	10	2	2	6	*	2	NA	10	14	150
Potato Chips, Ketchup and French Fry Flavor (Buckeye)	1 oz	2	*	10	2	*	6	*	2	230	11	14	160

		% U.S. RDA											
Potato Chips, No Salt Added (Wise)	1 oz	2	*	10	*	2	6	*	*	20	10	14	150
Pretzels (Mister Salty)	5	4	*	6	6	6	6	4	*	NA	1	20	100
Pretzels (Mister Salty Dutch)	2	4	*	2	2	2	2	2	*	NA	1	22	110
Pretzels (Mister Salty Little Shapes)	19	4	*	2	*	*	2	2	*	NA	1	22	110
Pretzels (Mister Salty Sticks)	94 (1 oz)	4	*	6	8	8	8	6	*	NA	1	22	110
Pretzels (Rokeach Baldies or No Salt Dutch)	1 oz	4	*	*	*	*	*	*	*	30	0	20	110
Pretzels (Rokeach Party)	1 oz	4	*	*	*	*	2	*	*	NA	1	23	110
Pretzels, Butter (Pepperidge Farm Butter Nuggets)	25	4	0	2	0	2	0	2	0	790	2	27	140
Pretzels, Butter (Pepperidge Farm Thin Sticks)	30	4	0	2	0	2	0	4	0	780	2	28	140
Pretzels, Butter (Pepperidge Farm Tiny Twists)	15	4	0	2	0	2	0	2	0	820	2	22	110
Sesame Chips (Flavor Tree)	1 oz	4	*	2	*	2	6	2	2	410	10	13	150
Sesame Nuts (Flavor Tree)	1 oz	8	*	8	4	6	6	6	6	185	14	8	180
Sesame Sticks (Flavor Tree)	1 oz	4	*	2	*	2	6	2	2	405	10	13	150
Sesame Sticks w Bran (Flavor Tree)	1 oz	6	*	4	*	4	6	4	4	370	11	11	160
Sesame Sticks, No Salt Added (Flavor Tree)	1 oz	4	*	2	*	2	6	2	4	10	11	12	160

| Snacks | Amt. | | | | % U.S. RDA | | | | | Sodium (mg) | Fat (g) | Carbohydrate (g) | Calories |
		Protein	A	C	B_1	B_2	Niacin	Calcium	Iron				
Sour Cream and Onion Sticks (Flavor Tree)	1 oz	4	*	*	2	*	2	6	2	415	10	13	150
Tortilla Chips (Nabisco)	1 oz	2	*	*	2	*	2	4	2	NA	7	19	150
Tortilla Chips (Old El Paso Nachips)	10 chips	3	0	0	*	*	2	4	4	111	10	17	169
Tortilla Chips, Nacho Cheese Flavor (Lite-line)	1 oz	2	*	*	*	*	2	4	2	165	5	19	130
Tortilla Chips, Nacho Cheese Flavor (Nabisco Buenos)	1 oz	2	*	*	2	2	2	4	2	NA	8	17	150
Tortilla Chips, Nacho Cheese Flavor (Wise Bravos)	1 oz	4	2	*	*	*	*	6	2	NA	8	17	150
Tortilla Chips, Sour Cream and Onion Flavor (Nabisco Buenos)	1 oz	4	*	*	2	*	2	4	2	NA	7	18	150
Wheat Nuts (Flavor Tree)	1 oz	4	*	*	8	2	2	*	2	185	16	8	190
Wise Corn Crunchies	1 oz	2	*	*	*	*	2	2	2	NA	10	16	160
Soft Drinks													
Bitter Lemon (Schweppes)	6 fl oz	*	*	*	*	*	*	*	*	2	0	20	84
Club Soda (Schweppes)	6 fl oz	*	*	*	*	*	*	*	*	26	0	0	0
Cola (Coca-Cola)	6 fl oz	*	*	0	*	*	*	*	*	7	0	19	72

			% U.S. RDA											
Cola (Caffeine Free Coca-Cola)	6 fl oz	3	*	*	*	*	*	*	*	*	0	20	76
Cola (diet Coke)	6 fl oz	13	*	*	*	*	*	*	*	*	0	.1	0-1
Cola (Caffeine Free Diet Coke)	6 fl oz	13	*	*	*	*	*	*	*	*	0	.1	0-1
Cola (Like)	6 fl oz	0-1	*	*	*	*	*	*	*	*	0	20	81
Cola (Sugar Free Like)	6 fl oz	14	*	*	*	*	*	*	*	*	0	0	0-1
Cola (Pepsi-Cola)	8 fl oz	6	*	*	*	*	*	*	*	*	NA	26	105
Cola (Diet Pepsi)	8 fl oz	36	*	*	*	*	*	*	*	*	NA	.2	0-1
Cola (Pepsi Free)	8 fl oz	6	*	*	*	*	*	*	*	*	NA	26	105
Cola (Diet Pepsi Free)	8 fl oz	46	*	*	*	*	*	*	*	*	NA	.2	0-1
Cola (Pepsi Light)	8 fl oz	28	*	*	*	*	*	*	*	*	NA	.1	0-1
Cola (RC 100 Caffeine Free)	6 fl oz	.3	*	*	*	*	*	*	*	*	NA	19	78
Cola (Diet RC 100 Caffeine Free)	6 fl oz	11	*	*	*	*	*	*	*	*	NA	.1	0-1
Cola (Royal Crown)	6 fl oz	.3	*	*	*	*	*	*	*	*	NA	19	78
Cola (Diet Rite Salt Free)	6 fl oz	0	*	*	*	*	*	*	*	*	NA	.1	0-1
Fresca	6 fl oz	18	*	*	*	*	*	*	*	*	0	0	2
Ginger Ale (Fanta)	6 fl oz	14	*	*	*	*	*	*	*	*	0	16	63
Ginger Ale (Schweppes)	6 fl oz	11	*	*	*	*	*	*	*	*	0	16	66
Ginger Ale (Schweppes Sugar Free)	6 fl oz	20	*	*	*	*	*	*	*	*	0	0	2
Ginger Beer (Schweppes)	6 fl oz	14	*	*	*	*	*	*	*	*	0	17	72

271

| | | % U.S. RDA | | | | | | | | | | | |
Soft Drinks	Amt.	Protein	A	C	B₁	B₂	Niacin	Calcium	Iron	Sodium (mg)	Fat (g)	Carbohydrate (g)	Calories
Grape (Fanta)	6 fl oz	*	*	*	*	*	*	*	*	7	0	22	86
Grape (Hi-C)	6 fl oz	*	*	60	*	*	*	*	*	6	0	20	78
Grape (Nehi)	6 fl oz	*	*	*	*	*	*	*	**	8	NA	22	87
Grape (Schweppes)	10 fl oz	*	*	*	*	*	*	*	*	25	0	40	161
Lemon (Hi-C)	6 fl oz	*	*	60	*	*	*	*	*	6	0	18	75
Lemon Dry (Schweppes)	10 fl oz	*	*	*	*	*	*	*	*	51.6	0	25.9	104
Mello Yello	6 fl oz	*	*	*	*	*	*	*	*	14	0	22	86
Mineral Water (Schweppes)	6 fl oz	*	*	*	*	*	*	*	*	3	0	0	0
Mountain Dew	8 fl oz	*	*	*	*	*	*	*	*	21	NA	29	118
Mr. PiBB	6 fl oz	*	*	*	*	*	*	*	*	10	0	19	71
Mr. PiBB, Sugar Free	6 fl oz	*	*	*	*	*	*	*	*	19	0	.2	0-1
Orange (Fanta)	6 fl oz	*	*	*	*	*	*	*	*	7	0	23	88
Orange (Hi-C)	6 fl oz	*	*	60	*	*	*	*	*	7	0	20	77
Orange (Nehi)	6 fl oz	*	*	*	*	*	*	*	*	12	NA	23	93
Orange (Schweppes Sparkling)	10 fl oz	*	*	*	*	*	*	*	*	27	0	37	148
Punch (Hi-C)	6 fl oz	*	*	60	*	*	*	*	*	6	0	20	77
Red Creme (Schweppes)	10 fl oz	*	*	*	*	*	*	*	*	25	0	35	144
Rondo (Schweppes)	10 fl oz	*	*	*	*	*	*	*	*	22	0	33	127

		% U.S. RDA											
Rondo (Schweppes Sugar Free)	10 fl oz	*	*	*	*	*	*	*	*	36	0	0	0
Root Beer (Fanta)	6 fl oz	*	*	*	*	*	*	*	*	10	0	20	78
Root Beer (Nehi)	6 fl oz	*	*	*	*	*	*	*	*	9	NA	22	87
Root Beer (Ramblin')	6 fl oz	*	*	*	*	*	*	*	*	10	0	23	88
Root Beer (Sugar Free Ramblin')	6 fl oz	*	*	*	*	*	*	*	*	29	0	.2	0-1
Root Beer (Schweppes)	10 fl oz	*	*	*	*	*	*	*	*	25	0	32	131
7UP	6 fl oz	*	*	*	*	*	*	*	*	16	0	18	72
Diet 7UP	6 fl oz	*	*	*	*	*	*	*	*	18	0	0	2
Sprite	6 fl oz	*	*	*	*	*	*	*	*	23	0	18	71
Sprite, Diet	6 fl oz	*	*	*	*	*	*	*	*	21	0	0	1
Strawberry (Nehi)	6 fl oz	*	*	*	*	*	*	*	*	0	NA	22	87
TAB	6 fl oz	*	*	*	*	*	*	*	*	15	0	.2	0-1
TAB, Caffeine Free	6 fl oz	*	*	*	*	*	*	*	*	15	0	.2	0-1
Teem	8 fl oz	*	*	*	*	*	*	*	*	21	NA	25	99
Tonic Water (Schweppes)	6 fl oz	*	*	*	*	*	*	*	*	4	0	16	66
Tonic Water (Schweppes Sugar Free)	6 fl oz	*	*	*	*	*	*	*	*	37	0	0	1
Vichy Water (Schweppes)	6 fl oz	*	*	*	*	*	*	*	*	80	0	0	0

Soups

		% U.S. RDA											
Asparagus, Cream of (Campbell's)	8 fl oz prep	2	6	2	2	2	2	2	2	900	4	11	90

| | | \% U.S. RDA | | | | | | | | | | | |
Soups	Amt.	Pro-tein	A	C	B₁	B₂	Nia-cin	Cal-cium	Iron	Sodium (mg)	Fat (g)	Carbohy-drate (g)	Calories
Bean w Bacon (Campbell's)	8 fl oz prep	10	15	*	4	2	2	6	10	875	5	21	150
Bean 'n Ham, Old Fashioned (Campbell's Chunky)	11 fl oz	25	100	8	10	6	10	10	15	1180	9	37	290
Bean w Ham, Old Fashioned (Campbell's Soup for One)	11 fl oz prep	10	25	*	8	2	4	8	10	1405	7	30	210
Beef (Campbell's)	8 fl oz prep	8	20	2	*	2	4	*	4	855	2	10	80
Beef (Campbell's Chunky)	10¾ fl oz	25	120	10	4	10	10	2	10	1190	5	23	190
Beef Flavor (Lipton Cup-a-Soup Lots-a-Noodles)	7 fl oz prep	8	6	*	15	6	6	2	4	730	2	21	120
Beef Flavor (Lipton Cup-a-Soup TRIM)	6 fl oz prep	*	*	*	*	*	*	*	*	650	0	1	10
Beef and Mushroom (Campbell's Chunky Low Sodium)	10¾ fl oz	20	120	15	8	20	20	4	10	75	7	23	210
Beef Noodle (Campbell's)	8 fl oz prep	8	4	*	4	4	4	*	4	875	3	7	70
Beef Noodle, Homestyle (Campbell's)	8 fl oz prep	10	*	2	4	6	8	*	4	810	4	8	90
Beef, Stroganoff Style (Campbell's Chunky)	10¾ fl oz	25	50	*	8	15	15	6	15	1315	16	28	300
Beef Vegetable Noodle (Lipton Hearty)	8 fl oz prep	4	4	*	8	2	4	*	2	905	0–1	14	80

Food	Serving	% U.S. RDA									
Black Bean (Campbell's)	8 fl oz prep	8	6	2	2	2	10	995	2	17	110
Bouillon, Beef Flavor, Instant (Lite-line Low Sodium)	1 tsp	*	*	*	*	*	*	10	0-1	2	12
Bouillon, Beef Flavor, Instant (Wyler's)	1 tsp	*	*	*	*	*	*	930	0-1	1	6
Bouillon, Chicken Flavor, Instant (Lite-line Low Sodium)	1 tsp	*	*	*	*	*	*	5	0-1	2	12
Bouillon, Chicken Flavor, Cubes (Wyler's)	1 cube	*	*	*	*	*	*	850	0-1	1	8
Bouillon, Onion Flavor, Instant (Wyler's)	1 tsp	*	*	*	*	*	*	NA	0-1	1	10
Broth, Beef (Campbell's)	8 fl oz prep	4	*	*	2	4	*	875	0	1	16
Broth, Beef (Swanson)	7¼ fl oz	2	*	*	*	8	*	840	1	1	20
Broth, Chicken (Campbell's)	8 fl oz prep	2	*	*	2	6	*	810	2	3	35
Broth, Chicken (Campbell's Low Sodium)	1 can	4	*	2	6	10	8	100	2	3	40
Broth, Chicken (Lipton Cup-a-Broth)	6 fl oz prep	*	*	*	*	*	*	800	0-1	4	25
Broth, Chicken (Swanson)	7¼ fl oz	4	*	*	4	10	*	910	2	2	30
Broth, Chicken, and Noodles (Campbell's)	8 fl oz prep	2	10	6	4	6	2	865	2	8	60
Broth, Chicken, and Rice (Campbell's)	8 fl oz prep	2	8	*	*	2	*	880	1	8	50
Broth, Scotch (Campbell's)	8 fl oz prep	8	*	*	2	4	2	900	3	9	80

Soups	Amt.	% U.S. RDA Protein	A	C	B₁	B₂	Niacin	Calcium	Iron	Sodium (mg)	Fat (g)	Carbohydrate (g)	Calories
Celery, Cream of (Campbell's)	8 fl oz prep	2	4	*	*	*	*	2	*	875	7	8	100
Celery, Cream of (Rokeach)	10 fl oz prep	4	8	*	2	2	*	6	2	950	4	12	90
Celery, Cream of, Made w Milk (Rokeach)	10 fl oz prep	15	10	2	6	15	*	25	2	1020	9	19	190
Cheddar Cheese (Campbell's)	8 fl oz prep	4	10	*	*	6	*	8	*	885	8	10	130
Chicken Alphabet (Campbell's)	8 fl oz prep	6	15	*	4	4	6	*	4	870	3	10	80
Chicken, Cream of (Campbell's)	8 fl oz prep	4	10	*	*	2	2	2	*	860	7	9	110
Chicken, Cream of (Lipton Cup-a-Soup)	6 fl oz	2	*	*	*	*	*	*	*	850	4	9	80
Chicken, Cream of (Lipton Cup-a-Soup Lots-a-Noodles)	7 fl oz	6	10	*	10	4	4	4	4	750	5	22	150
Chicken 'n Dumplings (Campbell's)	8 fl oz prep	6	6	*	*	2	6	*	2	995	3	9	80
Chicken Flavor (Lipton Cup-a-Soup Lots-a-Noodles)	7 fl oz prep	8	20	*	10	6	4	*	4	810	1	23	120
Chicken Flavor (Lipton Cup-a-Soup TRIM)	6 fl oz prep	*	*	*	*	*	*	*	*	550	0	1	10
Chicken Gumbo (Campbell's)	8 fl oz prep	4	2	*	*	*	2	2	2	910	2	8	60

Product	Serving	\% U.S. RDA											Calories
Chicken, Hearty (Lipton Country Style Cup-a-Soup)	6 fl oz prep	6	6	*	6	2	6	2	*	970	1	10	70
Chicken Mushroom, Creamy (Campbell's)	8 fl oz prep	6	15	*	*	4	4	2	2	940	7	9	110
Chicken Noodle (Campbell's)	8 fl oz prep	4	6	*	4	2	6	*	2	935	3	8	70
Chicken Noodle (Campbell's Chunky)	10¾ oz	25	20	*	8	10	20	2	10	1210	8	20	200
Chicken Noodle (Lipton)	8 fl oz prep	4	*	8	*	2	4	*	2	900	2	9	70
Chicken Noodle, Homestyle (Campbell's)	8 fl oz prep	6	15	2	4	4	6	*	2	910	3	8	70
Chicken NoodleO's (Campbell's)	8 fl oz prep	6	6	*	4	2	4	*	4	860	2	9	70
Chicken w Noodles (Campbell's Low Sodium)	1 can	25	40	8	10	20	25	2	10	90	5	17	170
Chicken and Noodles, Golden (Campbell's Soup for One)	11 fl oz prep	10	25	*	8	6	10	2	6	1460	4	14	120
Chicken Noodle w Meat (Lipton Cup-a-Soup)	6 fl oz prep	4	*	*	4	2	4	*	2	770	1	6	45
Chicken, Old Fashioned (Campbell's Chunky)	10¾ oz	25	150	20	2	8	15	4	8	1365	5	21	170
Chicken Rice (Campbell's Chunky), 19-oz Size	½ can	20	160	4	*	4	15	2	4	1060	4	15	140

Soups	Amt.	Protein	A	C	B₁	B₂	Niacin	Calcium	Iron	Sodium (mg)	Fat (g)	Carbohydrate (g)	Calories
							% U.S. RDA						
Chicken w Rice (Campbell's)	8 fl oz prep	4	8	*	*	*	4	*	*	870	3	7	60
Chicken Rice (Lipton Cup-a-Soup)	6 fl oz	2	*	*	2	*	4	*	2	760	0-1	7	45
Chicken and Stars (Campbell's)	8 fl oz prep	4	6	*	2	2	4	*	2	935	2	7	60
Chicken Supreme (Lipton Country Style Cup-a-Soup)	6 fl oz	4	*	*	*	2	*	2	2	930	5	11	100
Chicken Vegetable (Campbell's)	8 fl oz prep	4	50	*	2	2	4	*	2	880	3	8	70
Chicken Vegetable (Campbell's Chunky), 19-oz Size	½ can	20	140	6	2	6	15	15	6	1115	6	19	170
Chicken Vegetable (Campbell's Chunky Low Sodium)	1 can	20	130	15	10	20	25	4	8	100	11	20	240
Chicken Vegetable (Campbell's Soup for One)	11 fl oz prep	8	90	4	*	2	6	2	4	1500	6	13	120
Chicken Vegetable (Lipton Cup-a-Soup)	6 fl oz	2	20	*	*	*	2	*	2	800	0-1	7	40
Chili Beef (Campbell's)	8 fl oz prep	10	10	2	2	*	2	2	6	900	5	17	130
Chili Beef (Campbell's Chunky)	11 fl oz	35	30	6	6	8	10	6	25	1155	7	37	290

		% U.S. RDA											
Clam Chowder, Manhattan (Campbell's)	8 fl oz prep	2	30	8	*	2	4	2	4	860	2	11	70
Clam Chowder, Manhattan (Campbell's Chunky)	10¾ fl oz	10	130	15	*	6	6	6	10	1255	5	24	160
Clam Chowder, Manhattan (Doxsee)	6 fl oz	8	*	*	*	*	*	2	4	545	0	9	50
Clam Chowder, Manhattan (Snow's)	7½ fl oz prep	4	40	2	*	4	4	4	4	635	2	9	70
Clam Chowder, New England (Campbell's)	8 fl oz prep	6	*	2	*	*	2	2	4	885	3	11	80
Clam Chowder, New England, Made w Milk (Campbell's)	8 fl oz prep	10	2	4	2	10	2	15	4	940	7	17	150
Clam Chowder, New England (Campbell's Chunky)	10¾ fl oz	10	*	20	4	4	8	4	10	1155	16	27	290
Clam Chowder, New England (Campbell's Soup for One)	11 fl oz prep	8	20	6	*	4	4	6	8	1365	4	19	130
Clam Chowder, New England, Made w Milk (Campbell's Soup for One)	11 fl oz prep	15	25	8	4	10	4	15	8	1420	8	24	200
Clam Chowder, New England (Doxsee)	6 fl oz	10	*	*	5	7	7	9	17	746	2	12	90
Clam Chowder, New England, Prep w Milk (Snow's)	7½ fl oz prep	15	2	*	2	10	2	15	4	665	6	13	140

Soups	Amt.	Protein	A	C	B₁	B₂	Niacin	Calcium	Iron	Sodium (mg)	Fat (g)	Carbohydrate (g)	Calories
								% U.S. RDA					
Clam Chowder, New England (Stouffer's)	8 fl oz	15	4	10	6	15	6	15	2	510	10	19	200
Consomme, Beef (Campbell's)	8 fl oz prep	6	*	*	*	*	2	*	*	785	0	2	25
Corn Chowder, New England, Prep w Milk (Snow's)	7½ fl oz prep	10	4	*	4	10	4	15	2	640	6	18	150
Fish Chowder, New England, Prep w Milk (Snow's)	7½ fl oz	15	2	*	2	10	2	15	2	620	6	11	130
Green Pea (Campbell's)	8 fl oz prep	8	25	2	4	4	6	*	4	970	4	11	100
Green Pea (Lipton Cup-a-Soup)	6 fl oz prep	6	*	*	30	2	2	2	*	680	4	16	120
Ham 'n Butter Bean (Campbell's Chunky)	10¾ fl oz	20	50	6	8	6	10	4	10	1190	10	33	280
Meatball Alphabet (Campbell's)	8 fl oz prep	8	25	2	4	2	6	*	4	970	4	11	100
Minestrone (Campbell's)	8 fl oz prep	4	50	2	2	2	4	2	2	930	2	11	80
Minestrone (Campbell's Chunky) 19-oz Size	½ can	6	100	6	2	4	4	6	6	985	5	21	140
Mushroom, Beef Flavor (Lipton)	8 fl oz prep	2	*	*	*	2	2	*	*	995	0–1	7	40
Mushroom, Beefy (Campbell's)	8 fl oz prep	8	*	*	*	2	4	*	2	990	3	5	60

Food	Serving	% U.S. RDA											
Mushroom, Cream of (Campbell's)	8 fl oz prep	2	2	*	*	4	2	2	*	825	7	9	100
Mushroom, Cream of (Campbell's Low Sodium)	1 can	4	15	4	4	10	4	4	10	60	13	16	190
Mushroom, Cream of (Lipton Cup-a-Soup)	6 fl oz prep	2	2	*	*	2	2	*	*	810	4	9	80
Mushroom, Cream of, Savory (Campbell's Soup for One)	11 fl oz prep	4	2	*	*	6	4	2	2	1495	13	14	180
Mushroom, Cream of (Rokeach)	10 fl oz prep	4	4	6	2	4	4	6	2	1050	10	13	150
Mushroom, Cream of, Prep w Milk (Rokeach)	10 fl oz prep	15	15	8	6	20	4	25	2	1170	15	20	240
Mushroom, Golden (Campbell's)	8 fl oz prep	2	2	*	*	4	4	*	2	910	3	10	80
Mushroom, Golden, w Chicken Broth (Lipton)	8 fl oz prep	2	2	*	*	*	*	*	*	900	2	8	60
Noodle, Beef Flavor (Lipton Cup-a-Soup)	6 fl oz prep	2	2	4	4	2	2	4	2	780	0–1	8	45
Noodle w Chicken Broth (Lipton)	8 fl oz prep	2	2	8	8	2	4	4	2	785	2	10	70
Noodle, Curly, w Chicken (Campbell's)	8 fl oz prep	6	25	*	4	2	6	6	4	960	3	9	70
Noodle, Giggle (Lipton)	8 fl oz prep	4	4	8	8	2	6	4	2	925	2	12	80
Noodles and Ground Beef (Campbell's)	8 fl oz prep	8	20	6	6	4	4	6	6	845	4	10	90

281

Soups	Amt.	% U.S. RDA								Sodium (mg)	Fat (g)	Carbohydrate (g)	Calories
		Pro-tein	A	C	B_1	B_2	Nia-cin	Cal-cium	Iron				
Noodle, Ring (Lipton Cup-a-Soup)	6 fl oz prep	2	*	*	6	4	4	*	2	760	1	9	50
Noodle w Vegetables and Chicken Broth (Lipton Hearty)	8 fl oz	4	4	*	6	2	4	*	2	925	2	12	80
Onion (Lipton)	8 fl oz	*	*	*	*	*	*	*	*	640	0-1	6	35
Onion (Lipton Cup-a-Soup)	6 fl oz prep	*	*	*	*	*	*	*	*	860	1	5	30
Onion, Beefy (Lipton)	8 fl oz	*	*	*	*	*	*	*	*	950	1	5	35
Onion, Cream of (Campbell's)	8 fl oz prep	2	6	*	*	2	2	2	*	835	5	12	100
Onion, Cream of, Made w Milk and Water (Campbell's)	8 fl oz prep	6	8	*	2	8	*	8	2	865	7	15	140
Onion, French (Campbell's)	8 fl oz prep	2	*	2	2	*	2	2	2	960	2	9	70
Onion, French (Campbell's Low Sodium)	1 can	2	*	15	6	10	15	2	8	60	5	7	80
Onion, Golden, w Chicken Broth (Lipton)	8 fl oz	2	*	*	*	*	*	*	*	995	1	10	60
Onion-Mushroom (Lipton)	8 fl oz	*	*	*	15	6	4	*	*	995	1	7	45
Oriental Style (Lipton Cup-a-Soup Lots-a-Noodles)	7 fl oz prep	8	*	*	15	6	4	2	6	860	2	20	120
Oyster Stew (Campbell's)	8 fl oz prep	4	*	10	*	2	2	*	8	845	5	5	70

Product	Serving											
		% U.S. RDA										
Oyster Stew, Made w Milk (Campbell's)	8 fl oz prep	10	2	10	2	10	2	8	905	10	10	150
Pepper Pot (Campbell's)	8 fl oz prep	6	20	*	2	2	2	4	960	4	9	90
Pea, Virginia (Lipton Country Style Cup-a-Soup)	6 fl oz prep	8	*	45	*	2	2	*	840	5	18	140
Potato, Cream of (Campbell's)	8 fl oz prep	2	2	*	*	*	*	*	935	3	11	70
Potato, Cream of, Made w Milk and Water (Campbell's)	8 fl oz prep	6	6	*	2	6	8	*	960	4	14	110
Ring-O-Noodle (Lipton)	8 fl oz	4	*	8	2	2	*	2	855	1	9	60
Seafood Chowder, New England, Made w Milk (Snow's)	7½ fl oz prep	10	2	*	10	2	15	2	690	6	11	130
Shrimp, Cream of (Campbell's)	8 fl oz prep	2	*	*	*	*	*	*	905	6	8	90
Shrimp, Cream of, Made w Milk (Campbell's)	8 fl oz prep	10	4	2	2	10	15	2	965	10	13	160
Sirloin Burger (Campbell's Chunky)	10¾ fl oz	25	100	15	10	15	2	10	1285	9	23	220
Spinach, Cream of (Stouffer's)	8 fl oz	10	60	10	20	2	25	4	885	15	17	230
Split Pea (Campbell's Low Sodium)	1 can	15	20	8	10	10	2	10	25	5	37	240
Split Pea 'n Ham (Campbell's Chunky)	10¾ fl oz	20	80	10	6	10	2	10	1130	6	33	230

Soups	Amt.	Protein	A	C	B$_1$	B$_2$	Niacin	Calcium	Iron	Sodium (mg)	Fat (g)	Carbohydrate (g)	Calories
					% U.S. RDA								
Split Pea w Ham (Stouffer's)	8¼ fl oz	20	*	*	10	4	6	*	6	695	3	27	190
Split Pea w Ham and Bacon (Campbell's)	8 fl oz prep	10	8	*	8	2	4	*	10	810	4	24	170
Steak 'n Potato (Campbell's Chunky)	10¾ fl oz	25	*	10	2	10	15	*	10	1265	5	24	200
Tomato (Campbell's)	8 fl oz prep	2	8	40	*	*	4	*	2	750	2	17	90
Tomato, Made w Milk (Campbell's)	8 fl oz prep	10	10	40	2	10	4	10	2	800	6	22	160
Tomato (Lipton Cup-a-Soup)	6 fl oz	*	10	4	*	*	2	2	2	650	1	17	80
Tomato (Rokeach)	10 fl oz prep	4	6	6	2	2	*	2	2	980	1	20	90
Tomato, Made w Milk (Rokeach)	10 fl oz prep	15	10	8	6	15	2	20	2	1059	6	27	190
Tomato, Beefy (Lipton Cup-a-Soup TRIM)	6 fl oz	*	*	*	*	*	*	*	*	420	0	2	10
Tomato Bisque (Campbell's)	8 fl oz prep	2	8	30	*	2	4	2	2	840	3	23	120
Tomato-Onion (Lipton)	8 fl oz prep	2	6	*	*	*	2	2	2	975	0–1	15	70
Tomato Rice (Rokeach)	10 oz prep	4	15	4	4	4	4	4	4	815	5	25	160
Tomato Rice, Old Fashioned (Campbell's)	8 fl oz prep	2	6	20	*	*	2	*	2	780	2	22	110
Tomato Royale (Campbell's Soup for One)	11 fl oz prep	4	15	10	2	4	8	2	4	1335	3	35	180

Food	Serving					% U.S. RDA							
Tomato w Tomato Pieces (Campbell's Low Sodium)	1 can	180	30	5	40	8	4	15	8	8	50	25	6
Tomato Vegetable (Lipton Cup-a-Soup Lots-a-Noodles)	7 fl oz	110	21	1	885	4	*	4	10	2	2	15	6
Tomato Vegetable Noodle (Lipton Hearty)	8 fl oz prep	80	15	1	930	2	*	4	8	8	6	10	4
Turkey Noodle (Campbell's)	8 fl oz prep	60	8	2	920	4	*	6	6	6	*	4	6
Turkey Vegetable (Campbell's)	8 fl oz prep	70	8	3	825	2	*	4	2	2	60	*	4
Vegetable (Campbell's)	8 fl oz prep	80	12	2	770	4	*	4	2	2	60	*	2
Vegetable (Campbell's Chunky)	10¾ fl oz	140	23	4	1125	8	6	6	4	2	170	4	6
Vegetable Beef (Campbell's)	8 fl oz prep	70	8	2	830	4	*	4	2	*	40	2	8
Vegetable Beef (Campbell's Chunky Low Sodium)	1 can	170	19	5	65	10	4	20	15	10	110	15	25
Vegetable Beef (Lipton Cup-a-Soup)	6 fl oz	50	8	0–1	930	2	*	2	2	6	*	*	2
Vegetable Beef, Old Fashioned (Campbell's Chunky)	10¾ fl oz	180	20	5	1060	10	4	10	10	2	120	10	25
Vegetable Beef & Bacon, "Burly" (Campbell's) Soup for One	11 fl oz prep	150	20	5	1480	10	6	8	6	4	40	8	10
Vegetable w Beef Stock (Lipton)	8 fl oz prep	50	9	0–1	995	2	*	2	*	2	10	6	2

Soups	Amt.	Pro-tein	A	C	B₁	B₂	Nia-cin	Cal-cium	Iron	Sodium (mg)	Fat (g)	Carbohy-drate (g)	Calories
		% U.S. RDA											
Vegetable, Country (Lipton)	8 fl oz prep	4	25	4	6	4	4	*	2	995	1	14	80
Vegetable, Garden (Lipton Cup-a-Soup Lots-a-Noodles)	7 fl oz	8	30	2	10	6	6	*	6	730	2	23	130
Vegetable, Harvest (Lipton Country Style Cup-a-Soup)	6 fl oz	2	25	4	4	2	4	2	4	620	0-1	20	90
Vegetable, Herb (Lipton Cup-a-Soup TRIM)	6 fl oz	*	*	*	*	*	*	*	*	535	0	1	10
Vegetable, Mediterranean (Campbell's Chunky), 19-oz Size	½ can	6	130	15	4	6	8	6	8	1040	5	24	160
Vegetable, Old Fashioned (Campbell's)	8 fl oz prep	2	60	2	*	2	2	*	2	925	2	9	60
Vegetable, Old World (Campbell's Soup for One)	11 fl oz prep	6	60	8	2	2	4	6	8	1495	4	18	130
Vegetable, Spanish-Style (Campbell's)	8 fl oz prep	*	40	6	2	*	2	2	2	595	0	10	40
Vegetable, Spring (Lipton Cup-a-Soup)	6 fl oz	2	8	*	2	2	4	*	2	910	1	7	40
Vegetarian Vegetable (Campbell's)	8 fl oz prep	2	50	2	2	2	4	*	2	755	2	12	70

						% U.S. RDA							
Vegetarian Vegetable (Rokeach)	10 fl oz prep	4	60	*	4	2	*	2	2	1055	3	15	90
Vegetable Soup for Dip (Lipton)	8 fl oz prep	2	20	6	4	2	2	2	2	995	0–1	8	45
Won Ton (Campbell's)	8 fl oz prep	4	*	*	2	2	6	*	2	875	1	5	40
Sugar and Syrups													
Cinnamon Sugar (French's)	1 tsp	*	*	*	*	*	*	*	*	0	0–.5	4	16
Molasses, Cane, Light (1st Extraction)	1 tbsp	*	*	*	*	2	*	4	4	3	0	13	50
Molasses, Cane, Blackstrap (3rd Extraction)	1 tbsp	*	*	*	2	2	2	15	20	19	0	11	45
Molasses, Unsulphured (Grandma's)	1 tbsp	*	*	*	*	2	*	2	4	10	0	15	60
Syrup, Corn, Dark (Karo)	1 tbsp	*	*	*	*	*	*	*	*	40	0	15	60
Syrup, Corn, Light (Karo)	1 tbsp	*	*	*	*	*	*	*	*	30	0	15	60
Syrup, Fruit (Smucker's)	2 tbsp	*	*	*	*	*	*	*	*	0–10	0	26	100
Syrup, Maple	1 tbsp	*	*	*	2	2	*	2	2	2	0	13	50
Syrup, Low Calorie (Cary's)	1 tbsp	*	*	*	*	*	*	*	*	0–10	0	2	6
Syrup, Pancake (Golden Griddle)	1 tbsp	*	*	*	*	*	*	*	*	20	0	13	50
Syrup, Pancake and Waffle (Karo)	1 tbsp	*	*	*	*	*	*	*	*	35	0	15	60
Syrup, Pancake (Mrs. Butterworth's)	3 tbsp	*	*	*	*	*	*	*	*	NA	.5	40	165

Sugar and Syrups	Amt.	Pro-tein	A	C	B₁	B₂	Nia-cin	Cal-cium	Iron	Sodium (mg)	Fat (g)	Carbohy-drate (g)	Calories
							% U.S. RDA						
Syrup, Reduced Calorie (Cary's Lite)	1 tbsp	*	*	*	*	*	*	*	*	0–10	0	8	30
Syrup, Sorghum	1 tbsp	*	*	*	2	2	*	*	15	NA	0	14	60
Sugar, Brown	1 c packed	*	*	*	2	4	2	20	40	66	0	211	820
Sugar, White, Granulated	1 c	*	*	*	*	*	*	*	2	2	0	200	770
Sugar, White, Granulated	1 tbsp	*	*	*	*	*	*	*	*	Trace	0	11	40
Sugar, White, Powdered, Unsifted	1 c	*	*	*	*	*	*	*	*	2	0	200	460
Tea													
Bag (Lipton)	1 c	0	*	*	*	*	*	*	*	0	0	0	2
Instant (Lipton)	8 fl oz	0	*	*	*	*	*	*	*	0	0	0	2
Canned, Lemon Flavored w Vitamin C (Lipton)	8 fl oz	*	*	25	*	*	*	*	*	15	0	20	80
Canned, Lemon Flavored Sugar Free w Vitamin C (Lipton)	8 fl oz	*	*	25	*	*	*	*	*	20	0	0	2
Iced, Mix, Lemon Flavored (Lipton Sugar Free)	8 fl oz	0	*	*	*	*	*	*	*	5	0	0	2
Iced, Mix, Lemon Flavored w NutraSweet (Lipton)	8 fl oz	0	*	*	*	*	*	*	*	0	0	0	4
Iced, Mix, Lemon Flavored w Sugar (Lipton)	8 fl oz	0	*	*	*	*	*	*	*	0	0	16	60

Food	Serving					% U.S. RDA								
Iced, Mix, Lemon Flavored (Wyler's)	8 fl oz	80	21	0	NA	*	*	*	*	*	*	*	*
Iced, Mix, Sugar Free (Crystal Light)	8 fl oz	4	0	0	20	*	10	*	*	*	*	*	*
Lipton Flavored Teas, All Flavors	1 c	2	0–1	0	0	*	*	*	*	*	*	*	*
Lipton Herbal Teas, All Flavors	1 c	4	1	0	0	*	*	*	*	*	*	*	*
Toppings													
Butterscotch (Smucker's)	2 tbsp	140	33	0	75	*	*	*	*	2	*	2	*
Caramel (Smucker's)	2 tbsp	140	33	0	110	*	*	*	*	2	*	2	*
Chocolate Fudge (Hershey's)	2 tbsp	100	14	4	30	2	*	*	*	2	*	2	*
Chocolate Fudge (Smucker's)	2 tbsp	130	31	1	50	2	*	*	*	2	*	2	*
Chocolate Syrup (Hershey's)	2 tbsp	80	17	1	20	*	*	*	*	2	*	2	*
Chocolate Syrup (Smucker's)	2 tbsp	130	27	2	40	*	*	*	*	2	*	2	*
Hot Caramel (Smucker's)	2 tbsp	150	28	4	75	2	*	*	*	*	*	2	*
Hot Fudge (Smucker's)	2 tbsp	110	18	4	60	*	*	*	*	2	*	2	*
Peanut Butter Caramel (Smucker's)	2 tbsp	150	29	2	120	4	*	*	*	2	6	2	*
Pecans in Syrup (Smucker's)	2 tbsp	130	28	1	0–10	2	*	*	*	6	*	2	2
Pineapple (Smucker's)	2 tbsp	130	32	0	0–10	*	*	*	*	*	*	*	*
Strawberry (Smucker's)	2 tbsp	120	30	0	0–10	*	*	*	*	*	*	*	*

Toppings	Amt.	Pro-tein	A	C	B$_1$	B$_2$	Nia-cin	Cal-cium	Iron	Sodium (mg)	Fat (g)	Carbohy-drate (g)	Calories
					% U.S. RDA								
Swiss Milk Chocolate Fudge (Smucker's)	2 tbsp	4	*	*	*	6	*	4	*	75	1	31	140
Smucker's Magic Shell	4 tsp	*	*	*	*	*	*	*	*	25	10	11	130
Walnuts in Syrup (Smucker's)	2 tbsp	2	*	*	2	2	*	*	22	0–10	1	27	130
Whipped (Cool Whip Extra Creamy Dairy Recipe)	1 tbsp	*	*	*	*	*	*	*	*	2	1	1	16
Whipped (Dover Farms)	1 tbsp	*	*	*	*	*	*	*	*	2	1	1	16
Whipped, Nondairy (Cool Whip)	1 tbsp	*	*	*	*	*	*	*	*	1	1	1	14
Whipped, Mix (Dream Whip)	1 tbsp prep	*	*	*	*	*	*	*	*	5	1	1	10
Whipped, Mix (D-Zerta)	1 tbsp prep	*	*	*	*	*	*	*	*	5	1	0	8
Vegetables													
Artichoke Hearts, Frozen (Birds Eye Deluxe)	3 oz	4	2	8	2	6	4	*	4	40	0	7	30
Asparagus, Green, Fresh, Cooked, Drained, Spears	4 (½" diam at base)	2	10	25	6	6	4	2	2	1	0–1	2	10
Asparagus, Green, Fresh, Cooked, Drained, Pieces	1 c	4	25	60	15	15	10	2	4	1	0–1	5	30
Asparagus, Canned, Cut (Green Giant)	½ c	4	6	25	2	6	2	0	4	450	0	2	20

Food	Serving	% U.S. RDA											
Asparagus, Canned, Green, Spears and Tips (Del Monte)	½ c	2	10	25	4	6	2	*	2	355	0	3	20
Asparagus, Canned, Green Tipped (Del Monte)	½ c	2	10	25	4	6	2	*	2	355	0	3	20
Asparagus, Canned, Spears (Le Sueur)	½ c	4	6	20	4	6	4	0	4	390	0	4	30
Asparagus, Frozen, Cut (Birds Eye)	3.3 oz	4	20	45	8	6	6	2	4	5	0	4	25
Asparagus, Frozen, Cut Spears in Butter Sauce (Green Giant)	½ c	4	15	45	10	8	6	2	6	725	4	6	70
Asparagus, Frozen, Spears (Birds Eye)	3.3 oz	4	15	50	10	8	6	2	4	5	0	4	25
Beans, Green, Fresh, Cooked, Drained	1 c	4	15	25	6	6	4	6	4	5	0–1	7	30
Beans, Green, Canned, Cut (Del Monte)	½ c	*	10	6	2	2	2	2	4	355	0	4	20
Beans, Green, Canned, Cut (Del Monte No Salt Added)	½ c	*	10	6	2	2	2	2	4	0–10	0	4	20
Beans, Green, Canned, Cut (1½" pieces) (Green Giant)	½ c	0	4	4	2	2	2	2	4	310	1	3	20
Beans, Green, Canned, French Style (Del Monte)	½ c	*	10	4	2	2	*	2	4	355	0	4	20

Vegetables	Amt.	Pro-tein	A	C	B₁	B₂	Nia-cin	Cal-cium	Iron	Sodium (mg)	Fat (g)	Carbohy-drate (g)	Calories
		% U.S. RDA											
Beans, Green, Canned, French Style (Del Monte No Salt Added)	½ c	*	10	4	*	2	*	2	4	0–10	0	4	20
Beans, Green, Canned, French Style (Green Giant)	½ c	0	4	4	0	2	0	2	4	270	0	3	18
Beans, Green, Canned, French Style, Seasoned (Del Monte)	½ c	*	10	4	*	2	*	2	2	355	0	4	20
Beans, Green, Canned, Italian, Cut (Del Monte)	½ c	*	8	15	2	4	2	2	4	355	0	6	25
Beans, Green, Canned, Kitchen Cut (Green Giant)	½ c	2	6	6	2	2	0	2	4	260	0	3	20
Beans, Green, Canned, Whole (Del Monte)	½ c	*	10	10	8	2	4	*	2	355	0	4	20
Beans, Green, Frozen (Green Giant)	½ c	0	6	10	0	2	0	2	2	5	0	4	20
Beans, Green, Frozen, Cut (Birds Eye)	3 oz	2	10	15	2	4	*	4	4	5	0	6	25
Beans, Green, Frozen, Cut (Green Giant Harvest Fresh)	½ c	0	8	8	2	4	0	2	2	175	0	4	25
Beans, Green, Frozen, French Cut (Birds Eye)	3 oz	2	8	15	4	4	*	4	4	5	0	6	25

Food	Serving			% U.S. RDA								
Beans, Green, Frozen, Whole (Birds Eye Deluxe)	3 oz	*	10	15	4	4	*	4	4	0	0	5	25
Beans, Green, Frozen, French Style, Cut, in Butter Sauce (Green Giant)	½ c	2	8	10	2	4	0	2	2	355	1	6	40
Beans, Green, Frozen, in Cream Sauce w Mushrooms (Green Giant)	½ c	0	10	15	10	6	2	4	2	280	4	10	80
Beans, Green, Frozen, French, w Toasted Almonds (Birds Eye)	3 oz	4	8	15	2	4	2	4	2	335	2	8	50
Beans, Green, Frozen, Italian (Birds Eye)	3 oz	2	8	25	4	6	2	4	4	5	0	7	30
Beans, Green, w Corn, Carrots, and Pearl Onions, Frozen (Birds Eye Farm Fresh)	3.2 oz	2	90	10	2	4	2	2	2	15	0	10	45
Beans, Green, French, and Cauliflower and Carrots, Frozen (Birds Eye Farm Fresh)	3.2 oz	2	90	30	2	4	*	2	4	20	0	6	25
Beans, Lima, Fresh, Cooked, Drained	1 c	20	10	50	20	10	10	8	25	2	1	34	190
Beans, Lima, Canned (Del Monte)	½ c	6	2	15	2	2	2	2	8	355	0	14	70
Beans, Lima, Frozen (Green Giant)	½ c	8	0	4	6	0	0	2	8	30	0	19	100

| | | % U.S. RDA | | | | | | | | | | | |
Vegetables	Amt.	Pro-tein	A	C	B₁	B₂	Nia-cin	Cal-cium	Iron	Sodium (mg)	Fat (g)	Carbohy-drate (g)	Calories
Beans, Lima, Frozen (Green Giant Harvest Fresh)	½ c	10	4	25	6	2	4	2	10	310	0	19	100
Beans, Lima, Baby, Frozen (Birds Eye)	3.3 oz	10	4	30	6	4	6	4	10	115	0	24	130
Beans, Lima, Frozen, Fordhook (Birds Eye)	3.3 oz	10	4	30	6	4	6	2	8	100	0	19	100
Beans, Lima, Frozen, Tiny (Birds Eye Deluxe)	3.3 oz	10	6	35	6	4	4	2	8	145	1	21	110
Beans, Lima, Frozen, in Butter Sauce (Green Giant)	½ c	8	4	25	4	2	6	2	8	445	2	20	120
Beans, Wax, Fresh, Cooked, Drained	1 c	2	2	10	2	4	2	6	10	4	0-1	6	30
Beans, Wax, Canned, Cut (Del Monte)	½ c	0	*	10	*	2	*	2	2	355	0	4	20
Beans, Wax, Canned, French Style (Del Monte)	½ c	0	0	6	*	2	*	2	4	355	0	4	20
Bean Salad, Canned (Green Giant Three Bean)	½ c	4	6	6	2	2	0	2	20	540	0-1	18	80
Bean Sprouts, Raw	1 c	6	*	35	10	8	4	2	8	5	0-1	7	35
Bean Sprouts, Cooked, Drained	1 c	6	*	15	8	8	4	2	6	5	0-1	7	35

The following table presents nutritional data (% U.S. RDA). The first column is the serving size.

Food	Serving													% U.S. RDA
Beet Greens, Fresh, Leaves and Stems, Cooked, Drained	1 c	4	150	35	6	15	2	15	15	110	0–1	5	25	
Beets, Fresh, Whole, Cooked, Drained	2 beets (2" diam)	2	*	10	2	2	2	2	2	43	0–1	7	30	
Beets, Fresh, Diced or Sliced	1 c	2	*	15	4	4	2	2	4	73	0–1	12	60	
Beets, Canned, Sliced, Whole, or Tiny Whole (Del Monte)	½ c	*	0	4	*	2	*	2	2	290	0	8	35	
Beets, Canned, Sliced (Del Monte No Salt Added)	½ c	*	0	4	*	2	*	2	2	100	0	8	35	
Beets, Canned, Pickled, Crinkle Sliced (Del Monte)	½ c	*	0	6	*	*	*	*	*	375	0	19	80	
Broccoli, Fresh, Stalks, Whole, Cooked, Drained	1 med	8	90	270	10	20	6	15	8	18	0–1	8	45	
Broccoli, Fresh, Cut (½" pieces), Cooked, Drained	1 c	8	80	230	10	20	6	15	6	16	0–1	7	40	
Broccoli, Frozen (Green Giant Fanfare)	½ c	4	25	60	8	4	4	2	4	455	1	14	80	
Broccoli, Frozen, Baby Spears (Birds Eye Deluxe)	3.3 oz	4	25	120	6	8	2	4	4	15	0	5	30	
Broccoli, Frozen, Chopped (Birds Eye)	3.3 oz	4	40	90	4	6	2	6	4	20	0	5	25	

Vegetables	Amt.	% U.S. RDA								Sodium (mg)	Fat (g)	Carbohydrate (g)	Calories
		Protein	A	C	B₁	B₂	Niacin	Calcium	Iron				
Broccoli, Frozen, Cut (Birds Eye)	3.3 oz	4	40	90	4	6	2	6	4	25	0	4	25
Broccoli, Frozen, Cut (Green Giant)	½ c	2	8	60	2	4	0	2	0	10	0	2	16
Broccoli, Frozen, Cut (Green Giant Harvest Fresh)	½ c	4	25	80	2	6	2	2	2	160	0	4	30
Broccoli, Frozen, Florets (Birds Eye Deluxe)	3.3 oz	4	25	100	4	6	2	4	4	20	0	5	25
Broccoli, Frozen, Minispears (Green Giant Frozen Like Fresh)	½ c	2	4	35	0	2	0	0	0	10	0	3	16
Broccoli, Frozen, Spears (Birds Eye)	3.3 oz	4	25	100	4	6	2	4	4	20	0	5	25
Broccoli, Frozen, Spears (Green Giant Harvest Fresh)	½ c	4	25	80	2	6	2	2	2	160	0	4	30
Broccoli, Frozen, Spears, in Butter Sauce (Green Giant)	½ c	4	8	30	2	4	2	2	0	325	1	5	40
Broccoli, Frozen, w Almonds (Birds Eye)	3.3 oz	6	35	80	4	6	2	6	6	215	3	6	50
Broccoli, Frozen, w Cheese Sauce (Birds Eye)	5 oz	8	60	80	6	10	2	15	4	505	7	13	120

Food	Serving												
		% U.S. RDA											
Broccoli, Frozen, in Cheese Sauce (Green Giant)	½ c	4	30	30	4	8	2	6	2	425	2	8	70
Broccoli, Frozen, in Cheddar Cheese Sauce (Stouffer's)	4½ oz	10	30	70	4	10	2	20	4	970	8	8	130
Broccoli, Baby Carrots, and Water Chestnuts, Frozen (Birds Eye Farm Fresh)	3.2 oz	4	90	70	2	4	2	2	4	25	0	6	30
Broccoli and Carrots, Frozen (Green Giant Fanfare)	½ c	2	50	70	2	4	0	2	2	20	0	5	25
Broccoli and Carrots, Frozen, and Pasta Twists (Birds Eye Blue Ribbon)	3.3 oz	4	150	40	4	2	2	2	2	270	4	11	90
Broccoli and Cauliflower, Frozen (Green Giant Medley)	½ c	2	40	80	4	4	4	2	2	470	1	10	60
Broccoli and Cauliflower, Frozen (Green Giant Supreme)	½ c	2	40	60	2	4	0	2	2	30	0	4	20
Broccoli and Cauliflower, w Red Peppers, Frozen (Birds Eye Deluxe)	3.3 oz	4	15	100	4	4	2	2	4	20	0	5	25
Broccoli, Cauliflower, and Carrots, Frozen (Birds Eye Farm Fresh)	3.2 oz	2	110	60	2	4	2	4	4	30	0	5	25
Broccoli, Cauliflower, and Carrots, Frozen, w Cheese Sauce (Birds Eye)	5 oz	6	120	70	4	10	2	10	4	400	5	12	100

Vegetables	Amt.	Pro-tein	A	C	B$_1$	B$_2$	Nia-cin	Cal-cium	Iron	Sodium (mg)	Fat (g)	Carbohy-drate (g)	Calories
		% U.S. RDA											
Broccoli, Cauliflower, and Carrots, Frozen, in Cheese Sauce (Green Giant)	½ c	4	80	50	4	8	2	6	0	465	2	8	60
Broccoli, Corn, and Red Peppers, Frozen (Birds Eye Farm Fresh)	3.2 oz	4	15	70	4	4	4	*	2	10	0	11	50
Broccoli, Green Beans, Pearl Onions, and Red Peppers, Frozen (Birds Eye Farm Fresh)	3.2 oz	2	20	70	4	4	2	4	4	15	0	5	25
Broccoli and Water Chestnuts, Frozen (Birds Eye)	3.3 oz	4	35	80	2	6	2	4	4	215	0	6	30
Brussels Sprouts, Fresh (1¼" × 1½")	7–8 (1 c)	10	15	230	8	15	6	4	10	16	1	10	60
Brussels Sprouts, Frozen (Birds Eye)	3.3 oz	6	15	110	6	6	2	2	4	15	0	7	35
Brussels Sprouts, Frozen (Green Giant)	½ c	2	6	25	2	4	0	0	2	15	0	5	30
Brussels Sprouts, Frozen, Baby (Birds Eye Deluxe)	3.3 oz	6	15	130	6	8	4	2	6	10	0	7	40
Brussels Sprouts, Frozen, in Butter Sauce (Green Giant)	½ c	4	15	90	6	4	2	2	2	275	1	9	60

Food	Serving												
		% U.S. RDA											
Brussels Sprouts, Frozen, in Cheese Sauce (Green Giant)	½ c	4	10	90	4	10	6	6	2	475	2	13	80
Brussels Sprouts, Frozen, Baby, w Cheese Sauce (Birds Eye)	4.5 oz	8	45	90	6	10	2	10	4	435	6	13	120
Brussels Sprouts, Cauliflower, and Carrots, Frozen (Birds Eye Farm Fresh)	3.2 oz	4	80	80	4	4	2	2	4	20	0	6	30
Cabbage, Fresh, Cooked, Drained	1 c	2	4	80	4	4	2	6	2	20	0–1	6	30
Cabbage, Raw, Shredded Coarsely	1 c	2	2	60	2	2	*	4	2	14	0–1	4	18
Cabbage, Raw, Shredded Finely	1 c	2	2	70	2	2	2	4	2	18	0–1	5	22
Cabbage, Chinese, Raw, Shredded Coarsely	1 c	2	2	30	2	2	2	4	2	17	0–1	3	10
Cabbage, Red, Raw, Shredded Coarsely	1 c	2	*	70	4	2	2	2	4	18	0–1	5	22
Cabbage, Savoy, Raw, Shredded Coarsely	1 c	2	2	60	2	4	*	4	4	15	0–1	4	18
Cabbage, Spoon or Pak Choy, Cooked, Drained	1 c	4	110	40	4	8	6	25	6	31	0–1	4	25
Carrots, Raw, in Strips (¼" × 2½–3")	6–8 (1 oz)	*	60	4	2	*	2	2	2	13	0–1	3	10

Vegetables	Amt.	Pro-tein	A	C	B₁	B₂	Nia-cin	Cal-cium	Iron	Sodium (mg)	Fat (g)	Carbohy-drate (g)	Calories
					% U.S. RDA								
Carrots, Raw, Grated or Shredded	1 c	2	240	15	4	2	4	4	4	52	0–1	11	45
Carrots, Fresh, Cooked, Sliced, Drained	1 c	2	330	15	6	4	4	6	4	51	0–1	11	50
Carrots, Canned, Sliced, Diced, or Whole (Del Monte)	½ c	0	300	6	*	*	2	2	2	265	0	7	30
Carrots, Frozen, Baby, Whole (Birds Eye De-luxe)	3.3 oz	*	300	10	2	2	4	2	4	45	0	9	40
Carrots, Frozen, Crinkle Cut, in Butter Sauce (Green Giant)	½ c	0	310	6	0	0	2	2	0	315	1	16	80
Carrots, Baby, Sweet Peas, and Pearl Onions, Fro-zen (Birds Eye Deluxe)	3.3 oz	4	190	15	6	2	4	2	4	60	0	10	50
Cauliflower, Raw, Sliced, Flowerbuds	1 c	4	2	110	6	4	4	2	4	11	0–1	5	25
Cauliflower, Fresh, Cooked, Drained, Flowerbuds	1 c	4	2	120	8	6	4	2	4	11	0–1	5	30
Cauliflower, Frozen (Birds Eye)	3.3 oz	2	*	80	4	4	2	2	2	20	0	5	25
Cauliflower, Frozen, Cut (Green Giant)	½ c	0	0	4	0	2	0	0	0	30	0	3	16

		% U.S. RDA									
Cauliflower, Frozen, Florets (Birds Eye Deluxe)	3.3 oz	2	*	80	4	4	2	2	15	0	5	25
Cauliflower, Frozen, w Almonds (Birds Eye)	3.3 oz	4	*	80	4	4	2	4	270	2	5	40
Cauliflower, Frozen, w Cheese Sauce (Birds Eye)	5 oz	6	40	70	4	10	2	2	505	7	12	120
Cauliflower, Frozen, in Cheese Sauce (Green Giant)	½ c	2	15	50	2	8	0	2	450	2	10	60
Cauliflower, Frozen, in White Cheddar Cheese Sauce (Green Giant)	½ c	4	0	80	4	6	0	4	415	3	7	70
Cauliflower and Carrots, Frozen (Green Giant Bonanza)	½ c	2	30	45	6	4	2	4	295	3	7	60
Cauliflower and Green Beans, Frozen (Green Giant Festival)	½ c	0	2	50	2	2	2	2	30	0	3	16
Cauliflower, Green Beans, and Corn, Frozen (Birds Eye Farm Fresh)	3.2 oz	2	4	45	4	4	2	2	10	0	8	35
Celery, Green, Raw (8" × 1½" at Root End)	1	*	2	6	*	*	2	*	50	0–1	2	8
Celery, Green, Raw, Diced or Chopped	1 c	2	6	20	2	2	4	2	151	0–1	5	20
Celery, Green, Diced, Cooked, Drained	1 c	2	6	15	2	2	4	2	132	0–1	5	22

Vegetables	Amt.	Pro-tein	A	C	B_1	B_2	Nia-cin	Cal-cium	Iron	Sodium (mg)	Fat (g)	Carbohy-drate (g)	Calories
		% U.S. RDA											
Chard, Swiss, Fresh, Leaves, Cooked, Drained	1 c	4	190	45	4	10	4	15	15	151	0–1	6	30
Chilies, Green, Canned, Whole or Diced (Del Monte)	½ c	0	4	80	*	*	2	6	4	690	0	5	20
Chilies, Green, Canned, Chopped (Old El Paso)	2 tbsp	*	0	22	*	*	*	4	3	69	0–1	1	7
Chilies, Green, Canned, Whole (Old El Paso)	1 chili	*	0	21	*	*	*	6	3	105	0–1	1	7
Collards, Fresh, Cooked, Drained	1 c	10	300	240	15	20	10	35	8	20	2	10	60
Corn, Fresh, Cooked	1 (5" × 1¾")	4	6	10	6	4	6	*	2	0	1	16	70
Corn, Fresh, Cooked, Kernels, Drained	1 c	8	15	20	10	10	10	*	6	0	2	31	140
Corn, Canned, Golden, Cream Style (Del Monte)	½ c	2	2	8	2	2	4	0	2	355	1	18	80
Corn, Canned, Golden, Cream Style (Del Monte No Salt Added)	½ c	2	2	10	2	4	4	0	2	0–10	1	20	80
Corn, Canned, Golden, Shoe Peg (Green Giant)	½ c	2	0	4	2	4	4	0	2	270	1	18	90
Corn, Canned, Golden, Vacuum Packed (Del Monte)	½ c	4	4	15	2	4	6	0	2	355	1	22	90

Food	Serving												
		% U.S. RDA											
Corn, Canned, Golden, Vacuum Packed (Del Monte No Salt Added)	½ c	4	4	15	2	4	6	0	2	0–10	1	22	90
Corn, Canned, Golden, Whole Kernel (Del Monte)	½ c	2	2	10	2	4	4	0	2	355	1	17	70
Corn, Canned, Golden, Whole Kernel (Del Monte No Salt Added)	½ c	2	2	10	2	4	4	0	2	0–10	1	18	80
Corn, Canned, White (Green Giant Vacuum Pak)	½ c	2	6	10	4	4	6	0	0	270	0	20	90
Corn, Canned, White, Cream Style (Del Monte)	½ c	2	0	10	*	4	6	0	2	355	0	21	90
Corn, Canned, White, Whole Kernel (Del Monte)	½ c	2	0	15	2	4	4	0	2	355	0	16	70
Corn, Canned, Whole Kernel (Green Giant Vacuum Pak)	½ c	2	2	10	2	2	4	0	2	230	0	20	90
Corn, Canned, Whole Kernel (Le Sueur)	½ c	2	8	8	0	2	0	0	2	285	0	18	80
Corn, Canned, Cream Style (Green Giant)	½ c	2	0	8	2	2	6	0	0	320	1	21	100
Corn, Canned, w Peppers (Mexicorn)	½ c	2	10	8	2	4	4	0	2	335	0	18	80
Corn, Frozen (Green Giant Harvest Fresh Niblets)	½ c	4	4	4	4	4	6	0	2	280	0	22	100

| | | % U.S. RDA | | | | | | | | | | | |
Vegetables	Amt.	Pro-tein	A	C	B₁	B₂	Nia-cin	Cal-cium	Iron	Sodium (mg)	Fat (g)	Carbohy-drate (g)	Calories
Corn, Frozen, Sweet (Birds Eye)	3.3 oz	4	4	8	4	4	8	*	2	5	1	20	80
Corn, Frozen, Tendertreat Sweet (Birds Eye Deluxe)	3.3 oz	4	4	8	4	4	8	*	2	5	1	20	80
Corn, Frozen, on Cob (Birds Eye)	1 ear	6	6	15	10	6	10	*	4	5	1	29	120
Corn, Frozen, on Cob (Birds Eye Big Ears)	1 ear	8	6	15	15	8	15	*	6	5	1	37	160
Corn, Frozen, on Cob (Birds Eye Little Ears)	2 ears	6	6	15	10	6	10	*	4	5	1	30	130
Corn, Frozen, on Cob (Green Giant Nibblers)	1 ear	2	2	10	4	6	6	0	0	10	1	16	80
Corn, Frozen, on Cob (Green Giant Niblet Ears)	1 ear	6	4	20	8	10	10	0	2	20	1	30	140
Corn, Frozen, on Cob (Ore-Ida)	4.5 oz	2	*	6	4	4	8	*	4	0–10	1	31	150
Corn, Frozen, in Butter Sauce (Green Giant Niblets)	½ c	4	0	10	4	2	6	0	2	280	2	18	100
Corn, Frozen, Cream Style (Green Giant)	½ c	4	2	8	6	2	2	0	0	315	1	25	120

Food	Serving					% U.S. RDA							
Corn, Frozen, in Cream Sauce (Green Giant Niblets)	½ c	4	4	8	10	6	6	2	0	295	5	18	130
Corn, Frozen, Golden and White (Green Giant Niblets and White Corn)	½ c	2	2	4	4	2	6	0	0	5	1	16	80
Corn, Frozen, White, Shoepeg, in Butter Sauce (Green Giant)	½ c	4	0	10	4	2	6	0	0	290	2	19	100
Corn and Broccoli, Frozen (Green Giant Bounty)	½ c	2	15	60	4	4	4	0	2	10	1	11	60
Corn and Green Beans, Frozen, w Pasta Curls (Birds Eye)	3.3 oz	4	8	15	4	4	4	6	2	280	5	15	110
Cowpeas, Blackeyed, Fresh, Cooked, Drained	1 c	20	10	45	35	10	10	4	20	2	2	30	180
Cress, Garden, Cooked, Drained	1 c	4	210	80	6	15	6	8	6	11	1	5	30
Cucumbers, Raw, Pared, Sliced (⅛" thick)	1 c	2	*	25	2	4	2	2	2	8	0–1	5	20
Cucumbers, Raw, Not Pared, Sliced (⅛" thick)	1 c	2	6	20	2	2	*	2	6	6	0–1	4	16
Dandelion Greens, Cooked, 1 c (not pressed down)	1 c	4	250	30	10	10	10	15	10	46	1	7	35
Eggplant, Fresh, Diced, Cooked, Drained	1 c	4	*	10	6	4	4	2	6	12	1	8	40

305

| | | % U.S. RDA | | | | | | | | | | | |
Vegetables	Amt.	Pro-tein	A	C	B₁	B₂	Nia-cin	Cal-cium	Iron	Sodium (mg)	Fat (g)	Carbohy-drate (g)	Calories
Endive, Curly, Raw, Cut	1 c	2	35	8	2	4	2	4	4	7	0–1	2	10
Kale, Leaves, w/o Stems, Cooked, Drained	1 c	8	180	170	8	10	8	20	10	47	1	7	45
Lettuce, Boston or Bibb (5″ diam head)	1 large leaf, 2 med, or 3 small	*	2	2	*	*	*	*	2	1	0–1	0–1	2
Lettuce, Iceberg	¼ head (4¾″ diam)	2	8	15	6	4	2	2	4	12	0–1	4	18
Lettuce, Iceberg, Chunks, Small	1 c	2	4	8	2	2	*	2	2	7	0–1	2	10
Lettuce, Iceberg, Shredded or Chopped	1 c	*	4	4	2	2	*	2	2	5	0–1	2	8
Lettuce, Looseleaf or Bunching, Chopped or Shredded	1 c	2	20	15	2	2	*	4	4	5	0–1	2	10
Mixed, Canned (Del Monte)	½ c	2	100	6	2	2	2	2	4	355	0	7	40
Mixed, Frozen (Birds Eye)	3.3 oz	4	110	15	6	4	6	2	4	45	0	13	60
Mixed, Frozen (Green Giant)	½ c	2	60	15	6	2	2	2	2	35	0	10	50
Mixed, Frozen (Green Giant) Harvest Fresh	½ c	4	50	15	8	4	6	2	6	220	0	13	60
Mixed, Frozen, in Butter Sauce (Green Giant)	½ c	4	80	15	6	2	4	2	4	345	2	12	80

Food	Serving	% U.S. RDA											
Mixed, Frozen, w Onion Sauce (Birds Eye)	2.6 oz	4	80	10	4	6	2	6	2	350	5	11	100
Mixed, Bavarian Style, w Beans and Spaetzle, Frozen (Birds Eye)	3.3 oz	4	10	8	2	4	*	4	4	420	6	11	110
Mixed, Chinese Style, Frozen (Birds Eye)	3.3 oz	4	25	30	2	2	*	2	4	360	5	8	80
Mixed, Chinese Style, Frozen (Birds Eye) Stir-Fry	3.3 oz	2	35	30	4	4	2	4	6	480	0	7	30
Mixed, Chinese Style, Frozen (Green Giant)	½ c	0	50	40	4	2	0	0	2	280	3	7	60
Mixed, Far Eastern Style, Frozen (Birds Eye)	3.3 oz	4	45	80	4	4	2	2	2	390	5	8	80
Mixed, Italian Style, Frozen (Birds Eye)	3.3 oz	4	15	40	2	4	2	4	4	575	7	11	110
Mixed, Japanese Style, Frozen (Birds Eye)	3.3 oz	4	15	60	2	4	*	2	2	505	6	10	100
Mixed, Japanese Style, Frozen (Birds Eye) Stir-Fry	3.3 oz	2	15	45	45	2	2	2	4	570	0	6	30
Mixed, Japanese Style, Frozen (Green Giant)	½ c	2	20	70	4	6	0	2	4	155	1	8	45
Mixed, Mexicana Style, Frozen (Birds Eye)	3.3 oz	6	8	40	6	4	6	*	6	465	6	16	120
Mixed, New England Style, Frozen (Birds Eye)	3.3 oz	4	15	15	4	4	2	2	2	410	7	14	130

Vegetables	Amt.	Pro-tein	A	C	B₁	B₂	Nia-cin	Cal-cium	Iron	Sodium (mg)	Fat (g)	Carbohy-drate (g)	Calories
		% U.S. RDA											
Mixed, San Francisco Style, Frozen (Birds Eye)	3.3 oz	4	10	15	4	4	2	2	2	395	5	11	100
Mushrooms, Raw, Sliced, Chopped, or Diced	1 c	2	*	4	4	20	15	*	4	11	0-1	3	20
Mushrooms, Canned (B in B)	2 oz	2	0	6	0	6	4	0	2	525	0-1	3	25
Mushrooms, Canned (Green Giant)	2 oz	2	0	4	0	6	2	0	2	260	0	2	14
Mushrooms, Canned, in Butter Sauce (Green Giant)	2 oz	2	0	6	0	6	4	0	2	335	1	4	30
Mushrooms, Frozen, in Butter Sauce (Green Giant)	½ c	6	0	0	6	25	15	0	2	240	4	5	70
Mustard Greens, Fresh, Cooked, Drained	1 c	4	160	110	8	10	4	20	15	25	1	6	30
Okra, Fresh, Sliced, Cooked, Drained	1 c	4	15	60	15	15	6	15	4	3	0-1	10	45
Okra, Frozen, Cut (Birds Eye)	3.3 oz	2	10	15	4	6	2	8	2	5	0	6	25
Okra, Frozen, Whole (Birds Eye)	3.3 oz	2	8	25	6	6	4	8	2	5	0	7	30
Onions, Raw, Chopped	1 tbsp	*	*	2	*	*	*	*	*	1	0-1	1	4
Onions, Raw, Sliced	1 c	2	*	20	2	2	*	4	4	12	0-1	10	45

		% U.S. RDA												
Onions, Cooked, Drained	1 c	4	2	25	4	4	2	4	4	4	15	0–1	14	60
Onions, Green, Raw	2 med or 6 small	*	*	10	*	*	*	2	2	*	2	0–1	3	14
Onions, Frozen, Chopped (Ore-Ida)	2 oz	*	*	2	*	*	*	*	*	*	30	0	4	20
Onions, Pearl, Frozen (Birds Eye Deluxe)	3.3 oz	*	*	15	*	*	*	4	2	*	10	0	8	35
Onions, Frozen, Small, Whole (Birds Eye)	4 oz	*	*	15	*	*	*	4	2	*	10	0	10	40
Onions, Frozen, Small, w Cream Sauce (Birds Eye)	3 oz	2	2	10	2	6	*	6	*	2	335	6	11	110
Onions, Frozen, Fried (Ore-Ida Onion Ringers)	2 oz	2	*	2	2	*	*	*	2	6	200	9	17	150
Onions, Frozen, Small, in Cheese Flavored Sauce (Green Giant)	½ c	4	0	10	0	2	2	6	2	*	400	5	9	90
Parsley, Raw, Chopped	1 tbsp	*	6	10	*	*	*	*	2	2	2	0–1	2	2
Parsnips, Diced, Cooked, Drained	1 c	4	*	25	8	8	6	6	4	*	12	1	23	100
Peas, Fresh, Cooked, Drained	1 c	15	15	15	30	10	20	4	15	20	2	1	20	110
Peas, Canned, Early June (Le Sueur)	½ c	4	10	10	8	4	2	2	6	2	375	0–1	11	60
Peas, Canned, Seasoned (Del Monte)	½ c	4	8	20	6	4	4	*	6	4	355	0	11	60

Vegetables	Amt.	% U.S. RDA								Sodium (mg)	Fat (g)	Carbohydrate (g)	Calories
		Protein	A	C	B₁	B₂	Niacin	Calcium	Iron				
Peas, Canned, Sweet (Del Monte)	½ c	4	8	20	6	4	4	2	6	355	0	10	60
Peas, Canned, Sweet (Del Monte No Salt Added)	½ c	4	8	20	8	4	4	2	6	0–10	0	11	60
Peas, Canned, Sweet (Green Giant)	½ c	6	6	8	8	4	4	2	6	375	0	11	60
Peas, Canned, Sweet, Mini (Le Sueur)	½ c	6	8	10	8	4	4	2	8	425	0	11	60
Peas, Canned, Sweet, Small (Del Monte)	½ c	4	10	25	8	6	4	*	8	355	0	9	50
Peas, Canned, Early Sweet, and Onions (Green Giant)	½ c	6	4	4	4	4	8	2	6	535	0–1	10	60
Peas, Canned, Sweet, and Onions (Green Giant)	½ c	4	10	10	6	4	8	2	6	665	0–1	11	60
Peas and Carrots, Canned (Del Monte)	½ c	2	190	10	4	4	2	2	4	355	0	10	50
Peas, Frozen, Early June (Green Giant)	½ c	6	10	30	15	4	4	2	4	25	0	10	60
Peas, Frozen, Early and Sweet, in Butter Sauce (Green Giant)	½ c	6	15	40	15	4	6	2	4	490	1	14	90
Peas, Frozen, Green (Birds Eye)	3.3 oz	8	15	30	20	6	10	2	8	130	0	13	80

Food	Serving					% U.S. RDA							
Peas, Frozen, Sweet (Green Giant)	½ c	6	10	30	15	4	4	2	4	25	0	10	60
Peas, Frozen, Sweet (Green Giant Harvest Fresh)	½ c	8	15	20	20	4	6	2	8	280	0	14	80
Peas, Frozen, Tiny (Birds Eye Deluxe)	3.3 oz	6	15	30	15	6	8	*	6	120	0	11	60
Peas, Frozen, in Cream Sauce (Green Giant)	½ c	6	10	20	35	6	6	4	6	320	4	12	100
Peas, Frozen, Green, w Cream Sauce (Birds Eye)	2.6 oz	6	10	20	10	10	6	4	2	440	7	14	130
Peas, Carrots, and Pearl Onions, Frozen (Birds Eye Farm Fresh)	3.2 oz	4	140	20	10	4	6	2	6	85	0	11	60
Peas, Green, and Pearl Onions, Frozen (Birds Eye)	3.3 oz	6	15	30	15	4	8	*	4	310	0	13	70
Peas, Mini, Onions, and Carrots, Frozen, in Butter Sauce (Le Sueur)	½ c	6	15	25	15	4	6	0	8	100	3	11	90
Peas, Mini, Pea Pods, and Water Chestnuts, Frozen, in Butter Sauce (Green Giant)	½ c	6	15	280	15	4	4	2	6	410	2	10	80
Peas and Pearl Onions, Frozen, w Cheese Sauce (Birds Eye)	5 oz	10	35	25	15	10	8	10	6	460	5	18	140

Vegetables	Amt.	Protein	A	C	B₁	B₂	Niacin	Calcium	Iron	Sodium (mg)	Fat (g)	Carbohydrate (g)	Calories
		% U.S. RDA											
Peas and Potatoes, Frozen, w Cream Sauce (Birds Eye)	2.6 oz	6	8	20	10	8	6	4	2	480	7	15	140
Peas, Sweet, and Cauliflower, Frozen (Green Giant Medley)	½ c	4	30	45	8	2	2	2	4	35	0	7	40
Peppers, Green, Sweet, Raw	1 (about 5 per lb)	2	6	160	4	4	2	*	2	10	0–1	4	16
Peppers, Green, Sweet, Sliced, Cooked, Drained	1 c	2	10	220	6	6	4	2	4	12	0–1	5	25
Peppers, Jalapeño, Canned, Whole or Sliced (Del Monte)	½ c	*	35	20	*	2	2	2	15	1690	1	6	30
Peppers, Jalapeño, Canned, Whole (Old El Paso)	2 peppers	*	0	16	*	*	*	*	*	478	1	1	12
Peppers, Jalapeño (Vlasic Mexican)	1 oz	*	2	*	*	*	*	*	2	380	0	2	8
Peppers, Red, Sweet, Raw	1 (about 5 per lb)	2	70	250	4	4	2	*	2	0	0–1	5	25
Pimientos (Dromedary)	1 oz	*	10	15	*	*	*	*	8	NA	0	2	10
Potatoes, Baked, in Skin	1 (4¾" × 2⅓")	6	*	50	10	4	15	2	6	6	0–1	33	150
Potatoes, Boiled, in Skin	1 med (2½" diam)	4	*	35	8	2	10	*	4	4	0–1	24	100
Potatoes, Boiled, in Skin, then Peeled, Sliced, or Diced	1 c	6	*	40	10	4	10	2	4	5	0–1	27	120

Food	Serving	% U.S. RDA											
Potatoes, Boiled, After Peeling	1 med (2½" diam)	4	*	30	6	2	6	*	4	2	0–1	16	70
Potatoes, Boiled, After Peeling, then Sliced or Diced	1 c	4	*	40	10	2	10	*	4	3	0–1	23	100
Potatoes, French Fried in Deep Fat, 2"×3½" piece	10	4	*	20	4	2	8	*	4	3	7	18	140
Potatoes, Canned, Sliced or Whole (Del Monte)	½ c	2	0	25	2	*	2	2	2	355	0	10	45
Potatoes, Frozen, Whole, Peeled (Birds Eye)	3.2 oz	2	*	8	4	*	6	*	*	6	0	13	60
Potatoes, Frozen, Small, Whole, Peeled (Ore-Ida)	3 oz	2	*	10	4	*	4	*	2	40	0	17	80
Potatoes, Frozen (Birds Eye Tiny Taters)	3.2 oz	2	*	6	2	*	4	*	2	280	12	22	200
Potatoes, Frozen (Ore-Ida Crispers!)	3 oz	4	*	2	2	*	6	*	4	560	15	25	240
Potatoes, Frozen (Ore-Ida Crispy Crowns!)	3 oz	2	*	4	4	*	4	*	2	370	8	18	150
Potatoes, Frozen (Ore-Ida Golden Patties)	2.5 oz	2	*	4	4	*	6	*	4	340	10	17	130
Potatoes, Frozen (Ore-Ida Potatoes O'Brien)	3 oz	2	*	8	*	*	4	*	2	50	0	17	80
Potatoes, Frozen, Au Gratin (Stouffer's)	3¹³⁄₁₆ oz	4	*	*	2	6	4	10	2	480	8	13	135

313

| Vegetables | Amt. | % U.S. RDA | | | | | | | | | | | Fat (g) | Carbohy-drate (g) | Calories |
		Pro-tein	A	C	B$_1$	B$_2$	Nia-cin	Cal-cium	Iron	Sodium (mg)				
Potato, Frozen, Baked, Stuffed w Cheese Topping (Green Giant)	5 oz	6	6	10	4	4	10	4	4	520		6	33	200
Potato, Frozen, Baked, Stuffed w Sour Cream and Chives (Green Giant)	5 oz	6	8	8	4	4	10	4	4	580		10	31	230
Potatoes, Frozen, Fried (Birds Eye Cottage Fries)	2.8 oz	2	*	6	2	*	6	*	2	15		5	17	120
Potatoes, Frozen, Fried (Birds Eye Crinkle Cuts)	3 oz	2	*	8	4	*	4	*	*	35		4	18	110
Potatoes, Frozen, Fried (Birds Eye French Fries)	3 oz	2	*	8	4	*	2	*	2	25		4	17	110
Potatoes, Frozen, Fried (Birds Eye Steak Fries)	3 oz	2	*	6	4	*	4	*	2	25		3	18	110
Potatoes, Frozen, Fried (Ore-Ida Country Style Dinner Fries)	3 oz	2	*	6	2	*	4	*	2	50		4	20	120
Potatoes, Frozen, Fried (Birds Eye TastiFries)	2.5 oz	2	*	8	4	*	6	*	*	270		7	17	140
Potatoes, Frozen, Fried (Ore-Ida Cottage Fries)	3 oz	2	*	8	2	*	4	*	2	40		6	21	140

314

Item	Serving												
		% U.S. RDA											
Potatoes, Frozen, Fried (Ore-Ida Golden Crinkles)	3 oz	4	*	6	2	*	4	*	2	40	5	20	120
Potatoes, Frozen, Fried (Ore-Ida Golden Fries)	3 oz	4	*	6	2	*	4	*	2	40	5	21	130
Potatoes, Frozen, Fried (Ore-Ida Pixie Crinkles)	3 oz	2	*	6	2	*	4	*	2	40	10	22	160
Potatoes, Frozen, Fried (Ore-Ida Tater Tots)	3 oz	2	*	4	2	*	4	*	2	550	8	21	160
Potatoes, Frozen, Fried, w Bacon Flavor (Ore-Ida Tater Tots)	3 oz	4	8	4	6	*	4	*	2	720	7	21	160
Potatoes, Frozen, Fried, w Onions (Ore-Ida Tater Tots)	3 oz	2	*	4	2	*	4	*	2	600	8	21	160
Potatoes, Frozen, Hash Brown (Birds Eye)	4 oz	2	*	6	4	*	4	*	2	55	0	17	70
Potatoes, Frozen, Hash Brown, Shredded (Birds Eye)	3 oz	2	*	6	4	*	4	*	*	20	0	13	60
Potatoes, Frozen, Hashbrowns (Ore-Ida Shredded Hashbrowns)	6 oz	4	*	14	4	2	6	2	4	50	0	29	130
Potatoes, Frozen, Hash Brown (Ore-Ida Southern Style)	3 oz	*	*	6	4	*	4	*	2	60	0	17	70

Vegetables	Amt.	% U.S. RDA								Sodium (mg)	Fat (g)	Carbohydrate (g)	Calories
		Protein	A	C	B$_1$	B$_2$	Niacin	Calcium	Iron				
Potatoes, Frozen, Puffs (Birds Eye TastiPuffs)	2.5 oz	4	*	10	4	2	6	*	2	400	12	19	190
Potatoes, Frozen, Scalloped (Stouffer's)	4 oz	4	*	*	2	6	2	8	2	450	7	14	125
Potatoes, Frozen, Shoestring (Birds Eye)	3.3 oz	4	*	15	4	*	4	*	4	50	6	20	140
Potatoes, Frozen, Shoestring (Ore-Ida)	3 oz	2	*	4	2	*	4	*	2	40	7	24	160
Potatoes, Frozen, Sliced (Ore-Ida Home Style)	3 oz	2	*	8	4	*	6	*	2	40	4	17	110
Potatoes, Frozen, Sliced (Ore-Ida Home Style Potato Planks)	3 oz	2	*	8	4	*	6	*	2	30	.5	18	110
Potatoes, Frozen, Sliced (Ore-Ida Potato Thins)	3 oz	2	*	8	2	*	4	*	2	40	6	18	130
Potatoes, Frozen, Sliced, in Butter Sauce (Green Giant)	1/2 c	2	10	6	0	0	4	0	0	470	2	14	80
Potatoes, Frozen, Wedges (Birds Eye Farm Style)	3 oz	2	*	6	4	*	4	*	2	25	3	18	110
Potatoes, Frozen, Wedges (Ore-Ida Home Style)	3 oz	2	*	8	4	*	6	*	2	20	4	17	100
Potatoes w Onions, Frozen (Ore-Ida Crispy Crowns!)	3 oz	2	*	4	4	*	4	*	2	480	10	19	170

		% U.S. RDA											
Potatoes and Sweet Peas, Frozen, in Bacon Cream Sauce (Green Giant)	½ c	4	0	10	8	2	6	2	0	400	4	15	110
Potatoes, Mix (Betty Crocker Potato Buds)	½ c prep	4	4	2	*	2	6	2	*	355	6	15	130
Potatoes, Mix, Au Gratin (Betty Crocker)	½ c prep	4	4	2	*	6	4	8	2	605	6	21	150
Potatoes, Mix, Au Gratin (French's Tangy)	½ c prep	4	2	2	*	6	2	10	*	525	4	25	150
Potatoes, Mix, Chicken 'n Herb (Betty Crocker)	½ c prep	4	2	*	*	2	4	2	2	585	4	19	120
Potatoes, Mix, Creamed, Oven (Betty Crocker)	½ c prep	6	4	*	*	8	6	6	2	415	8	22	170
Potatoes, Mix, Creamed, Saucepan (Betty Crocker)	½ c prep	8	6	*	*	8	6	8	2	425	8	23	180
Potatoes, Mix, Hash Brown, w Onions (Betty Crocker)	½ c prep	4	4	*	*	*	6	*	2	460	6	22	150
Potatoes, Mix, Hickory Smoke Cheese (Betty Crocker)	½ c prep	4	4	*	*	6	4	8	2	650	6	21	150
Potatoes, Mix, Julienne (Betty Crocker)	½ c prep	4	4	*	*	4	2	6	*	570	6	17	130
Potatoes, Mix, Mashed (Country Store)	⅓ c dry	2	*	*	*	*	4	*	2	NA	0	15	70
Potatoes, Mix, Mashed (French's Big Tate)	½ c prep	2	4	2	*	2	4	2	*	410	7	16	140

Vegetables	Amt.	% U.S. RDA								Sodium (mg)	Fat (g)	Carbohydrate (g)	Calories
		Protein	A	C	B₁	B₂	Niacin	Calcium	Iron				

Vegetables	Amt.	Protein	A	C	B₁	B₂	Niacin	Calcium	Iron	Sodium (mg)	Fat (g)	Carbohydrate (g)	Calories
Potatoes, Mix, Mashed (French's Idaho)	½ c prep	2	4	2	*	2	4	2	*	365	6	16	120
Potatoes, Mix, Mashed (Hungry Jack)	½ c	4	6	8	2	6	2	4	0	380	7	17	140
Potatoes, Mix, Scalloped (Betty Crocker)	½ c prep	4	4	*	*	2	4	2	2	570	6	19	140
Potatoes, Mix, Scalloped (French's Crispy Top)	½ c prep	4	4	2	2	6	4	10	*	520	5	25	160
Potatoes, Mix, Scalloped, Cheese (French's)	½ c prep	4	2	2	2	8	4	10	*	540	6	25	160
Potatoes, Mix, Sour Cream 'n Chive (Betty Crocker)	½ c prep	4	4	*	*	2	6	2	2	535	7	21	160
Potatoes, Mix, Sour Cream and Chives (French's)	½ c prep	4	2	2	2	6	4	10	*	660	7	24	170
Pumpkin, Canned (Del Monte)	½ c	*	600	8	*	2	2	2	4	0-10	0	9	35
Radishes, Raw, Red	10 med	*	*	20	2	2	*	2	2	8	0-1	2	10
Rutabagas, Fresh, Cooked, Drained, Cubed or Sliced	1 c	2	20	70	6	6	6	10	2	7	0-1	14	60
Sauerkraut, Canned (Del Monte)	½ c	*	0	15	*	*	*	2	2	775	0	6	25

	% U.S. RDA											
Sauerkraut, Canned (Vlasic Old Fashioned) 1 oz	*	*	*	*	*	*	*	2	280	0	1	4
Soy Beans, Sprouted Seeds, Raw 1 c	10	2	*	25	15	10	4	6	NA	2	6	50
Soy Beans, Sprouted Seeds, Cooked, Drained 1 c	10	2	*	8	15	10	6	4	NA	2	5	50
Spinach, Raw, Chopped 1 c	2	90	45	4	6	2	6	10	39	0–1	3	14
Spinach, Cooked, Drained 1 c	8	290	80	8	15	4	15	20	90	0–1	7	40
Spinach, Canned, Chopped or Whole (Del Monte) ½ c	2	110	20	*	6	*	10	8	355	0	4	25
Spinach, Canned, Whole Leaf (Del Monte No Salt Added) ½ c	2	110	20	*	6	*	10	8	35	0	4	25
Spinach, Frozen (Green Giant Harvest Fresh) ½ c	6	180	50	6	10	2	10	10	350	0	4	30
Spinach, Frozen, Chopped (Birds Eye) 3.3 oz	4	150	35	6	8	*	10	10	80	0	3	20
Spinach, Frozen, Whole Leaf (Birds Eye) 3.3 oz	4	150	45	6	8	2	10	10	90	0	4	20
Spinach, Frozen, Cut Leaf. in Butter Sauce (Green Giant) ½ c	4	190	40	8	15	2	10	8	465	2	6	50
Spinach, Frozen, Creamed (Birds Eye) 3 oz	4	100	20	4	6	*	6	2	275	3	5	60
Spinach, Frozen, in Cream Sauce (Green Giant) ½ c	4	90	15	4	10	0	8	6	395	3	8	70

Vegetables	Amt.	Protein	A	C	B₁	B₂	Niacin	Calcium	Iron	Sodium (mg)	Fat (g)	Carbohydrate (g)	Calories
								% U.S. RDA					
Spinach, Frozen, Creamed (Stouffer's)	4½ oz	6	100	20	4	10	*	10	8	855	15	9	190
Spinach and Water Chestnuts, Frozen (Birds Eye)	3.3 oz	4	130	35	6	8	2	8	10	275	0	5	25
Squash, Summer, Cooked, Drained, Diced	1 c	2	15	35	6	10	8	6	4	2	0–1	7	30
Squash, Winter, Baked, Mashed	1 c	6	170	45	6	15	6	6	8	2	1	32	130
Squash, Winter, Frozen, Cooked (Birds Eye)	4 oz	*	90	20	2	4	2	2	4	0	0	11	45
Stew Vegetables, Frozen (Ore-Ida)	3 oz	2	35	4	2	*	4	2	2	50	0	12	60
Sweet Potatoes, Baked, in Skin	1 med (5" × 2")	4	180	40	6	4	4	4	6	14	1	37	160
Sweet Potatoes, Boiled, in Skin	1 med (5" × 2")	4	240	45	10	6	4	4	6	15	1	40	170
Tomatoes, Raw, Unpeeled	1 (3" diam, 2⅛" high)	4	35	70	8	4	6	2	4	5	0–1	9	40
Tomatoes, Cooked	1 c	4	50	100	10	8	10	4	8	10	0–1	14	60
Tomatoes, Canned, Baby, Sliced (Contadina)	½ c	*	15	20	2	2	4	8	2	465	0	10	50
Tomatoes, Canned, Italian Style (Contadina)	½ c	*	10	20	2	*	4	2	2	395	0	5	25

Food					% U.S. RDA							
Tomatoes, Canned, Stewed ½ c (Contadina)	*	10	25	4	2	4	4	2	405	0	9	35
Tomatoes, Canned, Stewed ½ c (Del Monte)	*	10	30	2	*	2	2	2	355	0	8	35
Tomatoes, Canned, Stewed ½ c (Del Monte No Salt Added)	*	10	30	2	*	2	2	2	45	0	8	35
Tomatoes, Canned, Stewed 4 oz (Hunt's)	2	15	30	4	2	4	4	6	460	0	8	35
Tomatoes, Canned, Stewed 4 oz (Hunt's No Salt Added)	2	15	30	4	2	4	4	6	20	0	8	35
Tomatoes, Canned, Wedges ½ c (Del Monte)	*	10	25	4	*	2	2	2	355	0	8	30
Tomatoes, Canned, Whole 4 oz (Hunt's)	*	15	20	4	2	4	4	4	415	0	5	20
Tomatoes, Canned, Whole 4 oz (Hunt's No Salt Added)	*	15	20	4	2	4	4	4	15	0	5	20
Tomatoes, Canned, Whole, ½ c Peeled (Contadina)	*	15	30	4	*	4	4	2	390	0	6	25
Tomatoes, Canned, Whole, ½ c Peeled (Del Monte)	*	10	30	2	*	2	2	2	220	0	5	25
Tomato Paste, Canned 6 oz (Contadina)	10	90	80	15	10	30	4	10	135	0	35	150
Tomato Paste, Canned ¾ c (Del Monte)	8	90	60	15	15	15	6	15	110	1	34	150

Vegetables	Amt.	Protein	A	C	B₁	B₂	Niacin	Calcium	Iron	Sodium (mg)	Fat (g)	Carbohydrate (g)	Calories
					% U.S. RDA								
Tomato Paste, Canned (Del Monte No Salt Added)	6 oz	8	90	60	15	15	15	6	15	110	1	34	150
Tomato Paste, Canned (Hunt's)	2 oz	2	40	45	8	4	10	2	10	150	0	11	45
Tomato Paste, Canned (Hunt's No Salt Added)	2 oz	2	40	45	8	4	8	2	10	25	0	11	45
Tomato Paste, Italian, Canned (Contadina)	2 oz	2	20	10	4	4	8	2	4	710	1	12	70
Tomato Paste, Italian Style, Canned (Hunt's)	2 oz	2	40	45	8	4	10	2	10	525	0	11	50
Tomato Paste, Italian, w Mushrooms, Canned (Contadina)	2 oz	*	20	10	4	4	6	2	4	735	1	12	60
Tomato Puree, Canned (Contadina)	½ c	2	25	25	4	2	6	*	4	90	0	11	50
Tomato Puree, Canned (Hunt's)	4 oz	2	35	45	8	4	8	2	10	185	0	10	45
Tomato and Green Chilies, Canned (Old El Paso)	¼ c	*	0	*	*	*	3	*	2	273	.1	2.5	12.6
Turnips, Cooked, Cubed, Drained	1 c	2	*	60	4	4	2	6	4	53	0–1	8	35
Turnip Greens, Cooked, Drained	1 c	4	180	170	15	20	4	25	8	NA	0–1	6	30

Food	Serving														
		% U.S. RDA													
Watercress, Raw, Whole	about 10 sprigs	2	35	45	2	4	2	6	6	4	2	18	0-1	1	8
Watercress, Raw, Chopped Finely	1 c	4	120	170	6	10	6	20	10	10	6	65	0-1	4	25
Yams and Apples, Frozen (Stouffer's)	5 oz	*	2	10	4	2	2	4	4	6	2	225	3	31	160
Zucchini, Canned, in Tomato Sauce (Del Monte)	½ c	*	10	6	2	2	2	2	2	4	2	485	0	8	30
Zucchini, Frozen, Baby, Sliced (Birds Eye Deluxe)	3.3 oz	*	10	6	2	2	2	*	2	2	2	5	0	3	16
Vegetable Juices															
Tomato (Campbell's)	6 fl oz	2	15	35	2	2	6	*	6	2	2	625	0	8	35
Tomato (Hunt's)	6 fl oz	2	25	30	4	2	6	2	6	6	6	550	0	7	30
Tomato (Hunt's No Salt Added)	6 fl oz	2	25	30	4	2	6	*	6	6	6	30	0	7	30
Tomato (Welch's)	6 fl oz	2	15	20	4	2	4	*	4	2	2	550	0	7	35
Tomato and Chili (Del Monte Snap-E-Tom)	6 fl oz	2	15	10	4	2	6	2	6	6	6	980	0	7	40
V-8	6 fl oz	2	45	45	*	2	6	2	6	4	4	625	0	8	35
V-8, No Salt Added	6 fl oz	2	45	45	*	2	6	2	6	4	4	50	0	9	40
V-8, Spicy-Hot	6 fl oz	2	45	45	*	2	6	2	6	4	4	625	0	8	35
Yogurt															
Apple Cinnamon (Yoplait Breakfast Yogurt)	6 oz	15	*	*	6	20	*	20	2	2	2	95	5	40	240

Yogurt	Amt.	Protein	A	C	B_1	B_2	Niacin	Calcium	Iron	Sodium (mg)	Fat (g)	Carbohydrate (g)	Calories
		% U.S. RDA											
Berries (Yoplait Breakfast Yogurt)	6 oz	15	*	*	6	20	*	25	2	95	5	39	230
Cherry (Dannon)	1 c	20	*	*	2	20	*	35	*	70-125	3	49	260
Cherry Vanilla (Borden)	8 oz	20	*	*	2	20	*	30	*	160	2	54	270
Citrus Fruits (Yoplait Breakfast Yogurt)	6 oz	15	*	*	6	20	*	25	2	95	5	43	250
Coffee (Dannon)	1 c	25	2	*	4	20	*	35	*	70-90	4	32	200
Coffee (Yoplait Custard Style)	6 oz	15	2	*	4	20	*	25	*	110	4	30	180
Fruit Flavors, All Varieties (Y.E.S.)	6 oz	15	2	*	6	25	*	30	*	40-90	4	33	190
Fruit Flavors (Yoplait Custard Style)	6 oz	15	2	*	4	15	*	20	*	95	4	32	190
Fruit Flavors (Yoplait Original)	6 oz	15	*	*	6	20	*	25	*	105	4	32	190
Lemon (Borden)	8 oz	20	*	*	2	20	*	30	*	115	2	69	320
Lemon (Dannon)	1 c	25	2	*	4	20	*	35	*	70-90	4	32	200
Orchard Fruits (Yoplait Breakfast Yogurt)	6 oz	15	*	*	6	20	*	25	2	95	5	40	240
Peach (Dannon)	1 c	20	*	*	2	20	*	35	*	70-125	3	49	260
Pineapple (Borden)	8 oz	20	*	*	2	20	*	30	*	115	2	51	260

324

		% U.S. RDA										
Plain (Dannon)	1 c	30	2	*	4	30	40	*	115	4	17	150
Plain (Lite-line)	8 oz	25	2	*	4	20	35	*	145	4	24	180
Plain (Yoplait Original)	6 oz	20	2	*	6	30	35	*	135	5	14	130
Plain w Honey (Yoplait Custard Style)	6 oz	15	2	*	4	20	25	*	110	4	23	160
Strawberry (Borden)	8 oz	20	*	*	2	20	30	*	145	2	46	230
Strawberry (Dannon)	1 c	20	*	*	2	20	35	*	70–125	3	49	260
Strawberry (Meadow Gold Sundae Style)	1 c	20	2	*	2	20	35	*	NA	4	49	270
Tropical Fruits (Yoplait Breakfast Yogurt)	6 oz	15	*	*	6	20	20	2	95	5	43	250
Vanilla (Dannon)	1 c	25	2	*	4	20	35	*	70–90	4	32	200
Vanilla (Yoplait Custard Style)	6 oz	15	2	*	4	20	25	*	110	4	30	180
Frozen, Blueberry (Danny)	1 c	15	*	*	2	15	20	*	NA	2	42	210
Frozen, Chocolate (Danny)	1 c	20	*	*	4	20	30	*	NA	3	32	190
Frozen, Piña Colada (Danny)	1 c	15	*	*	*	15	20	*	NA	4	44	230
Frozen, Raspberry (Danny)	1 c	15	*	*	2	15	20	*	NA	2	42	210
Frozen, Strawberry (Danny)	1 c	15	*	*	2	15	20	*	NA	2	42	210
Frozen, Vanilla (Danny)	1 c	15	*	*	2	15	25	*	NA	2	33	180
Frozen, Bar, Boysenberry, Carob Coated (Danny)	1 bar	4	*	NA	*	4	6	*	NA	8	15	140

Yogurt	Amt.	Protein	A	C	B₁	B₂	Niacin	Calcium	Iron	Sodium (mg)	Fat (g)	Carbohydrate (g)	Calories
		% U.S. RDA											
Frozen, Bar, Chocolate, Chocolate Coated (Danny)	1 bar	6	*	NA	*	10	*	15	*	NA	8	12	130
Frozen, Bar, Chocolate, Uncoated (Danny)	1 bar	6	*	NA	*	6	*	10	*	NA	1	10	60
Frozen, Bar, Piña Colada, Uncoated (Danny)	1 bar	4	*	NA	*	4	*	8	*	NA	1	14	70
Frozen, Bar, Raspberry, Chocolate Coated (Danny)	1 bar	4	*	NA	*	10	*	10	*	NA	7	15	130
Frozen, Bar, Strawberry, Chocolate Coated (Danny)	1 bar	4	*	NA	*	10	*	10	*	NA	7	15	130
Frozen, Bar, Vanilla, Chocolate Coated (Danny)	1 bar	6	*	NA	*	10	*	13	*	NA	8	11	130
Frozen, Bar, Vanilla, Uncoated (Danny)	1 bar	6	*	NA	*	6	*	8	*	NA	1	11	60
Frozen, Soft, All Varieties (Danny-Yo)	3½ oz	10	*	*	*	10	*	15	*	NA	1	21	115

ABOUT THE AUTHOR

Jean Carper is a well-known authority on health and nutrition. She is a former senior medical correspondent for Cable News Network in Washington, D.C. and currently writes a nutrition column for the *Washington Post*. She is the author of fifteen books, most recently *The Food Pharmacy*.

Bantam's Best In Diet, Health And Nutrition

- ☐ 26326   All-In One Calorie Counter (rev) .... $4.95/5.95 Canada
- ☐ 27245   Anxiety Disease .... $4.95/5.95 Canada
- ☐ 25267   Brand-Name Nutrition Counter .... $3.95/4.95 Canada
- ☐ 26886   Complete Scarsdale Medical Diet .... $4.95/5.95 Canada
- ☐ 27775   Controlling Cholesterol .... $4.95/5.95 Canada
- ☐ 28033   Getting Well Again .... $4.95/6.50 Canada
- ☐ 27667   The Rotation Diet .... $4.95/5.95 Canada
- ☐ 28508   T-Factor Diet .... $4.95/5.95 Canada
- ☐ 27751   Yeast Syndrome .... $4.95/6.50 Canada
- ☐ 34712   Asthma Handbook .... $9.95/12.95 Canada
- ☐ 05771   Dr. Abravanel's Anti-Craving Weight Loss Diet .... $18.95/23.95 Canada
- ☐ 34524   The Food Pharmacy .... $9.95/12.95 Canada
- ☐ 34623   Healing Visualizations .... $8.95/11.95 Canada
- ☐ 34618   Jane Brody's Good Food Book ..... $13.95/17.95 Canada
- ☐ 34721   Jane Brody's Nutrition (Updated) .... $13.95/17.95 Canada
- ☐ 34350   Jean Carper's Total Nutrition .... $12.95/15.95 Canada
- ☐ 34556   Minding The Body, Mending The Mind .... $9.95/12.95 Canada
- ☐ 05395   Seasons Of The Mind .... $18.95/23.95 Canada

---